Notes for the MRCGP

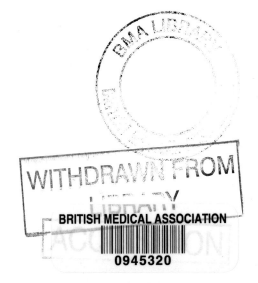

Notes for the MRCGP

A curriculum based guide to the AKT, CSA and WBPA

FOURTH EDITION

Keith Palmer

and

Nicholas Boeckx

Fourth edition fully revised by
Nicholas Boeckx

⟨W⟩WILEY-BLACKWELL

A John Wiley & Sons, Ltd., Publication

Blackwell Publishing was acquired by John Wiley & Sons in February 2007. Blackwell's publishing program has been merged with Wiley's global Scientific, Technical and Medical business to form Wiley-Blackwell.

Registered office: John Wiley & Sons Ltd, The Atrium, Southern Gate, Chichester, West Sussex, PO19 8SQ, UK

Editorial offices: 9600 Garsington Road, Oxford, OX4 2DQ, UK
The Atrium, Southern Gate, Chichester, West Sussex, PO19 8SQ, UK
111 River Street, Hoboken, NJ 07030-5774, USA

For details of our global editorial offices, for customer services and for information about how to apply for permission to reuse the copyright material in this book please see our website at www.wiley.com/wiley-blackwell

Library of Congress Cataloging-in-Publication Data
Palmer, K. T.
   Notes for the MRCGP / Keith Palmer, Nicholas Boeckx. – 4th ed.
      p. ; cm.
   Includes bibliographical references and index.
   ISBN 978-1-4051-5724-7 (alk. paper)
   1. Family medicine–Examinations, questions, etc.   2. Physicians (General practice)–Great Britain–Examinations–Study guides.   3. Royal College of General Practitioners.   I. Boeckx, Nicholas K.   II. Title.
   [DNLM: 1. Family Practice–Outlines. W 18.2 P174n 2010]
   RC58.P35 2010
   610.76–dc22
                                    2009029894

ISBN: 9781405157247

A catalogue record for this book is available from the British Library.

Set in 9.25 on 11.5 pt Minion by SNP Best-set Typesetter Ltd., Hong Kong
Printed and bound in Malaysia by KHL Printing Co Sdn Bhd

1   2010

Contents

Acknowledgements

I would like to thank my wife and dedicate this text to my daughter Charlotte. I would also like to thank all those who have contributed to the creation of this new edition, in particular: Dr Sophie Ball and Dr Sarah Westmore for reviewing and contributing to the CSA case chapters. Dr Joanne Kirby, Dr Christopher Wenham, Dr Amanda Latham and Dr Jill Boeckx for reviewing the book. I would also like to thank my practice partners, Dr Gillian Love, Dr Jonathan Darby, Dr Claire Halford and Dr Sarah Allen. Finally I would like to acknowledge the influence of Dr Gillian Love, Dr Amarjit Nagra, Dr Paul Farley, Dr Carol Griffiths, Dr Dominic Faux, Dr Manjeet Samra, Dr James Bullock and Dr Ian Reed.

N Boeckx
MBChB, MRCP, MRCGP

Preface

The aim of this book is to help prepare candidates for their MRCGP exams and to provide useful information for GPs starting their first year in practice. This text provides sample questions for the AKT, practice cases for the CSA and up-to-date topic summaries and hot topics. The chapters are mapped to the 16 sections of the RCGP curriculum. The range of clinical medicine covered by primary care is vast so the clinical topics covered here focus on the common exam topics and topical issues (e.g. HPV vaccine) most likely to appear in the exam. For those running out of time before the exam, the most improvement can be made from focusing on the areas in which your knowledge is poorest (provided that these carry a significant proportion of the marks). One way of identifying and targeting these areas is by taking the end-of-chapter MCQs first and starting revision in your lowest scoring areas.

This book contains summaries of the current evidence base including clinical guidelines. I have referenced the evidence sources in the text. In many cases the sources include evidence summaries themselves, e.g. Cochrane reviews, NICE & SIGN guidance. For practical purposes it has not been wherever possible to include all of the references, and I apologise for any omissions. If readers are searching for a source that has been omitted please first check national guidelines (NICE/SIGN) or those of national societies (e.g. British Thoracic Society, Diabetes UK). If you are unable to locate the reference you may contact me at bookenquiries@ halesowenmedicalpractice.com and I will try to assist you.

Dr N Boeckx

Abbreviations

AA	Attendance Allowance
ACE	angiotensin-converting enzyme
AKT	Applied Knowledge Test
AMHP	approved mental health professional
AMSPAR	Association of Medical Secretaries, Practice Managers, Administrators and Receptionists
AOM	acute otitis media
APMS	alternative provider of medical services
ARB	angiotensin receptor blocker
ARR	absolute risk reduction
ASW	approved social worker
BMA	British Medical Association
BMD	bone mineral density
BMI	body mass index
BNF	*British National Formulary*
BNP	B-type natriuretic peptide
BSE	breast self-examination
BTS	British Thoracic Society
BV	bacterial vaginosis
CBD	case-based discussion
CBT	cognitive–behavioural therapy
CCB	calcium channel blocker
CCT	certificate of completion of training
CDs	controlled drugs
CEX	clinical evaluation exercise
CHD	coronary heart disease
CI	confidence interval
CKD	chronic kidney disease
CKS	Clinical Knowledge Summaries (previously known as Prodigy)
CNS	central nervous system
COPD	chronic obstructive pulmonary disease
COT	consultation observation tool
CPA	care plan approach
CSA	Clinical Skills Assessment
CSR	clinical supervisors report
CVA	cerebrovascular accident
CVD	cardiovascular disease
DAFNE	dose adjustment for normal eating

DES	directed enhanced service
DESMOND	Diabetes Education and Self-Management for Ongoing and Newly Diagnosed
DEXA	dual energy X-ray absorptiometry
DLA	Disability Living Allowance
DM	diabetes mellitus
DOH	Department of Health
DOPS	direct observation of procedural skills
DTB	*Drugs and Therapeutics Bulletin*
DVLA	Driver and Vehicle Licensing Agency
DVT	deep vein thrombosis
DWP	Department of Work and Pensions
ED	erectile dysfunction
EEG	electroencephalogram
eGFR	estimated glomerular filtration rate
EMQ	extended matching questions
ENT	ear, nose and throat
EPS	electronic prescription service
ESR	erythrocyte sedimentation rate
FBC	full blood count
FEV_1	forced expiratory volume in 1 second
FVC	forced vital capacity
GMC	General Medical Council
GP	general practice
GUM	genitourinary medicine
HAD scale	Hospital Anxiety and Depression scale
HDL	high-density lipoprotein
HPV	human papillomavirus
HRT	hormone replacement therapy
HSE	Health and Safety Executive
ICE	ideas, concerns and expectations
IFG	impaired fasting glucose
IGT	impaired glucose tolerance
IMRAD	introduction, method, results, analysis, discussion
IMT	information management and technology
IV	intravenous
LABA	long-acting β agonist
LDL	low-density lipoprotein
LES	local enhanced service
LFT	liver function test
LIFT	local improvement finance trust
LMC	local medical committee
LMP	last menstrual period
LPA	lasting power of attorney
LVH	left ventricular hypertrophy
MAAG	medical audit advisory group
MAOI	monoamine oxidase inhibitor
MCQ	multiple-choice question

MeReC	Medicines Resource Centre (now part of the National Prescribing Centre)
MI	myocardial infarction
MIMS	monthly index of medical specialties
MMR	measles, mumps and rubella (immunisation)
MMSE	Mini-Mental State examination
MRCGP	Member of The Royal College of General Practitioners
MS	multiple sclerosis
MSF	multi-source feedback
MSU	mid-stream urine
NaTHNaC	National Travel Health Network and Centre
NES	National Enhanced Service
NHS	National Health Service
NI	National Insurance
NICE	National Institute for Health and Clinical Excellence
NNT	number needed to treat
NPC	National Prescribing Centre
NPCRDC	National Primary Care Research and Development Centre
NPDT	National Primary Care Development Team
NPSA	National Patient Safety Agency
NPV	negative predictive value
NRLS	National Reporting and Learning System
NRT	nicotine replacement therapy
NSAID	non-steroidal anti-inflammatory drug
NSC	National Screening Committee
NSF	National Service Framework
OCP	oral contraceptive pill
OOH	out of hours
OR	odds ratio
OT	occupational therapist
OTC	over the counter
PACT	prescribing analysis and cost
PALS	Patient Advisory and Liaison Service
PCG	practice commissioning group
PCT	primary care trust
PEFR	peak expiratory flow rate
PID	pelvic inflammatory disease
PMH	past medical history
POEM	psychological, organisational, educational and medicolegal
POMR	problem-oriented medical record
PPA	Prescription Pricing Authority
PPV	positive predictive value
PSA	prostate-specific antigen
PSQ	patient satisfaction questionnaire
PV	per vagina
QALY	quality-adjusted life-year
QMAS	quality management and analysis system
QOF	quality outcome framework

QPID	quality prevalence indicator database
RCGP	Royal College of General Practitioners
RCT	randomised controlled trial
RIDDOR	Reporting of Injuries, Diseases and Dangerous Occurrences Regulations
RMO	responsible medical officer
RR	relative risk
RRR	relative risk reduction
SBA	single best answer
SD	standard deviation
SEA	significant event analysis
SIGN	Scottish Intercollegiate Guidelines Network
SLS	selected list scheme
SMR	standardised mortality ratio
SSP	Statutory Sick Pay
SSRI	selective serotonin reuptake inhibitor
ST(1–3)	specialist training (year 1–3)
STI	sexually transmitted infection
TB	tuberculosis
TC	total cholesterol
TCA	tricyclic antidepressant
TFT	thyroid function tests
TIA	transient ischaemic attack
TOP	termination of pregnancy
U&E	urea and electrolytes
WHO	World Health Organization
WPBA	workplace-based assessment

1 The MRCGP examination

This chapter relates to curriculum statement 1 ('Being a general practitioner')
This chapter explains the new MRCGP exam format that followed the introduction of the RCGP curriculum (2006). It defines the skills and competencies required to pass and provides advice on exam technique with samples of the question formats (see www.rcgp-curriculum.org.uk).

Understanding the MRCGP exam

The new MRCGP exam consists of three parts:
1. Applied Knowledge Test (AKT)
2. Workplace-based Assessment (WPBA)
3. Clinical Skills Assessment (CSA).

   GP registrars must successfully complete each part to receive their Certificate of Completion of Training (CCT), necessary to work as a GP in the UK.

The Applied Knowledge Test

(www.rcgp-curriculum.org.uk/nmrcgp/akt.aspx)

Format
The AKT is a 3-hour exam consisting of 200 question stems. All questions are marked equally and each correct answer achieves one mark; there is no negative marking. It is computer based, i.e. each candidate sits in a booth and answers questions on a computer terminal. You are provided with a laminated sheet and pen for your workings out. There are three sittings of the exam each year. The question formats include single best answer (SBA), extended matching questions (EMQs), tables and algorithms (for completion), picture format questions, data interpretation ('interpretation of complex sets of data for patients with chronic conditions – risk tables included if appropriate') and seminal trials (familiarity with significant research, e.g. Anglo Scandinavian Cardiac Outcomes Trial [ASCOT]).

Notes for the MRCGP: A curriculum based guide to the AKT, CSA and WBPA, 4th edition. By K. Palmer and N. Boeckx. Published 2010 by Blackwell Publishing, ISBN: 978-1-4051-5724-7.

Examples of the question types are given at the end of this section. After each chapter there are AKT practice questions on the topics covered. Note that the clinical topics covered in the CSA chapter are also probable material for AKT questions so it is also worth reading this through when revising for the AKT.

The AKT can be taken at any point during GP specialist training and there is no limit on the number of attempts that a candidate can make to pass the exam. An exam pass is valid for 3 years.

Pass rate (Jan 2008)
- 83.7% overall
- 86% GP registrars/ST3
- 75% pre-registrar trainees/ST2.

The AKT tests a candidate's ability to apply knowledge and interpret information within a GP setting – hence GP registrars are at a slight advantage to pre-registrars and this is reflected in the pass rates.

Question setting
The questions are set by working GPs. The source material includes patients who have presented in surgery, practice issues and topical issues – so-called 'hot topics'. Hot topic items concern matters of current interest to GPs, the emphasis being on British general practice and British journals. A careful study of the last 2 years of major editorials and reviews in *The Lancet, British Medical Journal* and *British Journal of General Practice* is likely to yield a useful list of study items. This book summarises recent hot topics but look out for new topics arising; Pulse and Radio 4 health programmes often cover these.

The cases are referenced (usually to national guidance – NICE [National Institute for Health and Clinical Excellence], SIGN [Scottish Intercollegiate Guidelines Network], BNF [*British National Formulary*], DTB [*Drugs and Therapeutics Bulletin*], Cochrane, GMC [General Medical Council], GP curriculum) and reviewed by fellow case writers. Questions can be divided into three broad categories: common conditions, rare but high-impact conditions, e.g. child abuse, and topical issues.

AKT exam content
- 80% clinical medicine and problem-solving
- 10% critical appraisal and evidence-based clinical practice
- 10% ethical and legal issues, organisation and administration.

Organisation and administration covers knowledge of regulatory frameworks (primary care trusts or PCTs, etc.), legal aspects (Driver and Vehicle Licensing Agency or DVLA, etc.), professional regulation (GMC, etc.), ethical issues (mental capacity, etc.), business aspects (GP contract, etc.), prescribing (controlled drugs, etc.), appropriate use of resources (rationing, etc.) and health and safety (needle stick injury, etc.).

Marking

Every candidate gets feedback on their overall score, pass mark and performance in the three main subject areas.

MCQ technique

Understanding phrasing in the exam is important to correctly interpret questions. Some general pointers may be of use:
- Read the questions very carefully
- Invariably – 98% of cases
- Usually/Majority/Common >50% of cases
- Frequently/Often/Regularly – between 5% and 50% of cases
- Rarely/Unusually/Uncommonly/Infrequent/Occasional <5%
- Has been shown = proven in clinical trials
- Characteristic/Typical feature/Recognised feature – a finding with diagnostic/significance/therapeutic
- Always and never – usually false (but not always!!)
- May – usually true.

Example question types
Single best answer example
1. A 40-year-old white man is diagnosed with essential hypertension. Which is the agent of choice?
   a. Amlodipine
   b. Bendroflumethiazide
   c. Doxazosin
   d. Ramipril
   e. Losartan
   f. Bisoprolol

Extended matching question example
A Form Med 3
B Form Med 4
C Form Med 5
D Form Med 6
E DS 1500
F Mat B1
G Form RM 7
H Private certificate

For each patient, select the most appropriate certificate from the list of options above. Each option may be used once, more than once or not at all.
1. You see and examine a patient with a knee injury who has been off work for 10 days. She requests a certificate to cover her absence from work for the next 7 days. (Answer A)
2. You have been issuing medical certificates to a man complaining of back pain for 3 months and would like to request an independent assessment of his capability to work. (Answer E)
3. Etc.

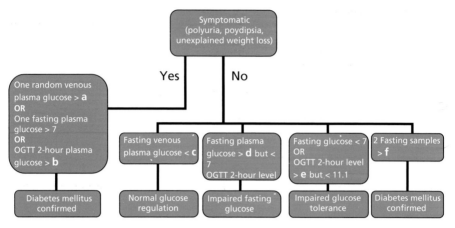

Figure 1.1 Diagnosing disorders of glucose regulation.

Tables/Algorithm question example
Diagnosing disorders of glucose regulation (Figure 1.1)
For each of the lettered gaps above, select ONE option from the list below to complete the algorithm. Each option may be used once, more than once or not at all.

Options
i. 11.1
ii. 7.1
iii. 7.0
iv. 6.8
v. 6.1
vi. 7.8

Answers based on the WHO criteria: (a) 11.1; (b) 11.1; (c) 6.1; (d) 6.1; (e) 7.8; (f) 7.0.

Data interpretation question example
The summary of a meta-analysis comparing the effects of β blockers on mortality is shown here (Table 1.1). Which study shows the most significant association between β blockers and reduction in mortality?

A Wilcox's (oxprenolol)
B Norris (propranolol)
C BHAT (propranolol)
D Multicentre (practolol)
E Multicentre (timolol)

Answer E – the only studies reaching significance are answers C and E (because the confidence intervals do not cross the line of no effect). E has the lowest ratio of crude deaths.

Table 1.1 Data for example question

Study	No. (%) of deaths in patients		β Blocker deaths		Ratio of crude death rates (99% CI) β Blocker: control
	β Blocker	Control	Logrank observed – expected	Variance of observed – expected	
Wilcox (oxprenolol)	14/157 (8.9)	10/158 (8.9)	2.0	5.6	
Norris (propranolol)	21/226 (9.3)	24/228 (9.3)	−1.4	10.2	
Multicantre (propranolol)	15/100 (15.0)	12/95 (12.6)	1.2	5.8	
Baber (propranolol)	28/355 (7.9)	27/365 (7.4)	0.9	12.7	
Andersen (alprenolol)	61/238 (25.6)	64/242 (26.4)	−1.0	23.2	
Balcon (propranolol)	14/56 (25.0)	15/58 (25.9)	−0.2	5.5	
Barber (practolol)	47/221 (21.3)	53/228 (23.2)	−2.2	19.5	
Wilcox (propranolol)	36/259 (13.9)	19/129 (14.7)	−0.7	10.5	
CPRG (oxprenolol)	9/177 (5.1)	5/136 (3.6)	1.1	3.3	
Multicentre (practolol)	102/1533 (6.7)	127/1520 (8.4)	−13.0	53.0	
Barber (propranolol)	10/52 (19.2)	12/47 (25.5)	−1.6	4.3	
BHAT (propranolol)	138/1916 (7.2)	188/1921 (9.8)	−24.8	74.6	
Multicentre (timolol)	98/945 (10.4)	152/939 (16.2)	−27.4	54.2	
Hjalmarson (metoprolol)	40/698 (5.7)	62/697 (8.9)	−11.0	23.7	
Wilheimsson (alprenolol)	7/114 (6.1)	14/116 (12.1)	−8.4	4.8	
■ Total*	640/7047 (9.1)	784/6879 (11.4)	−81.6	310.7	

0   0.5   1.0   1.5   2.0

Reduction 23.1% (SE5.0) P < 0.0001

β Blocker better   β Blocker worse

Heterogeneity between 15 trials: $\chi^2 = 13.9$; df = 14; P > 0.1.

Treatment effect P < 0.0001

*95% confidence interval as shown for the odds ratio.

From Lewis and Clarke. *BMJ* 2001;**322**:1479-80.

Seminal trial example

Which of the following trials investigated optimal blood pressure targets for the management of hypertension?

A. ISIS
B. ASCOT
C. CARE
D. CURE
E. HOT

(Answer E)

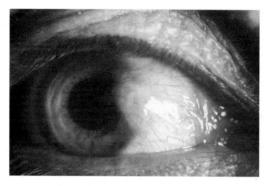

Figure 1.2 From www.cehjournal.org/images/ts020018.jpg.

Picture format question example

A 42-year-old office worker has noticed a change in the appearance of her eye (Figure 1.2). Which is the SINGLE MOST likely diagnosis? Select ONE option only.

A Pingeculum
B Pterygium
C Scleritis
D Episcleritis
E Iris melanoma

(Answer B)

Workplace-based Assessment

WBPA is the assessment of the trainee throughout her or his vocational training scheme (VTS) placements. It incorporates the trainer's report – the final year assessment in a general practice post. The trainee has to gather evidence of progress over the 3-year programme and store it on the web in an 'e-Portfolio'. During the process the trainee has 6-monthly reviews to evaluate progress. The WBPA assesses competencies in 12 areas (a subdivision of the six core areas of competency in the RCGP curriculum):

1. **Communication and consultation skills:** effective communication and the use of recognised consultation techniques

2. **Holistic care**: physical, psychological, socioeconomic and cultural dimensions, taking into account feelings as well as thoughts
3. **Data gathering and interpretation**: the gathering and use of data for clinical judgement, the choice of physical examination and investigations, and their interpretation
4. **Structured decision-making**
5. **Clinical management**: the recognition and management of common medical conditions in primary care
6. **Managing medical complexity and promoting health**: management of co-morbidity, uncertainty, risk and the approach to health rather than just illness
7. **Primary care administration and information management technology** (**IMT**): the appropriate use of primary care administration systems, effective record keeping and information technology for the benefit of patient care
8. **Working with colleagues and in teams**: working effectively with other professionals
9. **Community orientation**: health and social care of the practice population and local community
10. **Maintaining performance, learning and teaching**: continuing professional development
11. **Ethical approach to practice**: practising ethically with integrity and a respect for diversity
12. **Fitness to practise**: awareness of when his or her own performance, conduct or health, or that of others, might put patients at risk and the action taken to protect patients.

The assessment tools
Case-based discussion (CBD)
- Discussion of prepared cases.
- One of two prepared cases is selected for discussion in years ST1 and ST2 and two of four in year ST3. (How many are required? Six in years ST1 + ST2 and 12 in year ST3.)
- Evidence: an assessment form is uploaded to the e-Portfolio.

Consultation observation tool (COT)
- In primary care only
- Video consultations (requirements 12 in ST3)
- Evidence: rated against COT criteria and feedback uploaded to e-Portfolio.

Multi-source feedback (MSF)
- Trainee selects five colleagues
- Colleagues log on to the e-Portfolio of the trainee and answer questions on professional behaviour and clinical performance.

Patient satisfaction questionnaire (PSQ)
- In primary care only.

Direct observation of procedural skills (DOPS)
- In hospital post or GP posts, e.g. breast examination
- There are eight different procedures that require assessment for competency.

Clinical evaluation exercise (CEX)
- The hospital equivalent of a COT, e.g. evaluation of history-taking skills
- Six in ST1 and ST2.

Clinical supervisor's report (CSR)
- At the end of each hospital post
- Assessment of knowledge, practical skills and professional competency related to the post.

There is no pass/fail for these tools – just a judgement on whether the evidence satisfies competence or there is need for further training.

Preparing a case-based discussion

CBD is used to assess multiple competencies (Table 1.2). A structured approach to preparing cases can help identify the relevant issues which may be chosen for discussion. To avoid being questioned on areas for which you have not prepared consider whether the following issues apply to your case.

1. Consultation issues (mnenomic: The Essential Consultation Issues)
   Time management
   Ethics (beneficence, autonomy, non-maleficence, justice)
   Communication (rapport, empathy, cultural and religious aspects, use of consultation techniques)

Table 1.2 Sample trainer marking grid

	Proposed questions	Evidence obtained	Competency
Holistic practice			
Data gathering and interpretation			
Clinical management			
Making diagnosis/decisions			
Example	*How do you justify your decision?*	*Evidence base for decision, e.g. NICE guideline*	*Competent*
Managing medical complexity			
Primary care admin and IMT			
Working with colleagues			
Community orientation			
Ethical approach			
Fitness to practise			

IMT, information management technology.

Context (putting the condition in context, i.e. the impact physically, psychologically and socially at home and work)

Clinical (data gathering – red flags, choice of examination, investigation and management options, evidence-based decision-making, safety netting, housekeeping, co-morbidity)

ICE (**i**deas, **c**oncerns and **e**xpectations of patients)

2. Practice issues (mnemonic: **P**ractice **C**osts **M**oney **N**othing's **F**ree)

Professional responsibilities (safety of patients, DVLA, legal aspects, notifiable diseases)

Care of colleagues (GMC *Good Medical Practice* guidance)

MDT or **M**ultidisciplinary team (team working, delegation, coordination of care)

National/local issues (revalidation, appraisal, local PCT issues)

Finances (rationing, service provision, cost-effective prescribing)

Assessors review the prepared cases before the discussion and prepare questions about the issues. Cases are usually discussed in an informal atmosphere. The questions raised will help you to demonstrate competence in the 10 areas assessed by CBD. The assessor will upload evidence of the CBD to your e-Portfolio describing your level of competence ('excellent, competent, needs further development or insufficient evidence') for each of the areas covered by the case. Not all 10 areas are covered on each CBD. The assessor will cover as many areas as possible relevant to the case within the time allowed. To get an idea of the kind of questions that you may be asked, there are some sample assessors' questions mapped to the different areas available to download at the RCGP website CBD resources section. Twenty minutes are allocated to each CBD with a further 10 minutes for feedback.

Some useful models, frameworks, evidence and concepts applicable to CBD are summarised by topic throughout this book.

Preparing a consultation observation tool

Record consultations and select your best for use in a discussion, or get the trainer to sit in on a consultation. In all cases, valid written consent must be given by the patient beforehand. As a rule of thumb, recordings should not exceed 15 minutes. The COT assessment is based on the old MRCGP video criteria (with a few tweaks). It may be helpful to have a list of the criteria on your surgery wall to prompt you (out of sight of the camera)!

COT criteria

The candidate demonstrates the ability to:

1. Encourage the patient at appropriate times
2. Respond to cues (that lead to a deeper understanding of the problem)
3. Put the condition in the context, e.g. 'How is … affecting your daily activities/work?'
4. Explore the patient's health understanding (ICE, e.g. 'What do you think the problem might be?')
5. Ask questions to include or exclude likely diagnoses

6. Examine appropriately to test your diagnosis or address a patient concern
7. Make an appropriate working diagnosis
8. Explain the problem or diagnosis in appropriate language
9. Confirm the patient's understanding of the diagnosis and take steps to enhance his or her concordance:
    (a) Sometimes I don't explain things as well as I would like so could you explain back to me your understanding of the problem and the plan that we have agreed OR
    (b) How would you explain that to your wife/daughter, etc.?
10. Make an appropriate management plan (safe and in line with guidelines)
11. Involve the patient in a choice of treatment (shared decisions)
12. Explore the patient's understanding of their treatment and take steps to enhance concordance
13. Arrange follow-up.

For an in-depth guide go to RCGP COT resources (detailed guide to the performance criteria).

The COTs should be taken throughout the registrar year and demonstrate a range of presentations across the disease spectrum. At least one case must be of a child under 10, one an adult over 75 and one a mental health case. The consultation is reviewed with the trainer and assessed against the COT criteria. The trainer then formulates a global judgement for the overall consultation and offers formal feedback on the consultation with recommendations for further work and development. Evidence is uploaded to the e-Portfolio

Which tools assess which competencies?

Table 1.3 Tools for assessing competencies

Competence area	MSF	PSQ	COT	CBD	CEX	CSR
Communication and consultation skills	X	X	X		X	X
Practising holistically		X	X	X		X
Data gathering and interpretation	X		X	X	X	X
Making a diagnosis/decisions	X		X	X	X	X
Clinical management	X		X	X	X	X
Managing medical complexity				X	X	X
Primary care admin and IMT				X		
Working with colleagues and in teams	X			X		X
Community orientation				X		X
Maintaining performance learning and teaching	X				X	X
Maintaining an ethical approach	X			X		X
Fitness to practice	X			X		X

MSF, multi-source feedback; PSQ, patient source feedback; COT, clinical observation tool; CBD, case-based discussion; CEX, clinical evaluation exercise; CSR, clinical supervisor's report.

A fairer exam – but more work

The advantage of WBPA is that it assesses the application of knowledge and attitudes in real situations in a way that cannot be accurately simulated in the exam environment. It also helps to reveal areas of deficiency early in training and prompt learning to address them. The WBPA should make the MCRGP assessment fairer and more robust through a process called triangulation. Triangulation is the use of evidence gathering from multiple sources to demonstrate competency, e.g. competency in communication and consultation skills may be evidenced through the CSA, AKT and five of the WBPA tools (see Table 1.3).

The disadvantage is that there is a lot of administrative work for the candidate and the trainers.

The Clinical Skills Assessment

The CSA exam is discussed in Chapter 9.

The RCGP curriculum and being a GP

The RCGP curriculum draws on two important documents: the European Definition of General Practice/Family Medicine and the GMC's (2006) *Good Medical Practice* guidance (page 47):

> Set within a framework for a structured educational programme (VTS), the RCGP curriculum is designed to address the wide-ranging knowledge, competences, clinical and professional attitudes considered appropriate for a doctor intending to undertake practice in the contemporary UK National Health Service.
>
> (www.rcgp-curriculum.org.uk)

The new MRCGP exam specifically tests skills and knowledge in the six areas of competence and three essential features identified by the curriculum. These are summarised in Tables 1.4 and 1.5. The full curriculum is

Table 1.4 The RCGP six domains of core competencies

1. Primary care management	Managing problems with a primary care focus (knowledge of epidemiology and presentation of disease, prevention and health promotion, cost-effective management and communication)
2. Person-centred care	Sharing knowledge and the management of problems with patients
3. Specific problem-solving skills	Context specific skills (e.g. applying guidelines, focused data gathering and investigation, use of problem-solving consultation models)[a]
4. A comprehensive approach	Dealing with acute and ongoing problems in the consultation
5. Community orientation	Understanding local health needs (impact of poverty, ethnicity, local epidemiology, rationing and health economics)
6. A holistic approach.	Caring for the whole person (physical, psychological and social) in context of their experiences, beliefs, values and expectations

[a]'GPs in solving problems have to tolerate uncertainty, explore probability and marginalise danger, whereas hospital specialists have to reduce uncertainty, explore possibility and marginalise error' (Marinker and Peckham 1998).

Table 1.5 The RCGP's three essential features

1. Contextual aspects	Having an understanding of the impact of the local community on patient care (including socioeconomic and workplace factors)
	Being aware of the impact of overall workload on the care given to the individual patient and the facilities (e.g. staff, equipment) available to deliver that care
	Having an understanding of the financial and legal frameworks in which health care is given at practice level
	Having an understanding of the impact of the doctor's personal housing and working environment on the care that he or she provides
2. Attitudinal aspects	Being aware of own capabilities and values
	Identifying ethical aspects of clinical practice (prevention, diagnostics, therapy, factors that influence lifestyle)
	Having an awareness of self: an understanding that own attitudes and feelings are important determinants of how they practise
	Justifying and clarifying personal ethics
	Being aware of the interaction of work and doctor's own private life, and striving for a good balance between them
3. Scientific aspects	Being familiar with the general principles, methods and concepts of scientific research and the fundamentals of statistics (incidence, prevalence, predicted value, etc.)
	Knowledge of scientific backgrounds of pathology, symptoms and diagnosis, therapy and prognosis, epidemiology, decision theory, theories of forming hypotheses and problem-solving, preventive health care
	Assessing medical literature, reading and assessing it critically and putting the lessons from the literature into practice
	Developing and maintaining continuing learning and quality improvement

available on the RCGP website (www.rcgp-curriculum.org.uk) and contains a useful map of the curriculum with links to learning resources. It is a detailed document. This book covers the entire RCGP curriculum mostly in order. Each chapter heading highlights the relevant curriculum statements covered.

References

General Medical Council. *Good Medical Practice*. London: GMC, 2006.

Lewis S, Clarke M. Education and debate Forest plots: trying to see the wood and the trees. *BMJ* 2001;**322**:1479–80.

Marinker M, Peckham PJ (eds). *Clinical Futures*. London: BMJ Books, 1998.

2 The general practice consultation

This chapter relates to curriculum statement 2 ('The general practice consultation')
The consultation is a complex process and the basis of the clinical skills assessment (CSA). It has the potential to address many issues. When consultations fail to meet their potential it can be hard to know the cause because there are so many different factors to a successful consultation. Is it a result of a failure to complete the tasks set by the doctor or the patient? Has the doctor lacked the skills to elicit important findings, or failed to understand the emotional, psychological or social behaviour of the patient? Consultation models are a tool to provide insights into the strengths and weaknesses of our consulting. A plan can then be made to address perceived problems and tested in future consultations. Consulting such as this (the dreaded word 'reflection' applies here) helps to build up clinical, and communication skills and reduce the number of 'heartsink' (see later in chapter) patients. Ultimately this can be a satisfying way of working with benefits for doctors and patients.

This chapter considers the importance of communication skills and the consultation models. It summarises different models, their advantages and disadvantages, and how consultation techniques can be improved. Knowledge of different consultation models are assessed in the AKT and demonstration of competency in consulting skills in the CSA. Use of a consultation model in the CSA to display your consulting skills at their best is recommended (see Chapter 9 and 'Needs model' later in chapter). The chapter concludes with sections on prescribing and the referral of patients for secondary care, plus some sample AKT questions.

Communication skills

Good communication skills are vital to being an effective consulter. They are the lynchpin that all consultations and consultation models rely on. The good news is that there is plenty of evidence that communication skills can be learnt – just like any other skill. The Toronto Consensus Statement 1991 is probably the best known of all documents on communication skills in medicine (Simpson et al. 1991):

Notes for the MRCGP: A curriculum based guide to the AKT, CSA and WBPA, 4th edition.
By K. Palmer and N. Boeckx. Published 2010 by Blackwell Publishing,
ISBN: 978-1-4051-5724-7.

> Effective communication between doctor and patient is a central clinical function … the physician's interpersonal skills … *largely* determine the patient's satisfaction and compliance and positively influence health outcomes ….

There is now overwhelming proof to support this (Aspegren K. *Medical Teacher* 1999;**21**:563–70). Evidence suggests that effective communication consists of a repertoire of learned behaviours that may be identified and taught. Three different purposes of communication have been recognised in the medical context, namely: (1) creating a good doctor–patient relationship; (2) exchanging information; and (3) making treatment-related decisions (Hoos and Lammes. *Soc Sci Med* 1995;**40**:903–18). These factors form the building blocks of many of the consultation models and have been identified through research into the consultation.

The methods used to observe the consultation include:

- audio taping
- videotaping
- the use of two-way mirrors
- sitting in on colleagues' consultations
- role-play.

No single method has proved entirely satisfactory: audiotapes miss important non-verbal information and contain uninterpretable pauses; role-play is to some extent artificial; and the presence of a video camera, or a second doctor, or the knowledge that there are observers, may modify the behaviour of doctor or patient or both. Despite these problems, much useful descriptive information has been obtained. Taped consultations may be replayed and subjected to peer review and small group analysis, or dissected into their various social, linguistic and psychological components.

Consultation models

There are many different models, the most useful and popular of which are summarised here (with useful memory aids). They can be divided into two broad categories: task-based models and behaviour-based models. It is worth learning the central structure, a few key facts and some of the strengths/weaknesses because they often appear in the exam (and can help improve your consultation skills and job satisfaction).

Task-based models

Advantages

- Provide a simple structure to analyse the consultation
- Can be used as a framework to plan out your routine consultations (aide memoir)
- Encourage lateral thinking (e.g. health promotion, investigation of health beliefs)
- Easy to apply (most models).

Disadvantages

- Not all consultations fit into a prescribed framework
- Several consultations may be required to achieve the tasks set

- Trying to shoehorn inappropriate tasks into a consultation may lead to ineffective use of time and resources and damage the patient–doctor relationship.

The biomedical model
Tasks
1. Observe (take history and examination)
2. Hypothesise (make a differential diagnosis)
3. Deduce (investigate the differential diagnosis and come to a conclusion).

This is a hypotheticodeductive method of problem-solving (adapted from Elstein et al. 1978).

Studies show that GPs make a number of hypotheses – about three to six – and use key questions to test and discount these. Investigation can then help to confirm or narrow the differential diagnosis further.

Advantages
- Logical approach to clinical problem solving (but misses the human element).

Disadvantages
- Doctor centred and a tendency to oversimplify complex problems
- Does not involve the patient's emotional, social and environmental circumstances
- Ignores the patient's health beliefs, ideas, concerns or expectations.

MEMORY BOX: The biomedical model
- Hypotheticodeductive
- Published in 1978

Byrne and Long (1976)
Consultation phases
1. Establish relationship
2. Find why they come
3. Take history and examine
4. Consider the condition
5. Decide on further investigation/treatment
6. End consultation.

Byrne and Long (1976) analysed 2500 audiotaped consultations. Their model describes six consultation 'phases'. They identified the doctor-centred (in which the patient's input is minimal and often ignored) and patient-centred consultation styles. The GMC (General Medical Council) and RCGP focus heavily on patient-centred consulting. Candidates should strive for this shared approach to care.

Advantages
- Raises awareness of the locus of control (i.e. doctor vs patient centredness)
- Provides the consulting structure on which many later models are based.

Disadvantages
- Not comprehensive (early model).

MEMORY BOX: Byrne and Long
- **B**ug and **L**isten (2500 audiotaped consultations)
- Doctor centred vs patient centred
- Six consultation 'phases' (tasks)
- Published in 1976

Pendleton's model
Tasks
1. Identify the *main problem* for the patient's attendance, including the patients ideas, concerns and expectations (ICE) about the problem
2. Consider *other problems*, e.g. chronic disease management points, risk factors
3. Choose *action* for each *problem*
4. Achieve shared understanding
5. Share responsibility
6. Use time and resources appropriately
7. Maintain relationship (to help achieve the above).

This model was devised by Pendleton, Tate and Havelock but is commonly referred to as Pendleton's model (Pendleton et al. 1984). Although Pendleton suggests this model as a comprehensive framework to be applied to any consultation, the wider needs of the practice and business are not well defined in this model. They can, however, be considered under the sixth task. This is better described and easier to recall in a new comprehensive model called the 'needs model'. The MRCGP's Workplace-based Assessment (WPBA) video assessment criteria are based around Pendleton's model. Pendleton also developed consultation mapping – use of a grid to identify the tasks completed within a recorded consultation.

Advantages
- Patient centred
- Easy to apply in practice
- Covers many issues.

Disadvantages
- Despite covering many issues this model is not comprehensive.
- Behavioural insights do not feature prominently in this model.

> **MEMORY BOX:** Pendleton's model
> • Seven tasks – problems and actions
> • Published in 1984 and revised in 2003

Neighbour's model

1. Connect (establish a rapport with the patient)
2. Summarise (eliciting the patient's problems, ICE, and summarising them)
3. Handover (agree a shared management plan)
4. Safety net (contingency plans, follow-up)
5. Housekeep (preparing for the next consultation by clearing your mind of the negative psychological effects of the previous consultation).

Neighbour (1987) describes the consultation as a 'reflective conversation with the situation'. The doctor *facilitates* change by processing raw information from the patient into useable data with which to present a solution. This is achieved by using constant questioning of the current situation (who, what, where, what does this mean?) to develop an understanding of the patient's needs. The tasks or 'checkpoints' aid this process and 'ensure no serious disease or concerns are missed'.

Advantages
• Patient centred
• Easy to apply
• Acknowledges the role of the emotions of the doctor and patient within the consultation
• Encourages safe practice via safety netting.

Disadvantage
• Management of continuing problems, practice needs and health promotion among other issues are not considered explicitly in this model.

> **MEMORY BOX:** Neighbour's model
> • Housekeeping
> • Published 1987

Stott and Davis

Tasks
1. Identify and manage presenting problem
2. Manage continuing problems
3. Modify help-seeking behaviour
4. Opportunistic health promotion.

Stott and Davis list four areas that can be addressed in each consultation. They recognised that patient contact allows the doctor not only to deal with the immediate and continuing health problems but also to offer health promotion to prevent disease and reduce the burden of sickness on the community. This model has become increasingly relevant as the profile of health promotion for lifestyle diseases such as obesity and diabetes rises.

(In 2001 a fifth of adults were clinically obese with a rising trend. This has led to the NICE guidance in December 2006 on obesity management.)

> **MEMORY BOX:** Stott and Davis
> - Health promotion + help-seeking behaviour
> - Published 1979

Behaviour-based models

Advantages

Provide insights that improve our understanding of patients' behaviour and have the potential to:
- enhance communication skills
- increase concordance with management plans
- improve health outcomes
- reduce doctor frustration/heart sinks.

Disadvantages
- Behavioural models can lack structure and be difficult to apply
- Some suggested interventions are time-consuming (Balint's long consultation).

Helman

Helman is a medical anthropologist (the study of human behaviour). His work provides insights into the cultural factors in health and illness. He suggests that a patient with a problem comes to a doctor seeking the answer to six questions:

1. What has happened?
2. Why has it happened? $\Big\}$ *Ideas*
3. Why to me?
4. Why now? $\Big\}$ *Concerns*
5. What would happen if nothing was done about it?
6. What should I do about it/whom should I consult $\Big\}$ *Expectations*
   for further help?

Applying this model helps develop understanding of patient behaviour and promotes a patient-centred approach. It can be summarised by the mnemonic **i**deas, **c**oncerns and **e**xpectations (ICE, first coined by Pendleton 1983; summarising Balint (1957) it encapsulates this model well and is quoted in Neighbour's model).

> **MEMORY BOX:** Helman
> - Life questions (ICE)
> - Behavioural model
> - Published 1981

Balint

Michael Balint is a psychoanalyst, who started to research the GP–patient relationship in the 1950s. Balint found that patients' problems cannot be divided into physical and psychological categories because the two always coexist to some degree. Psychological problems often manifest physically, and physical diseases usually have psychological consequences. The Balint approach established that doctors are active rather than passive participants in the consultation, and showed how the doctor's feelings need to be identified and made use of in the consultation. Several important concepts have come out of their work:

- The flash: where the doctor becomes aware of his feelings and feeds this back to the patient in a way that can give insight into the problems that are presented, e.g. If the patient angers the doctor is he having same reaction with others?
- Doctor as drug: Balint suggested that doctors act as a drug that the patient takes periodically to improve their health (this differs to Neighbour where the doctor is a facilitator not the drug or 'change agent').
- The long consultation: Balint (1986) promoted the use of the 'long consultation' to investigate the underlying psychosocial causes behind heartsink patients (e.g. frequent attendees, long-term problems lacking satisfactory outcome). A single long session (lasting up to an hour) can provide enough insight for the doctor, and support for the patient to lead to a resolution of the problem.
- Apostolic function: the doctor's tendency to have unrealistic expectations of the patient based on the doctor's own values, e.g. 'You should give up alcohol, I never touch it'.

MEMORY BOX: Balint
- Doctor as drug
- The flash
- Mutual investment bank (relationship invested in by doctor and patient)
- Balint group (discussion of cases with colleagues focusing on the doctor–patient relationship)
- The long consultation
- The apostolic function
- Published 1957

Transactional analysis (Berne)

Eric Berne's model describes three 'ego' states (Parent, Adult and Child). During the consultation the doctor and patient each assume one of these states. Those in the parent role act paternalistically, directing the consultation. The child role is 'accepting and unquestioning' and the adult logical and questioning. Correct combinations communicate in transactions occurring in a predictable way and leading to a predictable outcome (rituals). Sometimes transactions are *crossed* (when, for example, the doctor talks like a parent and the patient adopts the role of subservient child – doctor centred), or *oblique* (when an ulterior message is aimed at another ego state in the recipient). A familiar example is the 'Why don't you? –Yes but …' ritual in which the doctor plays the parent ('I can make you grateful for my help, whether you want it or not') and the patient plays the child who always wins ('You go ahead and try …'). The 'ideal' consultation is between a doctor and patient both in the adult role sharing decisions. Being aware of the roles that you and your patient adopt can help steer towards this ideal and break out of unproductive cycles of behaviour.

MEMORY BOX: Berne
- Parent, Child, Adult
- Published 1964

Six-category intervention analysis (Heron)

In the 1970s the psychologist John Heron developed a model for the different of interventions that a doctor (counsellor or therapist) could use with the patient. Within an overall setting of concern for the patient's best interests, the doctor's interventions fall into one of six categories:

1. Prescriptive: giving advice or instructions, being critical or directive
2. Informative: imparting new knowledge, instructing or interpreting
3. Confronting: challenging a restrictive attitude or behaviour, giving direct feedback within a caring context
4. Cathartic: seeking to release emotion in the form of weeping, laughter, trembling or anger
5. Catalytic: encouraging the patient to discover and explore his or her own latent thoughts and feelings
6. Supportive: offering comfort and approval, affirming the patient's intrinsic value.

Each category has a clear function within the total consultation. Use of this model does not inevitably lead to long consultations. Simple actions like offering a tissue may be enough to precipitate the release of emotion and hence be cathartic. When a consultation 'gets stuck' use of one of the 6 interventional techniques may reveal insights which lead to a shared plan and solution.

MEMORY BOX: Six Category Analysis
- Six interventions
- Published 1975

The health beliefs model (Rosenstock, Becker and Maiman)

Patients vary in their health motivation, perceived vulnerability, the perceived seriousness of a problem, and the perceived costs and benefits; they behave rationally and consistently in the light of their own beliefs, which are fostered by a variety of cues, and modified by different outcomes.

One variation of this model (Rotter 1966) proposes that patients can be subdivided into those who explain what happens to them in terms of their own actions (i.e. have an internal locus of control) and those who explain everything as if they have little control (i.e. have an external locus of control). This aspect of the patient's psychological make-up influences outcome – thus, internal controllers are more likely to accept advice, keep appointments and take their prescriptions.

> **MEMORY BOX:** The health beliefs model
> - Behaviour of a patient is controlled by their health beliefs
> - Locus of control
> - Published 1966

The non-verbal model

More information is conveyed by non-verbal cues than by speech; doctors and patients read one another's non-verbal messages and sometimes acknowledge and act on them, but non-verbal messages that are inconsistent with spoken ones hinder communication.

A combined task/behaviour model

The Needs model is a current and practical model for use in the CSA and daily consultation. It builds on many of the aspects covered by previous consultation models by considering the needs of four key agents (all start with P).

Needs model (Boeckx)

Patient
- Manage clinical needs:
  - establish a rapport
  - identify the presenting problem and consider ongoing problems
  - consider ICE to achieve a shared understanding of the problems
  - consider the patient's behaviour (Adult, Child, Parent) and try to move towards an Adult–Adult consultation
  - discuss treatment options, jointly choose actions and share responsibility
  - consider opportunities for health promotion
  - safety net.

Practice
- Manage practice needs:
  - address repeat prescribing issues, misuse of the practice service, failures to attend appointments, breakdowns in the ongoing doctor–patient relationship
  - update QOF (Quality Outcome Framework) points by appropriate coding of problems/investigations/results
  - reclaim costs (minor surgery, immunisations).

Public and Partners
- Consider wider public health needs:
  - implications for partners/family members
  - DVLA (Driver and Vehicle Licensing Agency) medical rules
  - contact tracing
  - immunisations (childhood/flu) herd immunity.

Practitioner
- Manage practitioner's personal needs:
  - ➤ medicolegal:
    - ◆ document the consultation clearly (including important positive and negative findings and plan of management/follow-up plans)
    - ◆ provide the patient with written information where appropriate
  - ➤ educational:
    - ◆ identify any personal learning needs (e.g. notes for a reflective diary)
    - ◆ appraisal (record cases that show personal development in the areas required for annual appraisal)
  - ➤ organisational: dictation of letters, referral forms, create a to-do list
  - ➤ psychological: housekeeping (Neighbour).

The patient comes first – deal with their clinical needs (the tasks set are a consolidation of Stott and Davis's, Helman's, Pendleton's, Neighbour's and Berne's models); then consider the practice needs. With the advent of QOF and practice-based commissioning addressing the administration and business needs of the practice in the consultation has become increasingly important (failing to meet QOF targets due to poor administration and business skills reduces your practice income, so less money is available to the practice to offer improved and new services to meet local patient needs). Next consider needs of the public and partners, e.g. support for carers, contact tracing, driving licence implications. Finally consider your needs as the practitioner. The practitioners' needs can be recalled by using the mnemonic POEM (**p**sychological, **o**rganisational, **e**ducational and **m**edicolegal – though logic suggests that they are best dealt with in the reverse order).

This is a brief overview but the Needs model can be used to explore many of the aspects described by the established models (a few examples are given under each heading). The main advantage is that the basic construct is easy to recall and allows a structure on which to base a comprehensive analysis of the consultation. Application of this model in the CSA should help you cover all the relevant consultation issues.

MEMORY BOX: Needs model
- Patient
- Practice
- Public
- Practitioner

Further reading
If you are interested in further reading on consultation models see the literature for each model. Other models of interest include the RCGP consultation model, problem-based interviewing (Scott et al. 1999), Gelat's (1962) problem-solving model and the disease illness model (Stewart et al. 1995).

Effective consulting – studying outcomes

Measures of the effectiveness of a consultation, i.e. outcome, are imperfect. It is extremely difficult, for example, to measure the average health, medical knowledge or prognosis of a doctor's list and to relate it to variations in his or her consultative approach. Some important outcomes that can be counted are discussed here. When the consultation is judged according to these criteria, it is clear that its potential is often not fully realised.

Compliance

Compliance (conformance of a patient with a treatment plan) is assessed in a variety of ways (by biological methods, subjective ratings, self-report, pill counts and direct observation). Whatever the method of evaluation, non-compliance rates are high – a review of literature (by The Royal Pharmaceutical Society of Great Britain) in 1995 shows that approximately 50% of patients fail to follow the terms of their prescription.

Compliance vs concordance (RPSGB 1997)

The avoidable illness and premature deaths that result from poor compliance have a high cost for patients, businesses and society. The public cost in terms of economic loss and increased health services expenditure is vast. Poor compliance has been attributed to failures to establish effective therapeutic partnerships between doctors and patients. The fault is thought to lie with the traditional compliance model of prescribing, which requires the patient to follow advice from the doctor irrespective of health beliefs. Compliance is poorest where doctor's and patient's views conflict and the patient's views are not adequately addressed by the doctor's treatment plan.

Research showed that improvements of 'compliance' could be achieved through educational and behavioural approaches. This has led to the currently favoured concordance model. The concordance model of prescribing involves a discussion of patients' and doctors' health beliefs. This includes an explanation of risks and benefits, with the aim of achieving a shared management plan compatible with what the patient desires and is capable of achieving (very much like Pendleton's consultation model tasks 4 and 5). The doctors professionally held health beliefs are used to inform and do not have priority over the patient's own health beliefs. Where the agreement falls short of what evidence-based medicine considers optimal treatment, the decision should be documented and an opportunity to review treatment agreed.

Franz Kafka (1919), in *A Country Doctor*, wrote 'To write prescriptions is easy, but to come to an understanding with people is hard' (quote in Marinker 1997).

Patient recollection

1. Numerous studies suggest that more than 50% of information has been forgotten when patients are interviewed within a few minutes of leaving the surgery.

2. The characteristics of memorable information are that:
   (a) the patient believes it to be important (often diagnosis rather than treatment)
   (b) the patient understands it
   (c) the information is given early in the consultation
   (d) not too much is given at once.

Important information should be backed up by written information (an excellent source of free, good quality, evidence-based patient information is available from www.patient.co.uk.)

Patient satisfaction

Communication is an aspect of care in which patients are historically most dissatisfied. In one hospital study (McGhee 1961) 65% of patients were dissatisfied with communication. As the impact of good communication skills on patient satisfaction, concordance and positive health outcome have become recognised, taught and assessed (via the patient satisfaction questionnaire of QOF), the levels of patient satisfaction have increased. The National Survey of Local Health Services (2006) shows that 82% of patients felt carefully listened to and 92% treated with respect and dignity (data from the Department of Health or DH). Perhaps politicians should consider their satisfaction levels before criticising doctors! in this regard we compare favourably with our political masters and mistresses.

Valid diagnosis

Shepherd et al. (1966) reported wide variations between London GPs in the level of psychiatric illness that they detected – from 38 per 1000 up to 323 per 1000, which is a ninefold discrepancy. It is likely that GPs had different thresholds for diagnosis of depression or used alternative diagnostic labels – anxiety, stress. It is impossible to say which was the more effective doctor – those diagnosing more or those diagnosing less. Such dilemmas make it difficult to assess effective performance. For example, NICE advocates use of a study in the *British Medical Journal* (2003) which carried out trials of a quick two-question screening tool for identifying depression in high-risk patients, e.g. chronic disease patients. This tool is integrated into the chronic disease QOF frameworks. A positive response to both questions is 97% sensitive and 67% specific for depression (Arroll et al. *BMJ* 2003;**327**:1144). But a Cochrane review of the evidence published two years later concluded that such screening for depression had small or no impact on patient outcomes (probably because most cases identified were mild and self limiting)! The strategies used by those diagnosing less may have been equally effective.

Improving consultation techniques

Consultation factors

Consultation analysis has suggested various explanations for the relative failure in communication observed in doctor–patient studies; for example:

1. Patient factors:
   (a) limited knowledge of illness (many misconceptions and folk models of illness)
   (b) diffidence in asking for clarification; this is class related – only 45% of hospital patients obtain the information that they want by asking, but 65% of class 1 ask, whereas only 40% of class 5 do (Cartwright 1964)
   (c) the negative effect of anxiety
   (d) the 'hidden agenda' – patients often legitimise their desire to consult over one matter by presenting with another one that they think is a more respectable reason in the eyes of their doctor. If their complaint is taken at face value, the 'hidden agenda' may remain hidden and the patient leaves the room dissatisfied.
2. Doctor factors:
   (a) professional and personal attitudes; doctors vary at the extremes from autocratic, high-status information withholders to egalitarian sharers of information who place emphasis on the patient's role
   (b) medical uncertainty and doubt – which doctors prefer to hide
   (c) inappropriately technical language
   (d) too much information too quickly
   (e) failure to establish what concerns the patient
   (f) non-verbal cues of uncertainty or doubt, at variance with what is said
   (g) interrupting the patient early in the consultation
   (h) short consultation length.
3. Doctor–patient relationship factors:
   (a) communication and concordance are better if there is doctor–patient rapport (usually a doctor who is perceived to be empathetic and a patient who conforms to the doctor's idea of a model patient!);
   (b) Social, cultural and language barriers between doctor and patient are important. There appear to be linguistic and other social factors that produce better communication if doctor and patient come from a similar background.

Consideration of these factors suggests that various techniques can be employed to improve such outcomes as diagnostic accuracy, patient satisfaction, communication and concordance.

Key factors associated with positive outcomes include:
- a good relationship (caring and confiding)
- establishing and giving due weight to the patient's concerns, beliefs and expectations
- giving information early in a consultation
- keeping the message simple and clear (and not imparting too much in one session)
- listening for 2 minutes without interruption at the start of a consultation
- repeating the message and stressing its importance
- providing specific information and concrete examples

- offering longer consultations
- giving written instructions as a reminder (patient leaflets see www. patient.co.uk).

For more information consult Ley et al. (1976), Korsch and Negrete (1972), Royal Pharmaceutical Society Review (1997), Langewitz et al. (2002) and Wilson and Childs (2002).

In addition:

- Even in a context of busy surgery or exam time constraints, 2 minutes of listening should be enough to obtain a fairly complete list of the patient's reasons for seeking consultation in almost 80% of cases. Patient satisfaction was heavily influenced by whether or not the patient felt listened to and is assessed annually in the national patient satisfaction survey (Langewitz et al. 2002).
- Wilson and Childs (2002) show that doctors who have large clinic numbers with shorter consultation times have a:
  - ➤ higher rate of drug prescription
  - ➤ higher rate of visits (12.9% vs 7.2%, $P < 0.001$) for new visits and (34.3% vs 28.5%, $P < 0.02$) for follow-up visits
  - ➤ higher consultation frequency
  - ➤ lower patient satisfaction rating
  - ➤ lower levels of health promotion and prevention.
- Recall and satisfaction are both enhanced when patients are asked to repeat and give feedback on the instructions that they are given – Bertakis (1977)
- Outcome is improved by the correct use of non-verbal cues (e.g. body posture can communicate concern; several studies have shown that good communicators smile more, look at the interlocutor more and have a different intonation when compared with less successful colleagues – see the non-verbal consultation model)
- Patient-centred behaviour (seeing illness through the patient's eyes and with his or her expectations) has been linked with higher patient satisfaction, better compliance with treatment, better treatment of chronic health problems and better recovery from ill-defined illnesses.
- Law and Britten (1995) report from videotape analysis that women doctors tend to be more patient centred than men; also that the highest 'patient centredness' scores are achieved between women doctors and women patients – the lowest being between male doctors and female patients.
- The structure of the consulting environment affects the amount of information exchanged (e.g. seating arrangements can reduce or enhance exchanges by a factor of six; Pietroni 1976).

One interesting paper has looked at the doctor himself as a therapeutic instrument in the consultation, and the extent to which this is enhanced by a positive, assertive approach. Thomas (1987) found that, in the 40–60% of consultations where no firm diagnosis can be made, patients feel better in the hands of a positive physician.

Tools to develop communication skills
The Calgary–Cambridge Guide Mark 2 (Kurtz et al. 2003)
The Calgary–Cambridge Guide is a teaching tool for developing communication skills referenced in the curriculum. It is an evidence-based approach to consulting, including only skills shown by research and theory to aid doctor–patient communication. A list of useful techniques included in the model is given here. Candidates should be familiar with their use for WPBA, COTS, CSA (Clinical Skills Assessment) and everyday consulting.

Evidenced-based consulting skills from the Calgary–Cambridge Guide
- Patient's narrative (encouraging the patient to tell the story in their own words)
- Question style: open to closed cone (start with open questions then closed down)
- Attentive listening (2 min without interruptions)
- Facilitative response (verbal and non-verbal encourages, repetition, interpretation)
- Picking up cues (verbal and non-verbal to identify a hidden agenda)
- Clarification
- Time framing (e.g. prioritisation – out of your list of problems which was your main concern?, temporisation – using follow-up consultations)
- Summary (to confirm correct understanding of the patient's narrative)
- Appropriate use of language (explains any jargon used)
- Ideas, concerns, expectations, feelings and thoughts.

A useful structured handout of the model is available at www.skillscascade.com.

Many of the communication skills listed and defined by research seem common sense and are shared by other types of professional encounter – especially in education. Equally important is developing appropriate underlying professional attitudes towards our patients and ourselves (Skelton 2005).

The difficult patient
In the MRCGP exam (and in real life), there is a special interest in how to handle the difficult patient, the non-compliant 'troublemaker', the addict who will not relinquish his tranquilliser, the liberated rebel giving birth in an unheated caravan, contraceptive and ethical conundrums, problem families, and so on. Essentially they are those patients who leave us with negative feelings (anger, frustration, inadequacy) on completion of the consultation.

At the simplest level the courses of action open, given a contentious request are: to agree, to disagree, or to refer/bargain/educate/counsel – and each will have predictable implications.

Table 2.1 Types of 'difficult' patient

Class	Features
1 The dependent clinger	Expresses excessive gratitude for doctor's actions, but seeks regular reassurance over minor problems
2 The entitled demander	Frequently complains about imagined shortcomings in the service received
3 The manipulative help-rejecter	Presents a series of symptoms that the doctor is powerless to improve
4 The self-destructive denier	The patient who refuses to accept his behaviour affects his disease and will not modify self-harming habits

At a slightly more sophisticated level, there have been several attempts to classify the so-called 'heartsink' patient (Cohen 1986).

Groves (1951) has defined four categories of difficult patient (Table 2.1).

Gerrard and Ridded (1988) define 10 categories of patient, from 'black holes' to 'secrets'. Others have found heartsink patients to be a disparate group of individuals, defying obvious classification and sharing in common only the ability to 'exasperate, defeat and overwhelm' (O'Dowd 1988). Certain patient factors and doctor characteristics lead to an increased risk of developing a heartsink relationship.

Patient factors
- Depression
- Psychosomatic illness
- Lower social class
- Female
- Thick clinical records
- Increasing age.

Doctor factors (Butler and Evans 1999)
- Inexperience
- Greater perceived workload
- Lower job satisfaction
- Lack of postgraduate qualifications
- Lack of training in communication skills.

The common response to such patients is unnecessary investigation or inappropriate referral, arising from a need to escape for a time from contact with the patient.

Coping strategies (Butler and Evans 1999) include:
1. Improving clinicians' self-awareness, counselling and consultation skills. However, providing reflective and effective counselling often requires more time than is available for typical general practice consultations.
2. Help from counsellors and psychologists (for the patient, or doctor, or both!).

3. Alternative sources of therapy – the extended family network, religious organisations, self-help groups.
4. The work of Balint groups.
5. Peer group meetings – within the practice or without for support, information sharing and sharing responsibility through team discussion.
6. The 'holding strategy' (such as that sometimes adopted in social work practice), whereby positive attempts to bring about change are abandoned in favour of simply listening to the patient without contradicting him or her. The doctor acts as a safety valve in the hope that changes will occur for other reasons at some time in the future. This defies medical inclinations to intervene actively, and there is a danger that it encourages dependence upon the 'drug' known as 'doctor', which may divert the patient from dealing with underlying social and personal problems.
7. Challenging (with tact and sympathy) inappropriate patient demands and, if necessary making, a contract with him or her, e.g. the 'allowed' frequency of attendance, or a hierarchical problem list, so that one query is handled at a time.
8. Improving doctors' working conditions to reduce stress and enable them to cope better with difficult situations.

Problem patients will occupy a disproportionate amount of our time, both within exams and outside them, and this is an area worthy of special preparation.

The consultation is *the* central process in the practice of medicine. It is not surprising therefore that attempts at raising standards have placed such an emphasis on consultation techniques. This chapter is a simple résumé of a large and complex body of literature. For a more comprehensive review the interested reader is referred to Pendleton and Hasler's *Doctor–Patient Communication* (see Further reading).

Prescribing

Is it all necessary?

At least 50% of all consultations end with a prescription being written, amounting to 23 000 scripts per GP per year. In 2006 736 million items were prescribed by GPs, costing over eight thousand million pounds.

Though large in absolute terms, the UK stands up well to international comparison (Figure 2.1). Yet we are all familiar with examples of unnecessary prescribing; for example, when:

- diagnosis is still in doubt
- ingredients are probably ineffective
- combinations and formulations are irrational
- the value of treatment is debatable (in obviously self-limiting illness).

This raises several issues:

1. Increased cost of unnecessary prescriptions to the NHS (rationing other treatments)

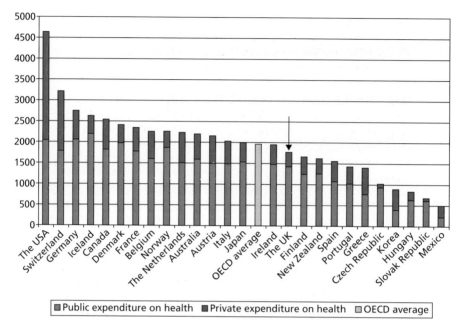

Figure 2.1 International comparison of prescribing. The Organisation for Economic Cooperation and Development, International comparison of prescribing, 2002. www.oecd.org/site/0,3407,en_21571361_33915056 _1_1_1_1,00.html

2. Suboptimal or harmful prescribing which fails to meet acceptable standards of care
3. Polypharmacy (this especially affects vulnerable groups such as elderly people who receive nearly half of all prescription items).

In prescribing surveys ingredient cost per item and prescribing rates vary considerably within a local area. Comparing patients within the locality means that variation cannot be accounted for solely in terms of variables such as patient demographics and mortality risk.

What factors affect doctors' prescribing?
(Carthy et al. 2000)

- GP knowledge: prescribers use a limited head-held drug formulary from which they prescribe. This learnt list of drugs is established early and is influenced by colleagues, patients and policies. Familiarity with a drug increases frequency of prescribing.
- Prescribing uncertainty:
  - ➤ due to: potentially severe adverse side effects (e.g. cytotoxics), ill-defined diagnoses, prescribing for children
  - ➤ reduced by: rapid access to prescribing guides.
- Prescribing support: the BNF (*British National Formulary*) and MIMS (*Monthly Index of Medical Specialties*) were identified as the most useful support materials influencing prescribing decisions.
- Peer influences: hospital consultants are viewed as a valuable source of advice and support; This is especially true in the use of new drugs.

- Prescribing policy.
- PACT data, and practice formularies: patient factors.
- Demanding and anxious patients/parents: prescribing costs.
- Influences of the pharmaceutical industry.

How can we improve prescribing habits?

Although it is relatively simple to collect prescribing statistics, it is not simple to interpret them. For example, it has been pointed out (Stott 1989) that doctors with above-average prescribing costs may:

- have expensive patients (e.g. those on growth hormone, domiciliary oxygen or fertility treatment)
- do more good (be more aware of the therapeutic possibilities; keep patients out of expensive hospital beds; keep them productive and at work, etc.)
- be more efficient in screening for (and then treating) latent problems such as hypertension or hyperlipidaemia.

The assumption that above-average prescribing is 'bad medicine' and below average is 'good medicine' has been challenged, because the process has not been related to outcome. Good prescribing could be better defined as prescribing based on the best available evidence and current guidelines.

How to prescribe rationally?

The choice of a drug is influenced by several considerations:

1. Is the diagnosis known?
2. Is a drug required?
3. Will it work?
4. Will it harm?
5. Is it the cost-effective choice?
6. Have all the alternatives been considered?
7. Is the likely benefit:risk ratio acceptable?

What to look for in a prescriber?

The responsible prescriber has several duties:

1. To ensure that the diagnosis is right.
2. To make a positive and correct decision that a drug is needed.
3. To choose a drug appropriate (evidence based) to the patient's needs.
4. To consult the patient, and to ensure that there is informed consent.
5. To explain the patient's role and to secure his or her cooperation.
6. To keep accurate prescribing records.
7. To oversee the course of treatment.
8. To terminate it when it is no longer needed.

Prescribing support

A number of initiatives provide advice and incentives to encourage rational prescribing and come under the heading prescribing support. They are aimed at changing prescribing patterns and recognise that publishing guidelines alone are not enough to establish change in practice. (Davis et al. 1995)

NICE (National Institute for Health and Clinical Excellence)

- Set up in 1999 (proposed in the 1997 White Paper 'The New NHS' – Department of Health 1997).
- NICE weighs up and provides guidance on the cost-effectiveness as well as the clinical effectiveness of treatments. Objectives:
  - ➤ faster uptake of new technologies
  - ➤ effective use of NHS resources
  - ➤ equitable access to treatments of proven clinical and cost-effectiveness.
- Since 1 January 2002 the NHS has had a statutory obligation to provide funding for NICE-approved technologies once a doctor has recommended it to his or her patient. This obligation falls on the primary care trusts (PCTs).
- NICE's guidelines have improved the uptake of new treatments and reduced ineffective practice, but only moderately. Uptake varies from treatment to treatment and area to area. NICE guidance influences clinicians' and PCTs' prescribing formularies and incentives. It also acts as a cost control or rationing mechanism.
- NICE blight: NICE has also had a negative impact on the speed of uptake of new treatments through a process that is known as NICE blight. This occurs when funding for treatments is withheld by trusts while an appraisal is in progress. As appraisals take an average of 12–14 months this can be a very serious source of delay, e.g. refusal of many PCTs to fund the cancer drug Herceptin during its appraisal.

Prescribing incentive schemes

Practices are rewarded financially by PCTs for achieving targets aimed at meeting local health needs, e.g. cost-effective prescribing of statins. Aims of the scheme:

- To encourage rational cost-effective prescribing based on the best available evidence
- Encouragement of generic prescribing
- Achievement of equity among and between practices.

Payments may be scaled depending on the level of achievement. Practices that overspend but show a budgetary improvement may qualify for incentive funding. PCTs may take into account factors beyond the control of the practice when awarding incentives (changes in list size, expensive drug prescribing, e.g. monoclonal antibody therapies). There are limitations on how incentive money can be used. Funds must be used for the benefit of patients of the practice, having regard to the need to ensure value for money. It cannot be used for the purchase of cars, land or buildings, drugs, dressings or the maintenance of equipment (but can be used to buy new equipment).

Practice/PCT formularies

Two-thirds of PCTs run formularies as well as a large number of practices. They promote rational prescribing habits and help keep prescribers up to date with the rapidly changing drug market.

PCT pharmacist support

PCT pharmacists aid practices in developing their own formularies, auditing prescriptions, achieving prescribing goals and may run their own medication review clinics. Use of a visiting pharmacist is known to improve GP prescribing (Carthy et al. 2000).

PACT

PACT (Prescribing Analysis and CosT) is a series of reports that tells GPs what they have prescribed and how much their prescribing has cost. The data are produced by the Prescription Pricing Authority (PPA) and give information on both individual GPs' and practices' prescribing costs, comparing them with other doctors in the same PCT and also nationally (Table 2.2).

IT-based resources

- Computerised prescribing systems (e.g. EMIS, vision), which promote generic alternatives to branded drugs, encourage use of formulary drugs, highlight polypharmacy and interactions, and suggest the most cost-effective preparation.
- Electronic Prescription Service (see page 105).
- BNF online (rapid access to drug information).
- *Drug and Therapeutics Bulletin* emails provide critical impartial reviews of medical and other treatments.
- MEREC bulletins from the National Prescribing Centre provide independent, evaluated reviews of newer medicines, ongoing reviews of key drug groups or treatment areas, and, occasionally, wider policy issues such as generic prescribing.

Table 2.2 The PACT scheme

PACT level	Format	Availability
1	The simplest level. A four-page report with basic information: • quarterly prescribing costs • average costs per item • relationship to list size • subdivision by therapeutic group • comparison with practice, local and national averages	All GPs receive this overview
2	More detailed information with special emphasis on the most expensive sections	On request. Also sent automatically to high-cost practices[a]
3	Full reports running to more than 100 pages with an index and technical guide	Only on request

[a]Practices with total costs exceeding PCT averages by at least 25% or where costs in one of the six major therapeutic categories are at least 75% above average.

- Cochrane reviews – evidence-based reviews of therapeutic interventions.
- GP Notebook – easily digestible evidence-based summaries of management guidelines and therapeutics.
- Clinical Knowledge Summaries (CKS – previously known as prodigy) evidence-based summaries for primary care from the NHS library for health.

Selected List Scheme (SLS) (Table 2.3)

A regulated list of drugs that can be prescribed on the NHS to a limited group of individuals, e.g. sildenafil for men with diabetes and erectile dysfunction. The prescription must be marked SLS. Drugs on this list are a possible exam question.

Social reasons for prescribing

Doctors often prescribe without proof of efficacy. Why should this be? Contributing factors include:

1. True variations in medical opinion (when the evidence is lacking or in contentious, e.g. the use of Lucentis (ranibizumab) for wet age-related macular degeneration).
2. The pressure of pharmaceutical advertising.
3. Habit, peer group recommendation and ignorance.
4. Patients' demands (there is evidence that this is overestimated and that a larger percentage leave a consultation with a prescription than those expecting one beforehand. Indeed, up to 20% of patients do not even have their scripts dispensed!).
5. Attempts at placebo prescribing (see below).
6. A variety of social reasons:
   (a) to play for time until the true picture becomes clearer or natural recovery occurs
   (b) to cover uncertainty, rather than admit it
   (c) because of medicolegal worries
   (d) to keep faith with patients, to justify their efforts and to demonstrate concern
   (e) to hasten the conclusion of a consultation
   (f) to avoid confrontation
   (g) to keep faith with their partners (hence the 'Friday afternoon antibiotic')
   (h) personal experience: we like to think we are scientific, but often base our prescribing on limited and subjective experiences with our own small patient samples.

Many patients are adept at securing social prescriptions, and use well-recognised ploys to obtain what they want (e.g. insistence, flattery, bargaining, comparison with other doctors).

Placebo prescribing

The response rate to placebos is high, of the order of 30–40%. According to some sources there are particular personality traits (e.g. extroversion,

Table 2.3 Selected List Scheme medications

Drug	Patient	Purpose
Clobazam	Any patient	Epilepsy
Cyanocobalamin tablets	A patient who is a vegan or who has a proven vitamin B_{12} deficiency of dietary origin	Treatment or prevention of vitamin B_{12} deficiency
Locabiotal Aerosol	Any patient	Treatment of infections and inflammation of the oropharynx
Niferex Elixir 30 ml Paediatric Dropper Bottle	Infants born prematurely	Prophylaxis in treatment of iron deficiency
Nizoral Cream	Any patient	Treatment of seborrhoeic dermatitis and pityriasis versicolor
Oseltamivir (Tamiflu)	[a]At-risk adult and child patients where: (a) It has been determined in accordance with a community-based virological surveillance scheme that influenza A or influenza B is circulating in the locality in which the patient resides or is present or was present at the time that the virus was circulating (b) The patient has an influenza-like illness (c) The patient can start therapy within 48 hours of the onset of symptoms	Treatment of influenza
	[a]At-risk patients aged 13 years and older where: (a) It has been determined in accordance with a community-based virological surveillance scheme that influenza A and influenza B is circulating in the locality in which the patient resides (b) The patient has been exposed to an influenza-like illness through being in close contact with someone with whom he lives who is or has been suffering from an influenza-like illness (c) The patient is not effectively protected by vaccination against influenza because: (i) he has not been vaccinated because vaccination is contraindicated (ii) he has not been vaccinated since the previous influenza season (iii) he has been vaccinated but it has yet to take effect (iv) he has been vaccinated but the vaccine is not well matched to the strain of influenza circulating in the locality in which the patient resides or is or has been present (d) The patient lives in a residential care establishment and another resident or member of staff of the establishment has an influenza-like illness (e) The patient can start prophylaxis within 48 hours of exposure to an influenza-like illness	Prophylaxis of influenza
Zanamivir (Relenza)	[a]At-risk adult patients where: (a) It has been determined in accordance with a community-based virological surveillance scheme that influenza A or influenza B is circulating in the locality in which the patient resides or is present or was present at the time that the virus was circulating (b) The patient has an influenza-like illness (c) The patient can start therapy within 48 hours of the onset of symptoms	Treatment of influenza

Continued

Table 2.3 *Continued*

Drug	Patient	Purpose

The following drugs for the treatment of erectile dysfunction:
Alprostadil (Caverject, MUSE, Viridal)
Apomorphine hydrochloride (Uprima)
Moxisylyte hydrochloride (Erecnos)
	(a) A man with erectile dysfunction who on 14 September 1998 was receiving a course of treatment under the Act, the National Health Service (Scotland) Act 1978(a) or the Health and Personal Social Services (Northern Ireland) Order 1972(b) for this condition with any of the following drugs:
	Alprostadil (Caverject, MUSE, Viridal)
	Apomorphine hydrochloride (Uprima)
	Moxisylyte hydrochloride (Erecnos)
	Sildenafil (Viagra)
	Tadalafil (Cialis)
	Thymoxamine hydrochloride (Erecnos)
	Vardenafil (Levitra)
	(b) A man who is a national of an EEA State who is entitled to treatment by virtue of Article 7(2) of Council Regulation 1612/68(c) as extended by the EEA Agreement or by virtue of any other enforceable Community right who has erectile dysfunction and was on 14 September 1998 receiving a course of treatment under a national health insurance system of an EEA State for this condition with any of the drugs listed in sub-paragraph (a)
	(c) A man who is not a national of an EEA State but who is the member of the family of such a national who has an enforceable Community right to be treated no less favourably than the national in the provision of medical treatment and has erectile dysfunction and was being treated for that condition on 14 September 1998 with any of the drugs listed in sub-paragraph (a)
	(d) A man who is suffering from any of the following:
	  diabetes
	  multiple sclerosis
	  Parkinson's disease
	  poliomyelitis
	  prostate cancer
	  severe pelvic injury
	  single gene neurological disease
	  spina bifida
	  spinal cord injury
	(e) A man who is receiving treatment for renal failure by dialysis
	(f) A man who has had the following surgery:
	  prostatectomy
	  radical pelvic surgery
	  renal failure treated by transplantation
		Treatment of erectile dysfunction

Drugs in column 1 of this part may be prescribed for persons mentioned in column 2, only for the treatment of the purpose specified in column 3. The prescriber must endorse the prescription with the reference 'SLS'.

Details of restricted availability appliances (vacuum pumps and constrictor rings for erectile dysfunction) can be found in Part IX of the *Drug Tariff* besides the listing for the relevant appliance.

[a] 'At risk' means an adult or child patient or a patient over the age of 13 who (a) has chronic respiratory disease (including asthma and chronic obstructive pulmonary disease); (b) has significant cardiovascular disease, excluding an adult or child patient who has hypertension only (c) has chronic renal disease; (d) is immunocompromised; (e) has diabetes mellitus; or (f) is aged 65 years or over.

sociability, neuroticism, awareness of autonomic function) that identify the placebo responder. However, other studies suggest no clear correlation and show that most people can respond given the correct situation.

Many conditions can be helped:
- Angina
- Anxiety and depression
- Arthritis
- Asthma
- Blood pressure
- Enuresis
- Hayfever
- Headaches
- Hyperglycaemia
- Hyperlipidaemia
- Insomnia
- Peptic ulcer
- Postoperative pain
- Premenstrual tension
- Social problems.

Note that the response is not entirely psychological: physiological changes have been observed, suggesting a 'real' effect, e.g. placebos have:
- reversed the motility effects of ipecacuanha
- lowered blood sugars
- lowered blood pressure
- reduced cholesterol (and mortality from ischaemic heart disease according to one study).

The time–response of placebo treatment also mimics the pharmacokinetics of active drugs.

Up to 40% of patients experience placebo side effects including: headache, anorexia, diarrhoea, nausea and vomiting, dry mouth, vertigo, lassitude, palpitations, dermatitis, even addiction!

Factors affecting the placebo response include:
- Pain levels – the more severe, the more likely is a placebo response
- Anxiety levels
- Tablet size, appearance and formulation; to be effective tablets should be:
  (a) very small or very large
  (b) unlike an everyday medicine in appearance
  (c) capsules or injections rather than tablets
  (d) bitter to taste
- Colour is also important (Table 2.4)
- Patient expectation
- High technology: attendance at outpatient clinics, radiographs and especially invasive investigations have a therapeutic effect.

The conviction of the prescriber, his or her charisma and the doctor–patient relationship probably also contribute. Male patients tend to respond more frequently than females, and higher social classes are especially prone.

Table 2.4 The effect of tablet colour on placebo response.

Colour	Best response in
Blue or green	Creams/ointments
Green	Anxiety
Red	Analgesia
Red or brown	Elixirs
Yellow	Depression

Ethical problems

Proponents of the placebo argue that:
- It is effective (what does the mechanism matter if the result is satisfactory?).
- It is reassuring, and helps morale in chronic/incurable disease.
- It fulfils patient expectations.
- There is no significant toxicity.
- There is evidence of an underlying physical basis (e.g. naloxone has been shown to reverse placebo pain relief, suggesting a possible endorphin-based mechanism).

Those against placebo prescribing argue that:
- It is deception and an abuse of a relationship of mutual trust.
- It may generate hurt and ill-feeling if the deception is uncovered.
- It delays true diagnosis.
- It reinforces the sick role.

Whatever the rights and wrongs, placebo prescribing is widely practised, and (if we admit it to ourselves) so is the habit of prescribing for largely social reasons.

Generic vs branded prescribing

There are a small number of drugs the release characteristics of which mean that patients should be maintained on the same product. Examples include theophylline, and modified-release preparations of nifedipine and diltiazem. Otherwise the only therapeutic rationale for prescribing by brand name is where there is a real risk that failure to maintain an individual patient on the same product could impair their adherence or understanding of therapy, and thus be detrimental to their health. Each year the PCTs are provided with information about their potential savings from increased generic prescribing.

Self-medication

A large number of over-the-counter (OTC) medicines are available.

Advantages
- An opportunity for patients to take more responsibility for their own health.
- An opportunity to save the cost, inconvenience and time involved in obtaining a prescription for doctors and patients.

Disadvantages and concerns
- Risk of drug interaction with prescription medicines.
- Increased risk of self-medication side effects.
- The risk of inappropriate self medication, e.g.:
  - self-medicating for a serious illness presentation of which is thereby masked or delayed
  - taking the wrong preparation or wrong formulation.
- A risk that a 'pills for all ills' culture will become fostered in consumers.
- Less chance to offer opportunistic health promotion activities.

Bradley et al. (1995) have pointed out that the trend to self-medicate has practical implications for GPs, who will need to:
- ask routinely about patients' use of non-prescription medicines (including complementary therapies) and consider the potential for drug interactions and side effects, e.g. St John's wort interacts with a large number of commonly prescribed items
- educate patients on responsible and safe use of OTC preparations
- forge close links with local pharmacists, who will increasingly be offering advice to their patients.

Referring

The present referral system from generalist to specialist arose historically from mid-nineteenth-century demarcation disputes of apothecaries, physicians and surgeons. Although this restrictive practice was intended to protect the livelihood of doctors, it has since been justified as a rational and effective basis for allocating healthcare resources.

Patients can only bypass the gatekeeper system in the case of urgent personal need (casualty), or public interest (sexually transmitted infection services). The GP as gatekeeper can:
- ration access according to need
- target care more specifically
- protect against over-investigation and over-medicalisation
- prevent the misuse of expensive high-technology facilities, and needless trafficking between specialisms.

Referral to outpatients generally falls into one of three categories:
1. Investigation/diagnosis
2. Treatment
3. Advice/reassurance for the patient and/or GP.

Criticisms of the present system
Critics point out that:
- GPs exercise a virtual monopoly in their control of access to secondary care in the UK.
- Other countries' healthcare systems function without such a restriction of choice.
- There is unacceptable variation in the performance standards of the gatekeepers, with expensive and potentially unfair consequences.

Effective referral practice
Referral rates
Significant variation in referral rates exists, at GP and practice level. Studies examining individual referral rates reported variation ranging from twofold to more than twentyfold (O'Donnell 2000). Many studies have tried to identify factors explaining the variation (Table 2.5). These can be categorised into:
- patient characteristics
- practice characteristics
- GP characteristics
- access to specialist care.

However, none of these factors can entirely explain the variation in referral. Of note variations in referral rates do not seem to correlate with the age of doctors, their use of investigations, postgraduate qualifications or experience in a specialty (which actually increases referrals to that specialty – (Reynolds et al. 1991).

How to make appropriate referrals
Whether a GP is a high, average or low referrer is less important than the percentage of appropriate referrals made. An appropriate referral can be defined as necessary for the individual patient, timely in the course of the disease, effective in achieving its objectives and cost effective (Coulter 1998). Judging appropriateness of a referral decision is complex. Guidelines exist (NICE/SIGN [Scottish Intercollegiate Guidelines Network]/local guidance) to help in this process. Four items are necessary to make an appropriate referral decision:
1. Clinical skills to elicit the patients signs and symptoms
2. Knowledge of clinical guidelines and current clinical practice
3. Knowledge of your patients health beliefs, ideas and expectations
4. An awareness of your competency and limitations.

Interestingly the use of clinical guidelines has lead to an increase in the absolute number of referrals (Fertig et al. 1993). This suggests that the variation in referral rates may result from under-referral. The take-home message is therefore that you should be less concerned about the quantity

Table 2.5 Factors influencing referral decisions

---

1 Distance from local hospitals
2 Availability of public transport
3 Family and social expectations
4 Community support services
5 Quality and quantity of available hospital services
6 Variations in morbidity, age–sex structure and other environmental factors within the population
7 The training, interests and experience of the GP
8 The GP's ability to abide uncertainty

---

of patients whom you refer and more concerned with making sure that your referrals are appropriate, i.e. necessary, timely and beneficial to the patient. Low referrers may have more reason for concern – particularly those with less experience, e.g. registrars/ST3 and newly qualified GPs.

AKT questions

Q1
Match the statements to the consultation models. Each option may be used once, more than once or not at all.
a   Byrne and Long
b   Balint
c   Helman
d   Neighbour
e   Pendleton
f   Stott and Davis
g   The biomedical model
h   The disease illness model

1. A task-based model focusing on identifying problems, choosing actions and sharing decisions.
2. The author(s) discussed the importance of preparing for the next consultation by dealing with the negative psychological impact of a previous consultation.
3. Analysis of 2500 consultations establishing a six-phase consultation model.
4. The positive health benefit that a patient receives through consultation is described as the doctor acting as a drug.
5. Raises the concept of opportunistic health promotion in his work 'The exceptional potential in each primary care consultation'.
6. Proposes that a patient presents to a doctor wanting answers to six questions.

Q2
Which of the following tools are recommended by NICE to screen for depression in patients with chronic disease? Select ONE option only.
a   PHQ9
b   Beck score
c   Two-question screen
d   Edinburgh questionnaire
e   FAST test

Q3
Identify the patient factor NOT associated with failures in doctor patient communication? Select ONE option only.
a   A limited knowledge of illness
b   Cultural similarity between the doctor and patient

c   Anxiety
d   Diffidence in asking for clarification
e   Hidden agenda

Q4

The following drug is prescribable under the selected list scheme. Select ONE option only.
a   Zoladex
b   Rifampacin
c   Oseltamivir
d   Infliximab
e   Lucentis (ranibizumab)

Q5

Shorter consultations times are NOT associated with: Select ONE option only.
a   Lower consultation frequency
b   Higher rates of drug prescription
c   Lower levels of health promotion
d   Lower levels of patient satisfaction
e   Higher numbers of home visits

Q6

The following are evidence-based techniques that facilitate effective doctor–patient communication EXCEPT. Select ONE option only.
a   Closed to open cone questioning
b   Facilitative response (verbal and non verbal encouragers)
c   Time framing (prioritisation of concerns)
d   Summarising
e   Cue identification (verbal and non-verbal)

Q7

All of the following are types of heartsink patient EXCEPT. Select ONE option only.
a   The manipulative help rejector
b   The recurrent non-attender
c   The entitled demander
d   The dependent clinger

Q8

Which of the following doctor factors are NOT associated with an increased number of heart sink patients? Select ONE option only.
a   Postgraduate qualifications
b   Low job satisfaction
c   Recent qualification
d   Lack of training in communication skills
e   Increased perceived workload

Q9

Feedback on prescribing data is regularly provided to GPs through what scheme? Select ONE option only.

a MEREC
b DTB
c Prescribing incentive scheme
d PACT
e QOF

Q10

Which of the following are NOT associated with improved patient satisfaction, communication and concordance? Select ONE option only.

a A caring and confiding relationship
b Repeating the message and stressing the importance
c Offering longer consultations
d Giving information late in the consultation
e Use of non-verbal clues
f Sharing decision-making

Answers

Q1

1. e
2. d
3. a
4. b
5. f
6. c

Q2 c

Q3 b

Q4 c

Oseltamivir is prescribable under SLS for the treatment and prophylaxis of influenza in at-risk adults and children, i.e. those with chronic disease, those who are immunocompromised and elderly people who present with flu-like symptoms and can be started on treatment within 48 hours of the onset of symptoms

Q5 a

Q6 a

Q7 b

Q8 a

Q9 d
PACT – Prescribing Analysis and CosT data is provided by the Prescription Pricing Authority.

Q10 d

References

Arroll B, Khin N, Kerse N. Primary care screening for depression in primary care with two verbally asked questions: cross-sectional study. *BMJ* 2003;**327**:1144–6.

Aspegren K. Teaching and learning communication skills in medicine: a review with quality grading of articles. *Medical Teacher* 1999;**21**:563–70.

Balint M. *The Doctor, His Patient, and the Illness*. New York: International Universities Press, 1957.

Balint M. *The Doctor, the Patient and the Illness*. Edinburgh: Churchill Livingstone, 1986. Available at: www.skillscascade.com/models.htm.

Bertakis KD. The communication of information from physician to patient. *J Fam Pract* 1977;**5**:217–22.

Bradley CP, Bond C. Increasing the number of drugs available over-the-counter: arguments for and against. *Br J Gen Pract* 1995;**45**:553–6.

Butler CC, Evans M. The 'heartsink' patient revisited. *Br J Gen Pract* 1999;**49**: 230–3.

Byrne PS, Long BEL. *Doctors Talking to Patients*. London: HMSO, 1976.

Carthy P, Harvey I, Brawn R, Watkins C. A study of factors associated with cost and variation. *Fam Practice* 2000;**17**(1):36–41.

Cartwright A. *Human Relations and Hospital Care*, London: Routledge & Keegan Paul, 1964.

Cohen J. Diagnosis and management of problem patients in general practice. *J R Coll Gen Pract* 1986;**36**:51.

Coulter A. Managing demand at the interface between primary and secondary care *BMJ* 1998;**316**:1974–6.

Davis DA, Thomson MA, Oxman, AD, Haynes RB. Changing physician performance: a systematic review of the effect of continuing medical education strategies. *JAMA* 1995;**284**:9.

Department of Health. *The New NHS*. London: DH, 1997.

Department of Health, Picker Institute Europe. *National Survey of Local Health Services*. Department of Health, Picker Institute Europe, 2006.

Elstein AS, Shulman LS, Sporafka SA. *Medical Problem Solving: An analysis of clinical reasoning*. Boston, MA: Harvard University Press, 1978.

Fertig A, Roland M, King H, Moore T. Understanding variation in rates of referral among general practitioners: are inappropriate referrals important and would guidelines help to reduce rates? *BMJ* 1993;**307**:1467–70.

Gelat HBJ. Decision making: a conceptual framework of reference for counselling. *Counselling Psychol* 1962;**9**:240–5.

Gerrard TJ, Riddell JD. Difficult patients: black holes and secrets. *BMJ* 1988;**297**: 1295–8.

Groves JE. Taking care of the hateful patient. *N Engl J Med* 1951;**298**:883–5.

Helman CG. Disease versus illness in general practice. *J R Coll Gen Pract* 1981;**31**: 548–62.

Hoos AM, Lammes FB. Doctor–patient communication: a review of the literature. *Soc Sci Med* 1995;**40**:903–18.

Kafka F. *Der Landarzt (A Country Doctor)*. Berkeley, USA: Counterpoint Publications, 1919. (Reprint 1945)

Korsch BM, Negrete VF. Doctor–patient communication. *Sci Am* 1972;**227**:66–74.

Kurtz S, Silverman J, Benson J, Draper J. Marrying content and process in clinical method teaching: enhancing the Calgary-Cambridge guides. *Acad Med* 2003;**78**: 802–9.

Langewitz W, Denz M, Keller A, Kiss A, Rüttimann S, Wössmer B. Spontaneous talking time at start of consultation in outpatient clinic: cohort study *BMJ* 2002;**325**:682–3.

Law SA, Britten N. Factors that influence the patient centredness of a consultation. *Br J Gen Pract* 1995;**45**:520–4.

Ley P, Whitworth MA, Skilbeck CE et al. Improving doctor–patient communication in general practice. *J R Coll Gen Pract* 1976;**26**:720–4.

McGhee A. *The Patient's Attitude to Nursing Care*. Edinburgh: E&S Livingstone.

Marinker M. Personal paper: writing prescriptions is easy. *BMJ* 1997;**314**:747.

Neighbour R. *The Inner Consultation*. Lancaster: MTP Press, 1987.

O'Donnell. Variation in GP referral rates: what can we learn from the literature? *Fam Pract* 2000;**17**:462–71.

O'Dowd TC. Five years of heartsink patients in general practice. *BMJ* 1988;**297**:528–30.

Pendleton D, Schofield T, Tate P, Havelock P. *The Consultation – An approach to learning and teaching*. Oxford: Oxford University Press, 1984 (2nd edn 2003).

Pietroni P. NVC in the GP surgery. In: Tanner B (ed.), *Language and Communication in General Practice*. Sevenoaks: Hodder & Stoughton, 1976: 162–79.

Reynolds GA, Chitnis JG, Roland MO. General practitioner outpatient referrals: do good doctors refer more patients to hospital? *BMJ* 1991;**302**:1250–52.

Rotter JB. *Generalized Expectancies for Internal versus External Control of Reinforcement*. Psychological Monographs. Stores, CT: University of Connecticut, 1966.

Royal Pharmaceutical Society of Great Britain. *From Compliance to Concordance*. London: RPSGB and Merck, Sharp & Dohme, 1997.

Scott J, Jennings T, Standart S, Ward R, Goldberg D. The impact of training in problem-based interviewing on the detection and management of psychological problems presenting in primary care. *Br J Gen Pract* 1999;**49**:441–5.

Shepherd J, Cooper B, Brown AC, Kalton GW. *Psychiatric Illness in General Practice*. Oxford: Oxford University Press.

Simpson M, Buckman R, Stewart M, et al. Doctor-patient communication: the Toronto consensus statement. *BMJ* 1991;**303**:1385–7.

Skelton J. Everything you wanted to ask about communication. *Br J Gen Pract* 2005;**55**:40-6.

Stewart M, Brown JB, Weston WW, McWhinney IR, McWilliam CL, Freeman TR. *Patient-centred Medicine: Transforming the clinical method*. Thousand Oaks, CA: Sage, 1995.

Stott P. Value for money. *Med Monitor* **9** June 1989, p. 13.

Stott NCH, Davies RH. The exceptional potential in each primary care consultation. *J R Coll Gen Pract* 1979;**29**:201–5.

Thomas KB. General practice consultations: is there any pointing in being positive? *BMJ* 1987;**294**:1200.

Wilson A, Childs S. The relationship between consultation length, process and outcomes in general practice: a systematic review. *Br J Gen Pract* 2002;**52**:1012–20.

Further reading

Becker MH, Maiman LA. Sociobehavioural determinants of compliance with medical care recommendations. *Med Care* 1975;**13**:10–24.

Berne E. *Games People Play*. London: Penguin, 1964.

Heron J. *Six Category Intervention Analysis*. Human Potential Research Project. Guildford: University of Surrey, 1975.

National Statistics. Obesity among adults: by sex and NS-SeC, 2001: *Social Trends* 34 and NICE guidance www.statistics.gov.uk/Statbase/ssdataset.asp?ulnk=7447& More=y.

Pendleton D, Hasler J, eds. *Doctor–Patient Communication*. St Louis, MI: Academic Press, 1983.

Rosenstock I. *Historical Origins of the Health Belief Model*, Vol. 2. Health Education Monographs. 1974;**2**:328–35.

3 Legal and ethical matters

This chapter relates to curriculum statement 3 (excluding 3.5 and 3.6):
- Ethics and values-based medicine
- Promoting equality and valuing diversity
- Clinical governance
- Patient safety
- Teaching, mentoring and clinical supervision.

The GMC

The General Medical Council (GMC) regulates doctors in the UK. Its statutory duties are:
- maintaining a medical register
- guidance on good medical practice (medical ethics)
- regulation of medical education to promote high standards (undergraduate, postgraduate and continuing professional development)
- regulation of doctors to ensure fitness to practise.

Under-performing doctors may be issued warnings or suspensions, or have restrictions placed on their practice, e.g. a supervision order.

(www.gmc-uk.org/about/role/index.asp)

Good medical practice (GMC 2006)
The *Good Medical Practice* document summarises the duties of a doctor and the seven areas of good clinical practice. Both are hot topics for the exam.

Duties of a doctor
- Make the care of your patient your first concern
- Protect and promote the health of patients and the public
- Provide a good standard of practice and care:
  - keep your professional knowledge and skills up to date
  - recognise and work within the limits of your competence
  - work with colleagues in the ways that best serve patients' interests

Notes for the MRCGP: A curriculum based guide to the AKT, CSA and WBPA, 4th edition. By K. Palmer and N. Boeckx. Published 2010 by Blackwell Publishing, ISBN: 978-1-4051-5724-7.

- Treat patients as individuals and respect their dignity:
  - ➤ treat patients politely and considerately
  - ➤ respect patients' right to confidentiality
  - ➤ respect and value equality and diversity
- Work in partnership with patients:
  - ➤ listen to patients and respond to their concerns and preferences
  - ➤ give patients the information that they want or need in a way that they can understand
  - ➤ respect patients' right to reach decisions with you about their treatment and care
  - ➤ support patients in caring for themselves to improve and maintain their health
- Be honest and open and act with integrity:
  - ➤ act without delay if you have good reason to believe that you or a colleague may be putting patients at risk
  - ➤ never discriminate unfairly against patients or colleagues
  - ➤ never abuse your patients' trust in you or the public's trust in the profession.

  You are personally accountable for your professional practice and must always be prepared to justify your decisions and actions. (GMC 2006)

Diversity is defined by the GMC guidance (diversity and equal opportunities) as 'the differences in the values, attitudes, cultural perspectives, beliefs, ethnic backgrounds, sexuality, skills, knowledge and life experiences of each individual in any group of people'. Promoting equality is about addressing inequalities to prevent discrimination against any individual or group. Some general principles should be applied in practice and the exam:

- Value beliefs and preferences where expressed
- Take care not to discriminate and act if you come across discrimination by others
- Be aware of cultural issues so that you can show respect, e.g. differences in attitudes to dress, diet, handling death, religious festivals and religious jewellery.
- Address patients/role players by their title and surname unless invited to do otherwise.

Good medical practice areas

There are seven areas of good medical practice (two in education and communication and three others). We suggest a mnemonic to recall them:
Excellent Health Care
Education (two areas):
- personal (keeping up to date, taking part regularly in education activity)
- teaching (doctors should contribute to colleagues medical education)

Health (register with a GP, avoid self-treating, seek help if illness may affect your practice)

Honesty (probity – act with integrity, justifying the trust of patients and public)

Communication (two areas):
- patients (act honestly and politely, treat patients with dignity; share decisions and admit errors*, obtain valid consent)
- team (respect and support colleagues, communicate effectively, regularly review performance, i.e. audit, protect patients from harmful colleagues, ensure continuity of care for patients when off duty)

Clinical care

take thorough histories and examinations and offer evidence-based treatments. Work within your limitations, and keep good records. Avoid treating anyone with a close personal relationship to you. Encourage self-care.

*If a patient under your care has suffered harm or distress, you must act immediately to put matters right, if that is possible. You should offer an apology and explain fully and promptly to the patient what has happened, and the likely short-term and long-term effects.

For more detail see www.gmc-uk.org.

Clinical governance

Clinical governance is the system through which NHS organisations are *accountable* for continuously improving the quality of their services and safeguarding high standards of care. This system was introduced in the 1997 government White Paper 'The New NHS, Modern, Dependable' (Department of Health or DH 1997). To demonstrate accountability clinical governance systems must collect evidence of quality standards. There are several tools for this in general practice.

Clinical governance tools in general practice
- Quality Outcome Frameworks (QOFs): a major clinical governance tool; it collects *evidence* of quality of care across a range of areas (clinical, organisational, etc.) and provides incentives through performance-related payment to improve standards
- Appraisal (see below)
- Audit (see below)
- Significant event reviews: regular meetings focusing on a near miss or event that is looked at in detail with the objective of using the lessons to improve patient safety and care. A significant event meeting can have several outcomes, for example recognition of good care already in place, an immediate response required to a problem, identification of a learning point, need for new protocols or guidelines.
- Complaints review
- Patient satisfaction surveys.

The RCGP curriculum describes 10 elements of clinical governance:
1. Quality improvement (including clinical audit)
2. Leadership
3. Evidence-based practice

4. Dissemination of good practice, ideas and innovation
5. Clinical risk reduction
6. Detection of adverse events
7. Learning lessons from complaints
8. Addressing poor clinical performance
9. Professional development
10. High quality data and record keeping.

Aids to clinical governance
Clinical aids
Guidance on clinical practice
- The National Institute for Health and Clinical Excellence (NICE)
- British Medical Association (BMA)
- GMC guidance on good conduct
- Medical defence organisations
- Societies and charities, e.g. British Thoracic Society, British Heart Foundation
- Cochrane reviews.

Feedback from colleagues
- Inside or outside the practice, primary or secondary care, medical or paramedical staff.

Non-clinical aids
Guidance on non-clinical practice
- AMSPAR (Association of Medical Secretaries, Practice Managers, Administrators and Receptionists)
- Department of Health advisory notes
- BMA reviews
- NHS Connecting for Health (IT advice).

Clinical guidelines
Clinical guidelines are tools designed to aid clinical judgement. They differ from clinical protocols (a set of mandatory rules) where no clinical judgement is required. For example, clinical trials use protocols to ensure a standardised approach. Failure to follow the protocol would lead to bias and a flawed trial. Clinical guidelines have been shown to improve health outcomes, promote an evidence-based approach, increase consistency of care, help keep doctors' practice up to date and increase public confidence. They are a vital tool in audit for comparing current and 'best' practice. Guidelines are not without flaws. They are only as good as the evidence on which they are based (and the authors that create the guidance). Also guidelines can make only a generalised judgement of risks/benefits at a population level. They cannot assess an individual's risks/benefits or account for patient choice. What is right for the majority may not be right for the patient in your clinic, e.g. a patient may be unfit for a surgical procedure even if recommended for one in a guideline as a result of their comorbidity.

(Woolf et al. 1999)

Nationally, the Healthcare Commission (previously called CHI) is responsible for ensuring that primary care trusts (PCTs) have adequate clinical governance systems in place.

Clinical governance practice requirements
- Each practice must have a named clinical governance lead.
- Practitioners and staff must carry out their obligations with 'reasonable skill and care'.
- Complaints procedures must be in accordance with the NHS complaints procedure and report details of complaints to the PCT.
- They must ensure that staff have appropriate qualifications and registration.
- They must have suitable premises for delivery of services and meet national standards, e.g. disability discrimination act.
- They must keep adequate patient records and have a named Caldicott Guardian (see Chapter 7) who leads on the practices and procedures for handling the confidentiality of patient records.
- They have a practice leaflet that is available to patients and annually updated.
- They have adequate infection control standards.
- They comply with all relevant legislation

MEMORY BOX
Clinical governance
- Quality control
- Introduced across the NHS in 1997 in its current format
- Measured through QOF, audit, complaints, patient satisfaction survey, significant event reviews and appraisal

---

Patient safety
Clinical governance involves managing risk and patient safety. In preparing for the MRCGP examination be aware of the tools and organisations involved in managing risk in primary care. Specifically, be aware of risk reduction steps (seven steps to patient safety – see below) and what to do in the event of an adverse event or near miss.

(www.npsa.nhs.uk)

The National Patient Safety Agency
This national organisation, set up in 2001, is responsible for improving safety and reducing risk to patients within the NHS.

The National Reporting and Learning System (NRLS)
This is a national system to collect confidential reports after near misses and adverse events, launched in 2004. Reports from GP practices can be made online via the National Patient Safety Agency (NPSA) website eform. The form gathers information about an incident in four steps:
1. When and where
2. What happened
3. Impact (actual harm/near miss and action taken)
4. Patient details.

The reports are analysed to identify common risks and improve safety through:

- Improved systems (e.g. clearer labelling of drugs)
- Raising awareness of specific risks through alerts (e.g. alert about manufacturing fault in medication or equipment)
- National initiatives (e.g. hand hygiene and cleaning)
- Staff education (development of a safety culture through work with The Royal Colleges and other training bodies).

Significant event analysis

This is a local form of risk analysis following a significant event (near miss or adverse event) and part of clinical governance in primary care. The event is analysed using a structured (much like critical analysis) format of questions to try to identify ways of preventing harm or improving care. The events do not automatically need to have a negative impact and significant event analysis (SEA) can be used to highlight and disseminate good models of care to colleagues. A more in-depth version called 'root cause analysis' should be used for events in which severe harm or death has resulted (available via the NPSA website – www.nspa.nhs.uk – and PCT clinical governance lead). GPs must show evidence of SEA for their annual appraisal.

SEA principles

- Involve the whole practice team (to encourage an open safety culture and share learning)
- Make it a regular event (similar to audit, SEA is an ongoing process)
- Use Pendleton's feedback criteria when discussing the case, i.e. feedback positive points first before criticism
- Avoid blame (to encourage reporting)
- Decide actions, and review implementation and effectiveness at the next meeting.

Risk management principles – seven steps to patient safety (NPSA) (Figure 3.1)

1. Build a safety culture: create an open and fair culture (avoid blame, which prevents colleagues reporting mistakes; make sure that the team knows what to do in the event of an incident).
2. Lead and support your staff: emphasise the importance of patient safety at work, have a lead member responsible for patient safety, usually a GP partner who runs the significant event analysis meetings.
3. Integrate your risk management activity: regular significant event meetings, proactive assessment and staff training about risks both:
   - clinical risk, i.e. confidentiality, record keeping, consent, complaints, prescribing
   - non-clinical risk, i.e. health and safety (maintenance of equipment and premises), care of drug stocks
4. Promote reporting: encourage reporting and facilitate it by making it easy to report locally (SEA) and nationally via the NRLS. Usually inci-

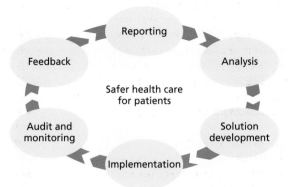

Figure 3.1 Seven steps to patient safety (National Patient Safety Agency).

dents will be reported to the GP partner leading on patient safety and significant event analysis.

5. Involve and communicate with patients and the public: patients should be informed of incidents promptly, fully and compassionately. This action reduces the trauma that patients experience and also reduces the risk of a formal complaint and compensation claim.
6. Learn and share safety lessons: share findings of significant event analysis and root cause analysis to collectively learn and prevent future incidents.
7. Implement solutions to prevent harm: act on the findings to make changes to practice, processes or systems.

Incidents in general practice

Near misses and adverse events can be valuable learning opportunities. All incidents should be reported and shared with the practice lead for patient safety and significant event analysis, who can provide guidance and support on the most appropriate action. In all cases:

- Immediate action should be taken to minimise any harm.
- If a patient may suffer as a result of the incident they should be:
  - informed promptly, fully and compassionately *and*
  - given details of the practice complaints procedure and the Patient Advisory and Liaison Service (PALS). PALS is based at the local PCT, which will support and guide patients if necessary while they make a complaint.

Options for reporting an event include:

- Yellow card system (for incidents involving medication side effects – yellow cards are available in the *British National Formulary* (BNF) or online at www.yellowcard.mhra.gov.uk)
- Reporting to the local PCT clinical governance lead (root cause analysis)
- Reporting to the NPSA through the NRLS
- In-house reporting – SEA.

Audit

Audit is a localised form of clinical governance. In 'Working for Patients' (DoH 1989) the government defined audit as: 'the systematic critical analysis of the quality of medical care. This includes procedures used for diagnosis and treatment, the use of resources and the resulting outcome and quality of life for the patients'. This implies a process more active than mere counting – there should be self-improvement through standard setting, measurement, change and re-measurement.

The scope of audit

Two major categories of activity are of consummate interest:

1. Audits of *process* (examining records, appointments, immunisation records, to see *how* patients are being treated)
2. Audits of *outcome* (mortality, morbidity, patient satisfaction – looking at the *results* of treatment).

The exercise often takes one of several popular forms:

- periodic random review of clinical records (with peer group discussion)
- the enumeration of process variables (workload, diagnosis, referral rates, waiting times, visiting rates, use of investigative facilities) and analysis of their trends
- significant event reviews (see above)
- outcome surveys
- patient satisfaction surveys
- peer group-structured practice inspections (of the sort undertaken for training approval).

The principal steps of the audit cycle

The essential steps in performing an audit are to do the following:

1. Define objectives (what needs to be measured and why)
2. Agree ideal performance standards (these may come from the consensus statements and guidelines of expert bodies or, where available, the conclusions of formal clinical trials)
3. Define methods (how the data are to be collected and analysed)
4. Perform the audit
5. Compare the outcome with performance criteria
6. Agree and implement change – to bring expected and actual performance closer together
7. Repeat steps 4–6, re-measuring and improving until the agreed standards are achieved.

This is the so-called virtuous cycle (Figure 3.2). Steps 4–7 are essential to 'close the feedback loop' and to effect beneficial change. In theory this should be continuous and never ending.

Audit comes of age

Doctors generally accept and the government now requires that self-improvement through self-examination should be an everyday part of medical practice. More specifically:

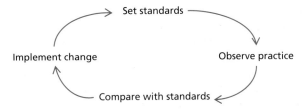

Figure 3.2 Virtuous circle.

- The GMC document *Duties of a Doctor* (GMC 2006) describes audit as an essential professional responsibility
- Audit forms part of annual appraisal
- The Royal Colleges and Faculties require evidence of audit when accrediting posts for specialist training.
  In practice several benefits have been forthcoming, e.g.:
- improved standards of medicine
- improved morale
- improved income
- improvements in practice management and planning of patient services.
  Several costs need to be counted as well. Audit demands:
- time and effort
- commitment (which may not be shared equally in a partnership)
- a willingness to be inspected
- a receptive attitude to constructive criticism and the flexibility to change.
  Notwithstanding these points, research and audit in primary care have helped to fill in many gaps in our knowledge, and have fostered in GPs a new willingness to improve by self-examination. The RCGP has been an instrumental force in this spirit of change.

Appraisal, revalidation and re-licensing

GP appraisal
An annual review of a doctor's performance through structured reflection, with planning to meet identified learning needs and aid professional development.

Documents and evidence required for annual appraisal
- Completed appraisal forms (can be filled in online at www.appraisals. nhs.uk and documents uploaded as evidence – a GP version of the e-Portfolio!). The appraisal forms require evidence of good practice in the seven areas of good medical practice as well as personal details, and details of any other work roles
- An ongoing professional development plan (jointly decided with the appraiser during the appraisal)

- The summary of your previous appraisal
- A significant event analysis
- Audit
- Two structured reflective case reviews
- Patient survey or multi-source feedback (360° appraisal) within the last 3 years.

(NHS Clinical Governance Support Team 2009)

Revalidation

Review of a doctor's fitness to practise 'to reassure the public that doctors are up to date' (GMC 2006) by 5-yearly re-licensing and specialist recertification. The details are yet to be finalised (July 2009).

The two components of revalidation:

- Re-licensing: 5-yearly licence to practise to include a summative component at annual appraisal and based on standards of practice set by the GMC. The licence to practise will be introduced in Autumn 2009.
- Recertification: an assessment likely to be at the same time as re-licensing to be run by the RCGP.

Removing a patient from your list
Relationships with patients

Patients may be removed from the practice list if they:

- register elsewhere
- move out of the practice area
- leave the country for more than 3 months
- get a 2-year prison sentence
- die
- are removed by the GP after an irretrievable breakdown in the doctor–patient relationship.

An irretrievable breakdown may be due to:

- violence or threatening behaviour (immediate removal)
- crime or deception (stealing from the surgery, fraudulently obtaining prescriptions)
- persistent unreasonable or inconsiderate behaviour.

Before you end a professional relationship with a patient, you must be satisfied that your decision is fair and does not discriminate e.g. on the basis of race, age, ethnicity. You cannot remove people who refuse to participate in screening, immunisation or activities contributing to QOF remuneration, or because they have made a complaint. You must be prepared to justify your decision and should inform the patient in writing. You should also inform the PCT and record the decision and reasons in the notes. Although patients can be removed without a warning, the GMS contract recommends that patients should receive a warning before removal.

(GMC 2006; DH 2004)

Complaints against GPs

The number of complaints against GPs is rising and at a faster rate than in other areas of medicine. In 2007 they increased by 12% compared with 2%

for other doctors (Iacobucci 2008). Most GPs will receive several complaints against them during their time in practice. A speedy response and apology where appropriate can reduce the stressful nature of a complaint for both patients and doctors, and prevent further escalation. The current complaints procedure (1996) aims to provide accessible, speedy and fair resolution locally. GPs are required to follow a specified procedure. A cause for concern is that patients may be resorting to alternative sources of complaint/retribution. A website (www.iwantgreatcare.org) rates doctors on trust, listening skills and whether you would recommend your doctor to others. GPs are concerned about its potential for malicious use.

Common causes for complaints
• Delay in or failure to make a diagnosis
• Removal of patients from the GP list
• Refusal to visit
• Prescribing errors
• Medical confidentiality.

The practice complaints procedure
Details
Publicised information should include a named practice complaints administrator, and outline the complaints procedure.
1. The complaints administrator should interview the complainant and explain:
   (a) how the complaint will be dealt with
   (b) the likely timetable
   (c) the rules of confidentiality
   (d) the availability of help from the local Community Health Council
   (e) the possible outcomes
   (f) the availability of PCT conciliation services
   (g) how to pursue the complaint with the PCT if still dissatisfied
   (h) the time limit for making a complaint (normally within 12 months).
2. The facts of the case should be established and recorded, together with a note of the action(s) taken.
3. The complaints administrator should share any findings with a designated partner.
4. The written explanation should:
   (a) summarise the complaint
   (b) explain the practice's view of the event
   (c) apologise, if appropriate
   (d) describe the outcome and steps taken
   (e) inform the complainant how to contact the PCT if still unhappy.
5. The complaints procedure itself should be periodically audited.
6. Complaint statistics and corrective actions must be included in the practice's annual report. It would also be wise to keep careful individual records, including a patients' complaint register.

If a complainant wishes to pursue the issue beyond this system, GPs are obliged to cooperate with PCTs in their complaints procedures.

> **MEMORY BOX:** Practice Complaints Procedure
> - The complaints procedure must be well publicised – a waiting room poster and information leaflet is adequate
> - Complaints must be acknowledged in writing within 2 working days
> - An explanation in writing to be provided within 10 days

The PCT complaints procedure

If called on, the PCT may conduct an independent review. This will first consider whether options for a practice-based resolution have been exhausted, whether to arrange conciliation or whether no more can be done. An independent review panel has three members: a lay chairperson, another lay representative (both nominated by the Secretary of State) and a convenor (non-executive director of the PCT). In clinical complaints the panel is helped by two local medical committee (LMC)-nominated clinical assessors.

There is no obligation to hold a formal hearing, or engage in lengthy evidence gathering, but, if dissatisfaction remains after the review, the complainant can make a further appeal to a Health Service Commissioner (Ombudsman).

Disciplinary hearings

If a GP is thought by the PCT to be in breach of his terms of service, a separate disciplinary investigation may follow. The panel for this hearing will include a legally trained chairperson, three lay members and three LMC-nominated GPs (from another area). The process will normally be completed within 6 weeks.

Medical confidentiality (GMC 2004)

Confidentiality has been a basic tenet of medical ethics for 2500 years and is embodied in the Hippocratic Oath, the International Code of Medical Ethics and the Declaration of Geneva (1947). There are several obvious *reasons* for confidentiality:

1. We set store by personal autonomy, the right of individuals to control their own lives and to control disclosures about them.
2. Consultations have an assumed privacy built into them. Indeed, although there are no legal precedents, there may be an implied *legal contract* of confidentiality, and patients could theoretically obtain redress for breaches through the courts or through the GMC Professional Conduct Committee.
3. Reciprocal respect and confidence are essential to obtain an honest history and meaningful doctor–patient relationship. This is to the mutual benefit of both parties and, in some cases, frankness may also serve the community best.

When can confidentiality be breached without consent?

There are three general circumstances in which confidentiality may be breached without consent. Patients should be informed about the disclosure but their consent is not required:

1. *When required by law.* Statutory disclosures include:
   - notifiable disease (Health Service and Public Health Act)
   - drug addiction (Misuse of Drugs Regulations)
   - births and deaths registration
   - coroners' cases
   - courts of law (and other bodies i.e. NHS tribunal, health and safety executive)
   - driving restrictions (see Driving rules, pages 68–70).
2. *When disclosure is in the public interest* – where the benefit to society outweighs the patient's right to confidentiality. If considering disclosing information under these circumstances always contact your medical defence body for advice. It is important to say this in the exam (CSA); it shows safe practice. Example: the hepatitis C patient having unprotected sex.
3. *When the patient is unable to consent:* where patients lack capacity to consent to treatment or disclosure you may disclose information provided that disclosure is in the patient's best interests:
   - Limit disclosure to relevant information
   - Tell the patient about the disclosure
   - Seek the views of an advocate or carer
   - Document your reasons clearly.

Protecting data and ensuring confidentiality

These are two important regulations regarding patient identifiable information. The Data Protection Act is concerned with the storage of data and the Caldicott principles regulate the transfer of data between health professionals.

The Data Protection Act 1984

Users of computer-held data must register with the data protection registrar. The term 'users' obviously includes GPs with a practice computer, but may also include computer services from PCTs or accountants, for example. The key point is the *control* of personal data, i.e. patient identifiable information.

Users need to comply with several principles. Data should be:

- obtained and processed lawfully
- held for a specific lawful purpose
- not otherwise used or disclosed
- no more than required for the purpose
- dispensed with when no longer necessary
- protected against unauthorised access
- kept accurate and up to date.

The Caldicott principles (1997)

The use of patient identifiable information was reviewed in 1997 in the Caldicott report. These principles apply to the transfer of patient identifiable information within the NHS and to non-NHS bodies. For example, when writing a referral letter you should:

• be ready to justify the purpose(s) for using confidential information
• only use it when absolutely necessary
• use the minimum that is required
• understand that access should be on a strictly need-to-know basis
• understand the responsibilities involved
• understand and comply with the law.

MEMORY BOX: Protecting data
• 1984 Data Protection Act – data storage
• 1997 Caldicott principles – data transfer

The management of confidentiality

Practices need to develop policies that safeguard the processing of confidential information, e.g.:

1. Store it in a secure fashion; restrict computer access to password holders.
2. Make sure that staff who have access to the records understand the principles above (write it into their contracts).
3. When assessing patient data for a third party (e.g. employer or insurance company) ensure that the patient provides written consent and understands at the outset the purpose of the assessment and that this may necessitate disclosure of personal information or a health opinion (with written consent).
4. Remember that the obligation continues after a patient's death.

Patient's access to medical reports and health records

Patients have the right to see medical reports written about them and the right to see their medical records. Doctors keen to avoid the pitfalls of these Acts need to modify their working practices, to ensure good clinical note keeping, e.g. maintain complete and accurate records, ensure that consent is in writing and recorded in the record, and avoid writing personal opinions. A good example of an inappropriate entry found by one of the authors in a patient record said – *Rash, otherwise well, GOK, see in a week* (GOK translates as God Only Knows)!

Access to Medical Reports Act 1988

• Patients have a right to view medical reports about them
• Twenty-one days are allowed for the patient to review the report
• Copies of the report must be kept for 6 months and provided on request.
Patients are allowed the opportunity to discuss the report with their doctors and to attach a codicil if they feel that the report is inaccurate. The GP, however, is not obliged to alter his or her comments if there is still a dif-

ference of view. Ultimately the patient can refuse to allow the report to be sent, so if access is requested a further consent should normally be obtained before dispatch.

Access to Health Records Act 1990
- Patients (over 16) have a right to view their medical notes.
- Access should be provided within 40 days of a written request for a nominal charge.
- GPs can withhold information from the patient if they believe that it is likely to risk serious physical or mental harm to the individual or others.

Note that this Act only applies to notes written after 1 November 1990.

The Mental Health Act (England and Wales) 1983/2007

Mental Health Act Sections

> **MEMORY BOX**
> **Powers of detention**
>
> | Section | Power |
> |---------|-------|
> | 2 | Assessment (28 days) |
> | 3 | Treatment (6 months) |
> | 4 | Emergency admission from community |
> | 5 | Inpatient temporary detention (72 hours) |
> | 135 | Courts power of detention |
> | 136 | Police holding power (72 hours) |
>
> **Other powers**
>
> | | |
> |---|---|
> | 7 | Guardianship |
> | 115 | Power allowing social workers to enter a client's house |

Changes to the Mental Health Act 2007 relevant to GPs
- The definition of mental health disorder has been simplified (previously there were different categories of disorder). In the new definition mental health disorder covers all disorders and disabilities of the mind. Drug and alcohol dependence remains excluded from the definition.
- Supervised community treatment has been introduced for patients discharged from hospital. This can ensure that patients continue treatment to prevent recurrent relapse and readmission ('the revolving door phenomenon').
- Patients' choice of nearest relative: patients can now apply to choose who acts as the nearest relative (NR). The NR has various powers such as the power to discharge the patient from compulsion, to apply for or block detention, to request a review of detention, and to receive certain information about the patient. Previously there was a hierarchical list.
- Treatability test: patients can be detained, or detention continued, only under sections 2 and 3 if treatment is currently available.

- Approved social worker and responsible medical officer roles can now be taken on by other trained health professionals, e.g. nurses, occupational therapists, psychologists. A health professional taking on the approved social worker (ASW) role is called an approved mental health professional (AMHP). Health professionals taking on the responsible medical officer (RMO) role are called the 'responsible clinician'. These titles are awarded to professionals with special expertise and training in mental health.

Principles
1. The *grounds* for admission under the various sections are similar, namely:
   (a) that the patient suffers from a mental disorder of a nature and severity that justify that particular section in the interests of the patient's own health and safety, and the safety of others
   (b) that treatment has to be in hospital.
2. The applicant must be an AMHP or NR.
3. Usually two medical recommendations are needed (an approved doctor and a doctor with prior knowledge of the patient), except in the event of emergency, when one signature gives limited powers of detention.
4. Admission has a limited tenure and there are prescribed discharge powers and rights of appeal.

The Mental Capacity Act 2005

The principles of the Mental Capacity Act:
- Presume capacity: every adult is presumed to have capacity unless proved otherwise
- Respect choice: an adult with capacity has the right to make eccentric or unwise decisions
- Support decision-making: a person must have been given appropriate help to make their own decisions
- Act in best interests: any action taken on behalf of a patient lacking capacity must be in their best interests
- Choose the least restrictive intervention: so that if capacity is regained their options will remain as broad as possible.

Assessing capacity
Capacity is specific to the question being asked, e.g. a patient with cognitive impairment may be incapable of deciding if major surgery is in their best interests but may well have capacity to consent to a blood test or examination. Hence you cannot generalise and label a person as 'incapable'.

Acting in the best interest
Best interests can be expressed by the patient in an advance statement, or through a lasting power of attorney (LPA). Advance directives are written

statements of the patient's wishes (see Advance directives, page 279). LPAs are people appointed to act on patients' behalf. They can be appointed to make decisions in two areas: (1) property and affairs *and* (2) health and welfare. Carers and family members also gain the right in this Act to be consulted. When acting in the best interest you must go through the following checklist:

• Consider whether capacity is likely to be regained
• Encourage involvement of the patient as far as is practicable
• Consider the patient's wishes using available knowledge of beliefs, values, and past and present wishes. Information should be sought from any written statements, family members, carers or LPA.

The Act introduces a new criminal offence of ill treatment or neglect of a person who lacks capacity; the penalty is up to 5 years' imprisonment.

Medical ethics

GMC *Good Medical Practice* guidance states that doctors should be willing and able to explain their decisions. Ethical frameworks can help us do just that. Although they won't be tested directly in the Applied Knowledge Test (AKT), they may feature in the Clinical Skills Assessment (CSA) and Workplace-based Assessment (WPBA). As part of WBPA and CSA, ethical frameworks may be useful to aid clinical decision-making, explain decisions to patients and as a tool for reflection (in case-based discussions or CBDs). They are an important life skill. There are many different frameworks but for the MRCGP it is probably enough to know the four principles of biomedical ethics and utilitarianism (Beauchamp and Childress 1977).

Mnemonic: **BAN Justice**
Beneficence
Autonomy
Non-maleficence
Justice

The terms are defined as:

Beneficence: acting in a way that you believe will benefit your patient.

Autonomy: respecting the right of individuals to make their own decisions and enabling them to do so by providing information in a way that patients can understand.

Non-maleficence: avoiding harm. There is risk with any treatment but on balance of risks there should be less risk of harm than benefit.

Justice: this refers to social justice – the fair distribution of limited resources. Similar patients should be treated equally.

In law patients with capacity cannot have their autonomous decisions overruled despite ethical arguments to the contrary.

Utilitarianism: acting in such a way to achieve the greatest benefits for that the greatest number with the resources available. This principle is important in rationing resources.

EXAMPLE

Mr Pink refuses referral for early suspected bowel cancer surgery because of a fear of not waking up after an anaesthetic.

Beneficence: on the balance of the evidence it is in the patient's best interests to be referred for potentially life-saving surgery, but this principle may conflict with the patient's autonomy.

Autonomy: if fully informed of the risks, benefits and consequences, the rights of the individual should be respected and the decision and discussion documented in the notes.

Non-maleficence: an attempt to coerce Mr Pink into surgery against his will may damage the doctor–patient relationship but this must be balanced against the potential harm resulting from delayed or untreated bowel cancer.

Justice: identification and treatment of early bowel cancer is more cost effective than treatment of more advanced disease (reduced complications, shorter hospital stay, less rehabilitation, shorter time off work). Delaying Mr Pink's treatment may deny resources to others.

For those wishing to read further, a useful resource are www.ethics-network.org.uk.

(www.gmc-uk.org/guidance/ethical_guidance/index.as;
www.ethics-network.org.uk)

Controlled drugs

MEMORY BOX: Controlled drugs
- CDs no longer have to be hand written
- Drug dependency is a notifiable condition
- The misuse of drugs regulations governs the use and storage of CDs

---

Much legislation now exists about the use and misuse of controlled drugs (CDs), e.g.:
- Dangerous Drugs, Notification of Addicts Regulations 1968
- Misuse of Drugs Act 1971
- Misuse of Drugs Regulations 2001
- Drugs Act 2005.

Under the 1971 Misuse of Drugs Act three categories of CDs were defined:

1. Class A: including opium, heroin, morphine, most opiates, pethidine, LSD and other hallucinogens, cocaine and methadone
2. Class B: including cannabis amphetamines and barbiturates
3. Class C: including, benzphetamine, chlorphentermine and diethylpropion.

These categories relate broadly to the degree of harm caused by misuse. The classification has limited significance for doctors and is used mainly in setting the penalties for unlawful possession and intent to supply.

Of greater importance to the medical profession is the Misuse of Drugs Regulations 2001 which defines five groups of drugs (Schedules 1–5) and describes those regulations governing import, export, production, supply, possession, prescribing and record-keeping of controlled drugs.

- Schedule 1: including drugs such as cannabis and LSD, which have no therapeutic use. Possession and supply are prohibited and availability is solely by Home Office licence for research purposes.
- Schedule 2: including the opiates and major stimulants. GPs can possess these drugs for approved medical use but there are strict rules regarding safe custody, record-keeping and the format of prescriptions (see below).
- Schedule 3: including barbiturates, diethylpropion and pentazocine. The format of the prescription is regulated and invoices must be kept for 2 years.
- Schedule 4: including benzodiazepines (except temazepam, which has been moved to Schedule 3). Control requirements are minimal.
- Schedule 5: CDs combined with other drugs in amounts so small that they are not liable to produce dependence. Invoices must be kept for 2 years and manufacture is regulated by the Home Office.

The other points of relevance to the GP are as follows:
1. A doctor must notify the Chief Medical Officer at the Home Office via the regional drug misuse database, within 7 days, if he or she attends a person addicted to narcotic drugs. Addicts are entered on the Home Office's central register.
2. Doctors need a special licence (issued by the Home Secretary) to prescribe heroin, morphine or cocaine in the treatment of drug addiction (a special prescription form, FP 10 (MDA), exists for this purpose).
3. Doctors must keep CDs within a locked compartment or, if on their person, within a locked receptacle. (Note that a locked car boot is insufficient; it must be a locked case in a locked boot.)
4. Doctors must keep a register of the use that they make of their CD supply, and the police have the right to inspect this register.
5. It is an offence to issue an incomplete prescription for a CD and the pharmacist will not dispense under these circumstances. The legal requirements are:
   - Date
   - Prescriber's signature (in indelible ink) and address
   - Name and address of the patient
   - The name, form (tablet/capsule) and strength of the drug
   - The total quantity in both words and figures or the number of dosage units
   - Dose frequency.
   Note that CDs no longer have to be hand written and may be printed (change in regulation from 2005).
6. If controlled drugs need to be disposed of, this should be done in the presence of a witness and formally recorded.
7. Controlled drugs cannot be prescribed for patients leaving the country, and doctors cannot carry CDs abroad unless endorsed by a licence from the Secretary of State.

Careless or improper use of drugs must also lay the GP open to a charge of professional misconduct or incompetence. Note that there is a black market for the resale of drugs obtained from GPs by deception, and also a black market for stolen blank scripts, which can be forged to obtain drug supplies.

Notifiable diseases

Under the Public Health (Control of Disease) Act 1984 and Public Health (Infectious Diseases) Regulations 1988, the following infectious diseases in England and Wales must be notified to the local authority's Medical Officer for Environmental Health:

Anthrax	Plague
Cholera	Polio
Diphtheria	Rabies
Dysentery (amoebic or bacillary)	Relapsing fever
Encephalitis	Rubella
Food poisoning	Scarlet fever
Lassa fever	Smallpox
Leprosy	Tetanus
Leptospirosis	Tuberculosis
Malaria	Typhoid fever
Marburg's disease	Typhus fever
Measles	Viral haemorrhagic fever
Meningitis	Viral hepatitis
Mumps	Whooping cough
Ophthalmia neonatorum	Yellow fever
Paratyphoid fever A and B	

There are some differences to this list in Scotland and Northern Ireland. A small fee is payable for each notification. AIDS is not notifiable by statute. However, doctors are urged to participate in a voluntary confidential reporting scheme.

The coroner

Notifiable deaths
Deaths that should be reported to a coroner include:
- all sudden or unexpected deaths, suicides and deaths where the cause is not known
- deaths that appear suspicious, violent or unnatural
- deaths where the doctor has not attended within the prior 14 days
- deaths within 24 h of hospital admission (in most areas – some personal variation)
- accidents and injuries
- industrial disease

- medical mishaps (specifically including anaesthetics, operations and drugs, either therapeutic or addictive)
- deaths arising from ill treatment, starvation or neglect
- poisoning
- abortions
- stillbirths (when there is doubt as to whether the child was born alive)
- service disability pensioners
- prisoners.

The Scottish system

In Scotland a slightly different system applies: deaths are reported to a procurator fiscal, in the same circumstances as for the coroner in England, with the addition of deaths of foster children and newborn babies.

The Abortion Act

A patient requesting a termination of pregnancy may present in the CSA (in which case the termination form HSA1 will be provided). Under the Abortion Act 1967 and the Abortion Regulations 1991 termination of pregnancy is allowable if there is a risk:

1. To the woman's life (greater than if the pregnancy were to continue)
2. Of grave permanent injury to the woman's physical or mental health
3. To her physical or mental health (greater than if the pregnancy were to continue)
4. To the physical or mental health of her existing children
5. Risk of a handicapped child (rubella damaged, Down's syndrome, etc.).

Clauses 3 and 4 are the most commonly used and can be employed only when the pregnancy does not exceed 24 weeks.

Two medical referees must sign the form (HSA 1).

The Abortion Act represents a middle ground between the extreme views of 'no abortion at all' and 'abortion on demand'. It does not place an absolute value on human life (human suffering coming higher in priority), but it places a *high* value – fetal destruction must be justified. Critics of the legislation point out that it is arbitrary and its application is inconsistent, e.g.:

- The 24-week time limit is based on notions of fetal viability which arguably occurs much sooner than this.
- Under clause 5, Down's syndrome pregnancies are routinely terminated, but in a legal test case a life-saving operation was ordered on Down's syndrome baby Alexandra against the parents' wishes.
- Clauses 3 and 4 are open to wide and subjective interpretation: practice varies widely throughout the country and from one doctor to another.
- The death rate from legal termination is lower than that for pregnancy, so it could be argued under clause 1 that *all* women should receive a termination on request.

Important issues to cover in a CSA:

- Calculate date of pregnancy from last menstrual period (LMP)
- Confirm reasons for wanting termination

- Consider alternative options, e.g. adoption
- Explain the procedure (medical termination – oral tablet followed 48 h later by a pessary, both taken on licensed premises; miscarriage will occur at home and is similar to a heavy period)
- Consider the need for time off work after the procedure – med3 form
- Fill in the certificate A form and send with the patient to the termination clinic
- Discuss contraception to prevent a recurrence of the event.

If for reasons of personal belief the candidate feels unable to arrange a termination of pregnancy, they must refer to a colleague without such conscientious objection.

A discussion of termination may form a useful CBD – an ethical framework will help you to explore the issues.

Medical advice on fitness to drive

Medical fitness to drive is a favourite examination topic. Some of the more important aspects are summarised in Table 3.1, which is adapted from the Driver and Vehicle Licensing Agency (DVLA) guidance.

Note that according to the law:
1. It is the duty of the *applicant* (not his doctor) to declare:
   (a) prescribed (relevant) disabilities, e.g. epilepsy and subnormality
   (b) intermittent or progressive disabilities that may become relevant (prospective disabilities).
2. Licence-holders are also obliged to notify the DVLA as soon as they develop relevant or prospective disabilities, and if a previously notified disability becomes worse.
3. Temporary disabilities (e.g. fractures) are excluded, if they are expected to last less than 3 months.

Failure of the licence holder to notify the DVLA places the doctor in an awkward position, because they may regard the physical safety of other road users to be at risk. This is one of the acknowledged circumstances under which breach of confidentiality may be justified.

The GMC driving guidance states:
1. The DVLA is legally responsible for deciding if a person is medically unfit to drive. They need to know when driving licence holders have a condition, which may, now or in the future, affect their safety as a driver.
2. Therefore, where patients have such conditions, you should:
   - make sure that the patients understand that the condition may impair their ability to drive. If a patient is incapable of understanding this advice, e.g. because of dementia, you should inform the DVLA immediately.
   - explain to patients that they have a legal duty to inform the DVLA about the condition.
3. If the patients refuse to accept the diagnosis or the effect of the condition on their ability to drive, you can suggest that the patients seek a second medical opinion, and make appropriate arrangements for the patients

Table 3.1 DVLA guidelines on fitness to drive

	Disease/Symptom	Group 1 – Standard licence	Group 2 – Heavy goods/buses
CARDIOVASCULAR	MI & Acute Coronary Syndrome	1 month ban[a]	6 week ban and negative exercise test
	Pacemaker	1 month ban[a]	6 week ban
	Angioplasty	1 week ban[a]	6 week ban and negative exercise text
	Angina	Ban if symptomatic at rest.[a] Restart when symptoms controlled.	6 week ban and negative exercise text
	Arrhythmia	Ban until cause identified and controlled for 1 month[a]	Ban until cause identified and controlled for 3 months
NEUROLOGICAL	First Fit	1 year ban[b]	10 year ban[b]
	Epilepsy	May drive if fit free for 12 months	May drive if fit free without medication for 10 years
	CVA/TIA	1 month ban Inform DVLA if residual neurological deficit	1 year ban
DIABETES	Insulin-treated diabetes	Inform DVLA – Limited Licence (1–3 yrs)	Total ban[c]
	Table-treated diabetes	Not limited[a]	Not limited
	Hypoglycaemia	Ban until symptoms controlled	
OTHER	Alcohol dependence	1 year ban	3 year ban
	Drug misuse	6 month ban minimum	1 year ban minimum
	Visual impairment	Must be able to read a licence plate at 20 m	Ban if acuity <6/9 in best eye
	Visual field defect	If impaired ban until field assessed as satisfactory (120° horizontal vision).	Ban if defect present
	Age	No limit	5-yearly review from 45, and yearly after 65

[a]DVLA need not be notified.
[b]If there is a clear provoking factor special consideration may be given.
[c]There are rare exceptions.

to do so. You should advise patients not to drive until the second opinion has been obtained.

4. If patients continue to drive when they are not fit to do so, you should make every reasonable effort to persuade them to stop. This may include telling their next of kin, if they agree you may do so.

5. If you do not manage to persuade patients to stop driving, or you are given or find evidence that a patient is continuing to drive contrary to advice, you should disclose relevant medical information immediately, in confidence, to the medical adviser at DVLA.

6. Before giving information to the DVLA you should inform the patient of your decision to do so. Once the DVLA has been informed, you should also write to the patient, to confirm that a disclosure has been made.'

The driving guidance is exhaustive and should be referred to when advising on specific conditions. However you may be expected to know the guidance for common conditions without reference.

For more details see the DVLA website, medical driving rules section.

Industrial injuries

(Included here for completeness but not a common exam topic.)

Patients can claim for injuries 'arising out of and in the course of their employment' even if due to their own foolhardiness or carelessness. The Industrial Injuries Act lays down over 40 'prescribed' industrial diseases that are recognised for compensation purposes, and a schedule for prescribed degrees of disablement from trauma. Importantly the benefits are not means tested and the individual does not need to give up their job to make a claim (partners can claim retrospectively).

Compensation becomes payable through:

1. The State Industrial Injuries Scheme: this contributes *disablement benefits* (on a 1–100% scale assessed by a medical board) and *industrial death benefits*
2. An individual's private action against his employer (if he can demonstrate negligence).

State claims can be made up to 5 years retrospectively.

In addition there are a group of diseases that are compulsorily *notifiable* by employers to the Health and Safety Executive when they occur in an industrial setting. Industrial diseases notifiable under the Reporting of Injuries, Diseases and Dangerous Occurrences Regulations (RIDDOR) 1995 include:

- poisoning by a number of industrial agents, e.g. arsenic, benzene, beryllium, cadmium, carbon disulphide, lead, manganese, mercury, phosphorus
- chrome ulceration
- skin cancers
- folliculitis and acne (induced by tar, pitch and oils)
- occupational asthma
- extrinsic allergic alveolitis
- pneumoconiosis
- byssinosis
- compressed air sickness
- vibration white finger
- a number of occupational infections, e.g. leptospirosis, tuberculosis, hepatitis, anthrax, work with human pathogens
- a number of occupational cancers (e.g. from ionising radiation or asbestos).

Notes

1. The lists of *reportable* and *prescribed* diseases associated with occupation are similar but not identical. They are drawn up for separate and quite distinct purposes: the one to allow investigation and enforcement under the Health and Safety at Work Act 1974, the other to allow state compensation under the industrial injuries provisions of the Social Security Act 1975.
2. The obligation to report under the RIDDOR Regulations falls on the employer, not the doctor (except in respect of his *own* staff). However, if the employer is to do so, the doctor must make the diagnosis clear to him.

AKT questions

Q1

The GMC 'duties of a doctor' include the following EXCEPT. Select ONE option only:

a Promote the health of patients
b Make care of patients your first concern
c Keep your professional skills up to date
d Recognise and work within the limits of your competence
e Perform annual appraisal

Q2

Which of the following is NOT a tool used in primary care for the purposes of clinical governance? Select ONE option only:

a Quality Outcome Frameworks
b Partners meeting
c Significant event meeting
d Complaints review
e Patient satisfaction survey

Q3

Which of the following is NOT one of the 10 areas of clinical governance described by the RCGP? Select ONE option only:

a Clinical risk reduction
b Professional development
c Leadership
d Prescribing incentives
e Learning lessons from complaints

Q4

At a PCT meeting you consider the request of local practices to remove patients from their practice lists. Which reason given is an inadequate ground for removal? Select ONE option only:

a Persistent inconsiderate behaviour
b Threatening behaviour
c Moving outside the practice area

d Leaving the country for more than 3 months
e Persistent refusal of immunisation and screening

Q5

John presented to the practice previously with a first fit and is awaiting an appointment with neurology. He has been informed not to drive until he is further assessed. Your receptionist noted that he drove to the surgery this morning. Choose the most appropriate course of action. Select ONE option only:

a Report John to the DVLA immediately without informing him.
b Inform John that he has been seen driving and you have a duty to report him to the DVLA. Advise him that he should arrange alternate transport home and for his car to be collected.
c Encourage John to inform the DVLA sharing the decision and discussing the risks and benefits of his continued driving. Ask him to arrange alternate transport home and for his car to be collected.
d As John has been advised to inform the DVLA of his first fit no further action is required.
e Call the police to inform them that your patient continues to drive despite advice not to in view of his medical condition.

Q6

Match the statements to the correct act. Each option may be used once, more than once or not at all:

a Access to Medical Records Act 1988
b Access to Health Records Act 1990
c Mental Capacity Act 2005
d Data Protection Act 1984
e Mental Health Act 1983 & 2007
f The Children's Act 2004
g The Public Health Act 1984

1. Directs doctors to choose the least restrictive action
2. Regulates against the unauthorised access to medical records
3. States that copies of a report must be kept for 6 months
4. Regulates the supervised community treatment of patients
5. States that access must be made available within 40 days of a written request

Q7

Match the sections of the mental health act to the statements. Each option may be used once, more than once or not at all:

a Section 2
b Section 3
c Section 4
d Section 5
e Section 7

f   Section 135
g   Section 136
h   Section 47

1. Used for temporary detention of an inpatient for up to 72 hours
2. A holding power used by the police
3. Used to hold a patient for assessment for up to 28 days
4. A power determining guardianship
5. A power used by courts to detain
6. Emergency power of admission

Q8

The GMC document *Good Medical Practice* lays out the following guidance EXCEPT. Select ONE option only:

a   You must act without delay to inform the PCT if you believe a colleague is putting patients at risk.
b   You must be prepared to justify your decisions and actions if questioned by a colleague or patient.
c   You do not need to provide emergency treatment to patients not registered at your practice.
d   You should act to minimise harm and offer an apology should a patient under your care suffer harm or distress.
e   You should contribute to colleagues' medical education.

Q9

A controlled drug prescription must meet the following requirements EXCEPT. Select ONE option only:

a   Written by hand
b   The form of the drug should be stated
c   Dose frequency should be stated
d   The total quantity must be in words and figures
e   The name and address of the patient must be clearly documented

Q10

Which one of the following deaths should be reported to the coroner? Select ONE option only:

a   A 76 year old with known COPD seen in clinic 10 days ago and started on steroids for an exacerbation.
b   A 32 year old with cystic fibrosis dies of pneumonia and was last seen in surgery 12 days before death and treated for a chest infection.
c   A 62 year old with heart failure is admitted to hospital and dies within 48 hours of admission.
d   A 7-day-old baby with severe metabolic disease under the care of the paediatricians.
e   An 84 year old with no significant past medical history or current medication last seen for a well man check by yourself 7 days ago.

Answers

Q1 e
The *Duties of a Doctor* document lays out general principles and does not stipulate the requirements for appraisal or revalidation.

Q2 b
Clinical governance tools must collect evidence of quality standards. The format of partners' meetings is unique to each practice and no record is required. As such they do not meet the requirements of clinical governance.

Q3 d

Q4 e

Q5 b
Confidentiality can be breached without consent where disclosure is required by law. Patients should be informed about the disclosure but their consent is not required.

Q6
1. c
2. d
3. a
4. e
5. b

Q7
1. d
2. g
3. a
4. e
5. f
6. c

Q8 c
You must offer all reasonable assistance and treatment to any person in an emergency irrespective of whether or not the patient is registered at your practice.

Q9 a
Since 2005 it is no longer a requirement for controlled drug prescriptions to be hand written.

Q10 e
Unexplained deaths should be reported to the coroner.

References

Beauchamp TL, Childress JF. *Principles of Biomedical Ethics*. New York: Oxford University Press, 1977.

Department of Health. *Working for Patients*. London: HMS, 1989.

Department of Health. *The New NHS, Modern, Dependable*. London: DH, 1997. Available at; www.dh.gov.uk/en/Publichealth/Patientsafety/Clinicalgovernance/DH_114.

Department of Health. *The General Medical Services Contract*. London: DH, 2004.

General Medical Council. *Confidentiality: Protecting and providing information*. London: GMC, 2004.

General Medical Council. *Good Medical Practice*. London: GMC, 2006.

General Medical Council. *Duties of a Doctor*. London: GMC, 2006.

Iacubucci G. GPs more likely to face GMC fitness to practise probes. Available at: www.pulsetoday.co.uk/story.asp?sectioncode=23&storycode=4119913&c=2.

NHS Clinical Governance Support Team, 2009. Available at: www.appraisalsupport.nhs.uk/default.asp.

Woolf SH, Grol R, Hutchinson A, Eccles M, Grimshaw J. Education and debate: Clinical guidelines potential benefits, limitations, and harms of clinical guidelines. *BMJ* 1999;**318**:527–30.

Further reading

Pringle M. General practice clinical governance in primary care: Participating in clinical governance. *BMJ* 2000;**321**:737–40. Available at: www.bmj.com/cgi/content/full/321/7263/737.

Pringle M. *Significant Event Auditing and Reflective Learning in Primary Care*. London: National Patient Safety Agency, 2007.

4 Statistics for the AKT

This chapter relates to curriculum statements 3.5 and 3.6 (research and academic activity; evidence-based practice)

Critical appraisal and evidence-based clinical practice account for 10% of the Applied Knowledge Test (AKT). Critical appraisal is defined as the systematic assessment and interpretation of research studies. In the exam this means that candidates are required to interpret research data, and demonstrate understanding of statistical tools and study models. This chapter has been difficult to write and, if unfamiliar, the concepts make for difficult reading. If you feel at sea and out of your depth, do not lose heart! The objective is to pass the MRCGP and in this context more information has been provided than is strictly necessary. For those struggling, stick to learning the risk calculations, sensitivity, specificity, positive predictive value (PPV), negative predictive value (NPV) and the interpretation of Forest plots. If you find the material straightforward the additional information may earn you an extra mark or two; it may even have stimulated your interest; if not there are other more important fish to fry!

This chapter begins with some brief advice on critical reading, and then proceeds to a simple overview of statistics and epidemiology for the uninitiated. For those requiring a more in-depth overview we would thoroughly recommend Trisha Greenhalgh's (2006) book *How to read a Paper*.

Digesting scientific material

An orderly approach to critical reading has much to commend it. Many journals organise their abstracts in a semi-structured manner; a similar model can conveniently be used by candidates for analysing and summarising published material. This is the IMRAD format. For example:
- *Introduction*: why did the author start?
- *Methods*: what did the author do?
- *Results*: what did the author find?
- *Analysis*: are the results statistically and clinically significant?
- *Discussion*: what does it mean?

In the same vein, the abstracts of papers in the *British Medical Journal* contain the following structured headings: objectives; design; setting;

Notes for the MRCGP: A curriculum based guide to the AKT, CSA and WBPA, 4th edition. By K. Palmer and N. Boeckx. Published 2010 by Blackwell Publishing, ISBN: 978-1-4051-5724-7.

subjects; interpretation; end-points; measurement and main results; and conclusions.

The findings need to be placed in context, and three useful supplementary questions will help:

1. What is the message and is it relevant to me? (For example, lowering cholesterol reduces heart attacks – an important message and relevant to general practice.)
2. Do I believe it? (That is, is the methodology sound?)
3. If true, how does it affect what I do at present? (There is no point in reading papers if you never alter your practice.)

Methodology

Flawed methods mean a flawed paper regardless of the results, so it is important to check some basic questions:

- If the study was a clinical trial was it randomised and controlled? Failure to do this may introduce bias and make results unreliable.
- Was the study type appropriate to address the question asked? Using the wrong study type can invalidate results – see Study designs below.
- Were the statistical tests used correctly performed? Examples of the commonly used statistical tests and how to perform and interpret them are given throughout the chapter. It is unlikely that you will have to comment on the choice of test; this is for a statistician!
- What population was studied (how many patients, age range, severity of disease)? If the population studied differs too much from the population of patients whom you see in practice the results may not be generalisable (and therefore not relevant to your population).
- How many withdrew? If large numbers of patients withdraw there may be bias in the results (unless data were analysed on an intention-to-treat basis – see below)
- What endpoints were used (and were they primary or secondary)? Primary endpoints, e.g. stroke, heart attack, or secondary endpoints e.g. lowering cholesterol, lowering blood glucose. Secondary (surrogate) endpoints are less reliable because they may not be a valid representation of the primary endpoint.

Intention-to-treat analysis

To avoid bias when analysing results of trials, studies should include results for all the patients who start the study **even** if patients in the intervention group stop their treatment during the trial. For example:

A trial looks at stroke events in two groups: one taking ACE inhibitors and a control. Five per cent of the ACE inhibitor group stop taking their ACE inhibitor during the study. There are three events in this subgroup. These events should be included in the analysis of the intervention group as though they had continued their treatment (thus ensuring that the intervention and control groups' randomisation is preserved to minimise confounding differences between the groups such as age, sex).

Epidemiology: basic definitions

1. *Epidemiology* is the study of the distribution and determinants of disease and other indices of health in human populations.
2. A *population* is a circumscribed group of individuals sharing one or more defined characteristic in common. Several groups may exist, e.g. epidemiology seeks to infer from the *particular* (study sample or population) to the *general* (target population). Whether it can do so depends critically on whether the study population is *typical* of the target population.

These groups	... are	... for example
The target population	All people everywhere who share diastolic blood pressures >100 mmHg	Men aged 40–50 years with the characteristic(s) defined
The study population	A fraction of the target population selected for study	All such men in region X
A study sample	The fraction of the study population sampled	All such men in practice Y from region X

3. A *measuring instrument* means (speaking epidemiologically) any technique used to collect data.
   (a) Examples might equally include:
      - blood samples
      - radiographs
      - spirometric graphs
      - questionnaires
      - agreed sets of diagnostic criteria.
   (b) Good measuring instruments must be:
      - *valid*, i.e. provide a true assessment of what they purport to measure
      - repeatable/*reliable*, i.e. provide the same result each time when re-measured (under the same conditions).
   (c) Validity is measured in terms of *sensitivity* and *specificity* (see below), compared with the gold standard of all measuring instruments.
   (d) Repeatability may be less than perfect because of:
      - *within-observer* variation (e.g. although the blood pressure is the same, I read it differently after a coffee break than I did before it)
      - *between-observer* variation (e.g. I tend to make the same blood pressure higher than you do)
      - *within-subject* variation (his blood pressure changes anyway).
   (e) Measuring instruments should be chosen, refined or tested by pilot study to ensure that they are as valid and repeatable as possible. (The best existing ones, e.g. the Medical Research Council Respiratory Questionnaire, have been developed in this way and should be used where appropriate and possible.)

Sensitivity, specificity, positive and negative predictive values
Sensitivity
The sensitivity asks what proportion of the studied population with disease is correctly identified by the test (true positives – TPs).

$$\text{Sensitivity} = \frac{(\text{No. of TPs that test identifies})}{(\text{No. of TPs in the sample population})}$$

Specificity
The specificity asks what proportion of the studied population without disease is correctly identified by the test (true negatives – TNs).

$$\text{Specificity} = \frac{(\text{No. of true TNs that test identifies})}{(\text{No. of true TNs in the sample population})}$$

Positive predictive value
PPV asks what proportion of patients testing positive really have the disease.

$$\text{PPV} = \frac{(\text{No. of true TPs that test identifies})}{(\text{No. that the test claims are positive})}$$

Negative predictive value
NPV asks what proportion of patients testing negative are really disease free.

$$\text{NPV} = \frac{(\text{No. of true TNs that test identifies})}{(\text{No. the test claims are negative})}$$

These definitions can be confusing without a 2 × 2 table to look at. By convention, always draw a 2 × 2 table in the same way, with the true disease status on top. If you draw the table this way sensitivity and specificity are calculations down the table columns and negative and positive predictive values are calculations across the rows.

	Disease, e.g. bowel cancer		
FOB test	Present	Absent	Total
Positive	2TP	18FP	20
Negative	1FN	182TN	183
Total	3	200	203

http://en.wikipedia.org/wiki/Positive_predictive_value
FOB, faecal occult blood; TP, true positive; FP, false positive; FN, false negative; TN, true negative
Sensitivity = 2/3 = 66%.
Specificity = 182/200 = 91%.
PPV = 2/20 = 10%.
NPV = 182/183 = 99%.

Interpreting the findings

From the 2 × 2 table you can see that sensitivity and specificity provide information at a population level, i.e. they are concerned with identifying the proportion of people in a *population* with or without disease that are correctly identified by the test. Predictive values give information at an *individual* level, i.e. for a positive result PPV tells me the probability that the positive result in front of me has correctly confirmed the condition for which I am testing.

A good example of interpreting findings posted on wikipedia is used here. A positive faecal occult blood (FOB) test result is poor at confirming the diagnosis of bowel cancer (PPV 10%) and so the patient needs further tests to confirm presence of disease. However, with a negative result I can be quite confident in reassuring the patient that they do not have cancer as the NPV is high (99%). Looking at the test on a population level (e.g. as a screening tool) the test will identify 66% of cancers (sensitivity) and is good at correctly identifying the absence of disease in the population as the specificity is high (91%).

Study designs

Longitudinal versus cross-sectional

1. A study in which events evolve and are enumerated over a period of time is said to be *longitudinal*: case–control and cohort studies are of this type.
2. A study that takes a representative sample of a target population to provide a snapshot picture of the state at a particular point in time is said to be *cross-sectional*, and is also known as a survey. This type of study is most appropriate for defining the prevalence of a disease.

Some examples should make the difference clear.

Longitudinal study

In a study from general practice, patients with backache were randomised between receiving an education leaflet or not. Over the next year the numbers presenting with backache were counted for the two groups.

Cross-section study

In another study doctors from practice X examined a randomly chosen selection of patient records to establish the proportion of patients currently being treated for backache.

Cohort versus case control

1. The cohort study (also called a prospective study) is a longitudinal study that follows forward over a fixed period of time two groups of people who have different exposures to an agent of interest, but are otherwise matched. Questions about the incidence of disease can be compared in the two groups. Example of a suitable study: does taking the oral contraceptive pill cause thrombosis?

2. The case–control study (or retrospective study) compares people who have a specific disease (cases) with those who do not (controls) to establish whether their past exposure to possible disease risk factors differed. Example of a suitable case control study: investigating the association between cholangiocarcinoma and exposure to oestrogens.

Both case–control and cohort studies look for an association between exposure to an agent and a disease. Case–control studies, because they are retrospective, provide lower quality evidence than cohort studies. However, they are the better choice for studying rare diseases. In these cases the disease incidence is too low for a prospective study to identify sufficient cases for useful statistical analysis.

The essential difference between cohort and case control studies is illustrated in Figure 4.1. Note particularly that groups in a cohort study are compared with respect to *disease*, whereas those in a case–control study are compared with respect to *exposure*. In other words, case-control studies cannot demonstrate causality – only an association.

Case reports

Although weak on the evidence front, case reports have an important role in highlighting topics that may require further investigation, e.g. a clinician using a new drug, madeupalol, notes two cases of thrombocytopenia. This is a rare condition, so the cases warrant further enquiry.

Which studies provide the strongest evidence?

The relative strength of evidence of the main study types are listed in order here. The higher up the list the more likely that the results will be valid and reliable. This does not mean that study types lower down the list are redundant. It may be impracticable or unethical to use a different study type e.g. case controls are more appropriate than cohorts for studying rare disease, you cannot double blind certain procedures.

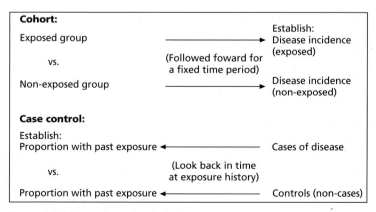

Figure 4.1 Cohort and control study designs.

1. Systematic reviews and meta-analyses   Strongest
2. Randomised controlled trials
3. Cohort studies
4. Case–control studies
5. Cross sectional studies
6. Case reports.   Weakest

So, it is important to choose the trial type that not only offers the strongest evidence but is appropriate to address the question that you are asking. This leads to the following inevitable question.

(www.shef.ac.uk/scharr/ir/units/systrev/hierarchy.htm)

Which study type for what question?

Question: Is a therapeutic intervention (e.g. drug treatment, procedure) effective?

Most appropriate study type: RCT (randomised controlled trial)

Question: Is a new diagnostic test valid (gives a true result) and reliable (provides the same result each time)?

Most appropriate study type: cross-sectional study (comparing the new test against a gold standard).

Question: Is a screening test effective (i.e. can test X identify presymptomatic disease in large populations)?

Most appropriate study type: longitudinal cohort.

Question: What is the prognosis of a disease after diagnosis?

Most appropriate study type: longitudinal cohort.

Question: Does exposure to an agent (drug, etc.) cause disease X?

Most appropriate study type: cohort (case control if the disease is rare).

(Swinscow 1997; Greenhalgh 2006)

Note that it is not ethical to randomise people to receive a suspected hazard. This has two consequences:

1. RCTs tend to be restricted to a situation of equipoise (not knowing which is best around questions of benefit).
2. Evidence on hazards (e.g. asbestos) comes from observational studies (observing what is already happening, rather than RCTs).

Randomisation, placebos and blind trials

1. If the purpose of a study is to compare two groups receiving different treatments (e.g. chemotherapy vs placebo), patients would ideally be randomised between the groups. This design would be called a randomised controlled trial.
2. If the patient does not know which treatment he is receiving but the doctor does, this is called single-blind randomisation.
3. If neither the patient nor the doctor knows which treatment is being given, this is called double-blind randomisation.

The purpose of randomisation is to iron out any chance differences that exist between the groups. The double-blind design removes one source of bias – that due to patient and doctor expectation.

Error and bias

These terms have distinct and separate meanings. *Bias* is a form of *systematic* error, leading to consistent over- or under-recording of the true situation. *Random error*, because of its chance nature, leads to neither.

This is a more important distinction than it seems. Random error leads to a less precise estimate of the study parameter, but the degree of imprecision can be statistically estimated, and the effect can be offset by making the study larger. The effect of bias is harder to estimate and its magnitude cannot be reduced simply by including more participants. A study beset with random errors may be salvaged; a biased study may not, unless the bias is recognised and removed.

Come common types of bias

- Selection bias: bias caused by a failure of randomisation leading to systematic differences between the groups randomised.
- Performance bias: a systematic bias in the way the groups are managed, e.g. in a depression trial offering longer appointments to those in the treatment group.
- Exclusion bias: systematic differences in withdrawals from the trial.
- Detection bias: bias resulting from systematic differences in the way that the groups are assessed (e.g. closer scrutiny of the treatment group by taking more samples).

Measuring rates

1. *Incidence*: the rate of occurrence of new cases. (Note that you need to exclude old cases at the outset of the study, because they must not be counted.)
2. *Prevalence*: the proportion of the population at risk affected at a given time (point prevalence = at a given point in time; period prevalence = within a stated period).
3. *Age standardisation*: age is such an important determinant of ill health that it would be very misleading to compare two study populations with different age structures. Suppose, for example, we suspected that the medical standards exercised in preventing cerebrovascular accidents differed in Bournemouth and Milton Keynes. We could attempt to test this hypothesis by comparing the incidence of cerebrovascular accidents in each population, but the comparison would be meaningless unless some account was taken of the age groups found in each community. Age standardisation is a technique that allows the comparison to be made (the details need not concern us). It is from this technique that the standardised mortality ratio (SMR) is derived.
4. *Expressing results*: in comparing the incidence rates of disease in exposed (Ie) and non-exposed (In) populations, we are asking: What is the risk in the one population compared with the other? This comparison can be expressed in several ways, e.g.:
   (a) the absolute difference between the rates (Ie−In)

(b) the proportionate difference in rates [(Ie–In)/Ie]

(c) the ratio of the rates (Ie/In).

The latter is usually chosen. It is called the *relative risk*.

The SMR is an important example. It is also a product of convenience: because of the expense and difficulty of following groups through a cohort study, convention allows the control group in mortality studies to exist only on paper, a reference population whose mortality experience can be looked up in tables of national statistics. After age standardisation the rates are compared:

$$SMR = \frac{\text{Observed deaths in study population}}{\text{Expected deaths in study population}} \times 100$$

Expected is understood in the sense of 'the number of deaths that would occur in the study population if it experienced the same age-specific mortality as the reference population'.

A mortality experience equivalent to that of the reference population gives an SMR of 100. If >100, the mortality experience was greater, and so on.

As the starting point in the design of a case–control study is quite different, we cannot calculate relative risk in quite the same way. The *odds ratio* (OR) is an approximation to relative risk suitable in interpreting the findings of case–control studies.

Its interpretation is broadly similar to that of the SMR.

Calculating risk

Absolute risk (AR): the risk of an event in a group.

Relative risk (RR): the ratio of risk of an event in one group compared with the other.

Relative risk reduction (RRR): the difference in risk between the two groups over the control group.

Absolute risk reduction (ARR): the difference (subtraction) between control and intervention group risk.

Number needed to treat (NNT): the number of people whom you need to treat to prevent one event (1/ARR).

Odds ratio: the ratio (or odds) of events/no events in the intervention group compared with the ratio in the control group.

Example

A trial looks at the number of stroke events in patients taking an ACE (angiotensin-converting enzyme) inhibitor (the intervention group) versus a control group over a 10-year period.

	Events	No events	Total
Control	338	1100	1438
Intervention	240	1200	1440

Absolute risk in the two sample populations

Risk in intervention group (240/1440 = 0.17 or 17% chance of a stroke in patients taking an ACE)

Risk in control group (338/1438 = 0.24 or 24% chance of a stroke in the control group).

Relative risk

Risk in intervention/risk in control (0.17/0.24)

Answer = 0.71 (or 71% risk of stroke in the intervention group compared to the control group).

Relative risk reduction

Difference in risk (0.24 − 0.17 = 0.07)/Risk in control group (0.24)

Answer = 0.29 (or 29% reduction in the risk of stroke as a result of the intervention).

Absolute risk reduction

Difference in risk between two groups (0.24 − 0.17)

Answer = 0.07 (or 7% reduction in the absolute risk of stroke).

Number needed to treat

1/ARR (1/0.07)

Answer = 14 (you need to treat 14 people with an ACE inhibitor to prevent one stroke).

Odds ratio

Odds in intervention group (240/1200 = 0.2 or 20%)

Odds in control group (338/1100 = 0.31 or 31%)

Odds ratio (0.2/0.31)

Answer = 0.65 (this demonstrates that the odds of having a stroke is lower in the intervention group).

Basic principles of medical statistics

Definitions

1. Statisticians divide their field into:
   (a) *descriptive statistics*: the summarising, enumerating and presenting of data in meaningful forms
   (b) *inferential statistics*: the use of data from study groups to draw inferences concerning target populations.
2. Statistical data can be:
   (a) *quantitative*: data to which an exact number can be ascribed (blood pressure, episodes of backache)
   (b) *qualitative* :data to which a quality can be ascribed but not an exact member (sex, blood group).

Quantitative data may be:

(a) *discrete*: assuming only certain discrete values (e.g. number of children)

(b) *continuous*: assuming any value along a continuum (e.g. serum cholesterol).

It is subject to the normal rules of arithmetic.

Qualitative data may be grouped into categories that have an order (ordinal data, e.g. clinical severity grading scales for breathlessness), but cannot be treated in a simple arithmetic way.

3. Data can be summarised in tabular or graphic form by means of contingency tables, bar charts or frequency histograms.

4. It is conventional in describing statistical data to measure central tendency and distribution or dispersion of the data points.

(a) Measures of central tendency include:

- the *mean*: the average value
- the *mode*: the most commonly occurring value
- the *median*: the middle observation when all the values are ranked in ascending or descending order.

The mean is the most widely used of these measures, because it can be mathematically manipulated. In a normal distribution all three have the same value.

(b) The most important measure of dispersion around the mean is called the *standard deviation* (SD).

(The square of the deviation from the mean is taken for each data point. The results are summed and averaged. The square root of this value is the SD.)

The SD has convenient properties where values are normally distributed (as in many biological systems):

- 66% of values lie within the range of $X \pm 1$ SD
- 95% of values lie within the range of $X \pm 2$ SD
- 99% of values lie within the range of $X \pm 3$ SD.

Qualitative research (the value of)

Qualitative research aims to answer different questions to those asked of quantitative studies. They are not about enumerating (i.e. identifying frequency, incidence, calculating relative risk) but investigate understanding of a clinical issue. The best way of demonstrating this is by looking back at the example study. The quantitative analysis tells us that 5% of patients withdrew from the intervention arm. A qualitative analysis can help provide an answer into why. Were the tablets bitter tasting? Did the patients find it difficult to follow the treatment regimen? Did the patients fail to see or understand benefits from the treatment? The answers given by qualitative studies provide valuable insights into problems that cannot be investigated through quantitative methodology. Qualitative studies use different methodologies and critical analysis of this type of study requires specialised knowledge. In addition to the standard three questions:

1. What is the message and is it relevant to me?
2. Do I believe it?
3. If true, how does it affect what I do at present?
   Two extra questions may be helpful:
4. Could this question have been answered using quantitative methodology (if so the choice of study design is flawed)?
5. Have the researchers tried to validate their data by collecting it using several different methods? For example, interviews, questionnaires, documents and texts (this is called triangulation).

(www.qual.auckland.ac.nz)

Correlation and regression

If we wished to assess the association between two quantitative variables (say height and blood pressure) we might start by plotting height against the blood pressure for each of the individuals studied. The variables height and blood pressure would be x and y coordinates on the graph and each participant would be represented by a single point. An immediate visual inspection of this graph (which is called a *scatter diagram*) might give the impression that a linear association existed. Correlation is the mathematical verification of this impression.

A *correlation coefficient* is a measure of the strength of linearity between two quantitative variables. It has a value on a scale of −1 to +1:
- +1 indicates a perfect direct association
- −1 indicates a precise inverse association
- 0 (and values close to it) indicate no association.

They process is a descriptive one.

Regression, by contrast, is a predictive process. The line of best fit in the scatter diagram is found mathematically, and used to *predict* the value of one variable given the value of another.

Notes

1. The processes are complementary. Regression can always find a line of best fit – even if the fit is very poor and in all probability no linear relationship exists. A high correlation coefficient tells us that there probably *is* a line there, so the regression result is credible.
2. For purposes of correlation, the variables can be used interchangeably on x or y axes. But, in regression, the one on the y axis must be chosen as the dependent variable and the one on the x as the predictor variable (weight depends on height but height does not depend on weight).
3. Strictly speaking these points relate to *linear* regression. Non-linear regression is also possible, but here the association is assumed to be non-linear and calculations are based on formulae describing the form of the relationship between the variables.

Sampling statistics: standard error of the mean

If we take a study sample and ascertain its mean and standard deviation, we have an approximation of the true population mean and standard deviation. If we took another sample and repeated the exercise we would probably end up with a slightly different estimate.

According to the theory of sampling statistics, if we take an infinite number of samples, our estimates of the population mean would show a normal distribution around the true mean. The standard deviation of this sampling distribution could in turn be described and is called the *standard error of the mean*.

This standard deviation of the sampling means gives us an idea of the dispersion of our estimates around the true value, and a better statement of the range in which the true value is likely to lie.

Significance tests

1. Tests of statistical significance, though varied, are based on a common line of reasoning. The so-called *null hypothesis* contends that no true differences exist between population groups in a study and that any apparent difference is the result of the effects of chance alone. This results, for example, in their sample means lying at different points on a single normal distribution of sample means.
2. The probability (P) of getting values as far apart as those observed, while still belonging to the same family of sampling means, can be deduced.
3. If the probability appears small ($P < 0.05$) we would contend that the null hypothesis is unlikely and that the two populations are indeed different; if the probability does not appear small enough ($P > 0.05$) we would contend that the null hypothesis could still be true and the differences observed could be due to chance alone. The value of P at 0.05 has been chosen arbitrarily, and is called the *significance level* of the test. Usually: $P < 0.05$ leads to rejection of the null hypothesis, indicating statistical significance, and $P < 0.01$ is regarded as *highly significant*.

Notes

1. Even if $P > 0.05$, the difference could still be genuine, but such a study would have failed to prove it so.
2. A statistically significant difference may not be a *clinically* significant one: although it is likely to be a genuine difference, the magnitude of effect may be small and the consequences clinically unimportant.

Type I and type II errors

Significance testing indicates only the balance of probabilities. A conclusion based on it can still be wrong:

1. A *type I error* occurs if the test leads us to conclude that there is a difference when one does not actually exist. The risk of this occurring depends on the significance level that we choose for the test: the lower it is, the more convinced we require to be and the lower the risk of a false positive.
2. However, if we are too strict we may miss a genuine difference between compared groups. As we insisted on a value of $P < 0.0001$ when we could only demonstrate $P < 0.01$, we draw a false-negative conclusion. This is a *type II error*.

3. Type II errors can be reduced by increasing the size (power) of the study. They are not normally quoted, but they are used beforehand by statisticians in this way to establish the minimum size worthy of study.

Power

The power of a study is a calculation. It estimates the size of the study required to demonstrate a difference between groups if it really exists. The calculation is complex and depends on several factors (the level of difference that constitutes a clinically significant effect, the level of statistical significance, etc. (Greenhalgh 2006). You will not be expected to calculate it. Most studies work on a power calculation of around 80–90% (i.e. 8–9 out of 10 studies will reveal a significant statistical difference at a predefined level e.g. $P < 0.05$ if one truly exists). Lack of power leads to a type 2 error – concluding that there is no difference between the groups when there really is one.

Confidence intervals

Most published articles report their findings using *confidence intervals* (CIs). The confidence interval is an estimate of how close the result calculated in a trial or study lies to the true result. Another way of thinking about this is that if you repeat the same trial several times you will get slightly different results. The confidence interval is an estimate of the distribution of these results. It gives an upper and lower value for this distribution. Bigger trials have narrower CIs because we can be surer that the results lie close to the true value.

For example, going back to our example stroke trial, the relative risk of a stroke in the intervention group was 0.71. If the CI was calculated to be (0.69–0.82) it would mean that the true relative risk could be as low as 69% or as high as 82%. CIs are usually expressed as the 95% CI. This means that we can be 95% certain the true value lies somewhere within the two values.

Confidence intervals that cross zero
Example
- Risk of death in control 21%
- Risk in intervention group 16%
- Improved survival in intervention group = 5% (95% CI −1.3 to +11).

If the CI crosses zero it means that the trial has not achieved statistical significance. Why? Well, in this example the intervention may improve survival (by 11%) but may also reduce survival (by −1.3%), i.e. the study is inconclusive. This could be because there really is no difference between the two groups compared or because the study is under powered.

Forest plots

Results from multiple trials are often pooled (meta-analysis) and displayed using a Forest plot (Figure 4.2). These often pop up in the AKT. Studies should be pooled, however, only when they measure the same thing, e.g. similar clinical endeavour employing the same treatment (do not mix apples with pears!)

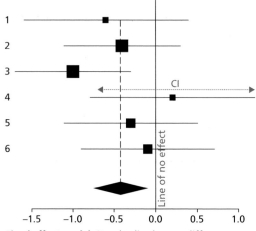

Fixed effect model Standardised mean difference

Figure 4.2 The *y* axis shows six separate trials – labelled 1–6. The horizontal lines passing through the central blobs indicate the confidence intervals of the separate trials. The size of the blob is proportionate to the numbers in the study (big study, big blob). The solid vertical line indicates the zero effect line. As you can see the confidence intervals (CIs) of trials 1, 2, 4, 5 and 6 all cross this line and therefore have not achieved statistical significance. The diamond blob at the bottom represents the pooled data. The width of the diamond is its CI. Larger studies have narrower CIs because we can be surer of the results. Hence the pooled data CI is much narrower than that of the component studies. As you can see it does not cross the line of no difference and has achieved statistical significance. This demonstrates the ability of a meta-analysis to provide a definitive result when component studies fail to reach significance by pooling the data to increase the power. (See www.childrens-mercy.org/stats/model/images/metaanalysis.)

Summary

The ability to read, comprehend, appraise and digest new findings is an important life-long skill for aspiring general practitioners. Aspects of critical appraisal and interpreting evidence may also be assessed in WBPA.

AKT questions

Q1
Define sensitivity. Select ONE option only:
a The proportion of patients testing positive who are correctly identified as having the disease.
b The proportion of the studied population without disease who are correctly identified by the test.
c The proportion of patients testing negative who are correctly identified as disease free.
d The proportion of the studied population with disease correctly identified by the test.
e The proportion of the studied population with disease.

Q2

Match the choices with the correct statistical tests. Each option may be used once, more than once or not at all.

	Disease		
Test	Present	Absent	Total
Positive	6	14	20
Negative	2	186	188
Total	8	200	208

a   14/20
b   6/8
c   186/200
d   186/188
e   6/20
f   14/200

1. Sensitivity
2. Specificity
3. Negative predictive value
4. Positive predictive value

Q3

You wish to investigate the possible causes of Goods' syndrome, a rare disease. Choose the most appropriate study design from the following. Select ONE option only:
a   Randomised control trial
b   Cohort
c   Case–control
d   Cross-sectional study
e   Case report

Q4

A trial assessing blood pressure lowering between two groups (standard treatment and a new agent Cintapril) measures blood pressure using electronic sphygmomanometers. If the blood pressure is raised on the first reading in the Cintapril group the trialists repeat the reading. A single reading is taken in the standard treatment group. This is an example of? Select ONE option only:
a   Exclusion bias
b   Selection bias
c   Monitoring bias
d   Performance bias
e   Detection bias

Q5

A new diagnostic screening test for prostate cancer has been developed. You have been asked to design a study to assess its use in practice. Choose the most appropriate. Select ONE option only:

a   Case–control
b   Randomised control trial
c   Non-randomised cohort
d   Cross-sectional study
e   Time series study

Q6

A trial looks at the number of COPD exacerbations in patients using a long-acting β agonist (LABA) compared with a control group on 'standard treatment'. The data set is shown below. Match the calculations to the correct statistical terms. Each option may be used once, more than once or not at all.

	Events	No. of events	Total
Control	102	488	600
LABA group	86	514	600

a $(86/600)/(102/600) = 0.82$
b $(102/600) - (86/600)$
c $(86/514)/(102/600)$
d $86/600$
e $(102/488)/(86/514)$
f $102/600$

1. Absolute risk in the LABA group
2. Relative risk
3. Odds ratio
4. Absolute risk reduction

Q7

A trial drug in the intervention group shows an absolute risk of 18%. The absolute risk in the control group is 22%. What is the number needed to treat? Select ONE option only:

a   10
b   4
c   25
d   82
e   8

Q8

The results of a meta-analysis are shown here. The mera-analysis compares the number of strokes on treatment 'x' compared to standard treatment. For each question select ONE option only.

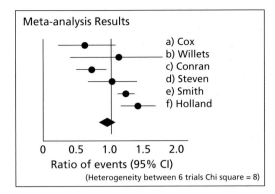

1. Which trial had the widest confidence interval?
2. Which trial showed the most significant benefit from treatment?
3. Which trial is likely to have been the largest?
4. Which trial showed the most significant harm from treatment?

Q9

In reference to the meta-analysis in Q8 choose the correct answer. Select ONE option only:

a All of the studies show significant findings.
b Overall the meta-analysis shows no significant benefit from treatment.
c The results from this group of trials are homogeneous.
d The confidence interval in the Willet's study indicates that it is the most significant individual study.
e More studies are needed before the results can be validated.

Q10

Match the statistical terms with the correct definitions. Each option may be used once, more than once or not at all:

a Mean
b Median
c Mode
d Negative predictive value
e Positive predictive value
f Sensitivity
g Specificity
h Absolute risk
i Relative risk reduction

1. The ratio of the absolute risk reduction to the absolute risk in the control group
2. The proportion of patients testing negative who are correctly identified as disease free
3. The middle value in a range
4. The most common value observed
5. The risk of an event in a group

Answers

Q1 d

Q2
1. b
2. c
3. d
4. e

Q3 c

Q4 e

Q5 d

Q6
1. d
2. a
3. e
4. b

Q7 c
NNT = 1/absolute risk reduction, i.e. 1/(22–18%), i.e. 1/0.04 = 25.

Q8
1. b
2. c
3. e
4. f

Q9 b
Regarding part (c), heterogeneity is a measure of the similarity of findings between trials. Confidence intervals that overlap closely are homogeneous. In this Forest plot some of the CIs of the trials do not overlap at all.

Q10
1. i
2. d
3. b
4. c
5. h

References

Greenhalgh T. *How to Read a Paper: The basics of evidence-based medicine*, 3rd edn. Oxford: Wiley Blackwell, 2006.

Swinscow TDV. *Statistics at Square One*, 9th edn (revised by MJ Campbell). London: BMJ Publishing Group, 1997.

5 Management and practice matters

This chapter relates to curriculum statement 4 (Management in primary care and Information management and technology)
The MRCGP exam tests your ability to problem solve in a UK GP setting, so an understanding of the structure of general practice is helpful for new GPs and GP registrars. Although awareness of the key resources, constraints and requirements is important, you are unlikely to be tested on the finer points of practice management. This chapter provides pertinent background information and is split into two sections: exam points (Part 1) and practice points (Part 2). Part 1 provides current information on practice matters that are more likely to turn up in your Acquired Knowledge Test (AKT) and Clinical Skills Assessment (CSA) exams. Part 2 provides useful background information for the WPBA (workplace-based assessment) to aid better understanding of the framework of general practice today.

PART 1 EXAM POINTS

The new GP contract ('the blue book')

The new GP General Medical Services (GMS) contract (also called 'the blue book') was introduced in April 2004 and replaced the old GP contract (called 'the red book'). There has been a change not just in primary colour, but also in the way that primary care services are run. The key differences are shown in Table 5.1.

Where does the money come from?
A proportion of taxation collected by the government is allocated to the Department of Health (DH). From this the DH allocates budgets to the primary care trusts (PCTs) to fund local services. PCTs receive approximately 75% of the overall NHS budget.

Practice income
Practices now receive income from four main areas:
1. The global sum
2. Enhanced services
3. Quality Outcome Framework (QOF) payments
4. Additional payments (seniority, premises).

Notes for the MRCGP: A curriculum based guide to the AKT, CSA and WBPA, 4th edition. By K. Palmer and N. Boeckx. Published 2010 by Blackwell Publishing, ISBN: 978-1-4051-5724-7.

Table 5.1 Key differences

The old red book	The new GMS contract (the blue book)
The contract is with the individual GP	The contract is with the GP practice
Patients register with an individual GP	Patients register with a practice (no individual GP lists)

Payment comes from:
• Items of service, i.e. practices charge the PCT (the body responsible for local health services) for virtually every service that the practice provides, e.g. minor surgery, antenatal services, health promotion, this is essentially bean counting
Plus
• Reimbursements (staff budget)
• Patient-based fees
• Capitation fees (number of patients on practice list)
• Health promotion payments
• Rural practice payments
• Practice allowances
• Basic practice allowance, postgraduate education allowance
	Payment comes from:
	• Limited items of service:
	  ➤ registration fees
	  ➤ temporary residents fees
	  ➤ emergency treatment fees
	  ➤ contraceptive fees
	  ➤ vaccination and immunisation fees
	• The majority of item of service fees are replaced by two new concepts:
	  ➤ essential, additional and enhanced services[a]
	  ➤ QOFs
	Plus
	• Reimbursements (staff budget)
	• Patient-based fees
	  ➤ capitation fees (no. of patients on practice list)
	  ➤ health promotion payments
	  ➤ rural practice payments
	• Practice allowances: basic practice allowance, postgraduate education allowance

GPs responsible for providing their own IT equipment (reimbursement for 50% of costs from the PCT)	PCTs responsible for providing all of the costs of IT (Purchasing and maintenance)
GPs responsible for providing out-of-hours services	GPs able to opt in or out of certain services (e.g. QOF and out-of-hours services)
Payment per item throughout the financial year.	Practices are given an individual budget called the 'global sum'
Old superannuation scheme.	Changes to the GPs superannuation (pension) scheme

[a]Essential services: every GP must provide basic services to their patients, and these are termed 'essential services'. They are loosely defined as the care of acutely and chronically ill patients.

Additional services: these include payment for travel immunisations, minor surgery, maternity services, contraceptive services, out-of-hours services, etc.

IT, information technology; PCT, primary care trust; QOFs, Quality Outcome Frameworks.

The global sum

The global sum includes payment for essential services, additional services, item of service payments, patient-based fees, reimbursements and practice allowances (see Table 5.1). It is calculated by the infamous Carr–Hill formula – this takes the number of patients and the payment per patient for providing the above services and multiplies this by the Carr–Hill factor, which tries to take into account factors in the locality that may affect the cost of caring for patients, e.g. patients' ages (older patients require more visits and cost more), number of newly registered patients (these generate more work), cost of living, rurality. In some areas the global sum payment, when calculated, was less than the payment GPs got under the old red book contract (this was obviously very unpopular). To rectify this practices were guaranteed a minimum of what they earned under the red book for those services covered by the global sum. This is called the minimum practice income guarantee (MPIG).

Enhanced services

There are three types of enhanced service: directed enhanced services (DES), national enhanced services (NES) and local enhanced services (LES).

DES

These are nationally agreed services that *all PCTs are obliged to provide* to their patients, e.g. childhood immunisations, flu vaccines for those aged 65 and over or at risk, care for violent patients.

NES

These are optional services that are commissioned by PCTs where there is a high population of patients with a particular health need that is of national importance, e.g. drug abuse service, alcohol misusers service, specialised care of patients with depression. (There are national specifications and benchmark prices for these services.)

LES

These are services that the PCT commissions to meet its local aims and targets (the arrangements are specific to the PCT) e.g. care of refugees.

Quality Outcome Frameworks

> The Quality & Outcomes Framework (QOF) is a system to remuner-
> ate general practices for providing good quality care to their patients,
> and to encourage further improvement of the quality of health care
> delivered. (DH 2007)

The simplest way of thinking about QOF is that it provides performance-related pay for GP services. If the surgery achieves certain criteria, points are awarded. The higher the number of points a surgery collects, the higher the practice income. There are four main 'domains' where you can pick up points:

1. Clinical services (2009–10 areas):
   - anxiety and depression
   - asthma
   - atrial fibrillation

- cancer
- cardiovascular disease
- chronic obstructive pulmonary disease
- chronic kidney disease
- dementia
- diabetes mellitus
- epilepsy
- heart failure
- hypertension
- hypothyroid
- learning disabilities
- mental health
- obesity
- palliative care
- sexual health – contraception
- smoking indicators
- stroke and transient ischaemic attacks (TIAs)

2. Organisational (five areas):
   - education and training
   - communication with patients
   - medicines
   - practice management
   - records and information

3. Additional (four areas):
   - cervical screening
   - child health surveillance
   - contraceptive services
   - maternity services

4. Patient experience (three areas):
   - patient survey
   - consultation length
   - access to appointments (assessed via patient survey).

The clinical services domain points are collected through the quality management and analysis system (QMAS). QMAS analyses the electronic records system in the practice (which PCTs are obliged in the new contract to provide) and sends data to a national database (called QPID – Quality Prevalence Indicator Database). Clinical QOF points are then adjusted depending on local disease prevalence to account for the extra workload in higher prevalence areas.

Practices are paid a proportion of their expected QOF achievement monthly ('aspiration payments'). The final 'achievement payment' is made at the end of the year.

Additional payments

Examples of additional payments are seniority (years of service), premises operating costs (business rates, water and sewage rates, clinical waste disposal), and cost of staff training for use of IT systems.

Advantages and disadvantages of QOFs

Advantages

- The promotion of well-researched evidenced-based management strategies through QOF areas should lead to improved standards of care.
- Health improvements from improved standards have physical, psychological, social and financial benefits for patients and society.
- Annual QOF targets promote audit and continuing professional development in the clinical areas measured.
- QOF recognises that management plans require tailoring to the individual. Not all patients tolerate or agree to the QOF prescribed management plans and so exception reporting of cases does not penalise the practice.

Disadvantages

- Focus on QOF areas may draw focus away from areas where achievement is less measurable but no less important, e.g. care in dementia, psychiatry and clinical skills (i.e. minor surgery).
- QOF increases the administrative cost of a practice, in some cases without health benefits (e.g. yearly questioning is required about smoking habit even if the patient stopped smoking many years previously).

MEMORY BOX: New GMS contract 2004
- QOF: 4 domains, 20 clinical areas (in 2009–10), payment through QMAS and QPID
- DES and NES: nationally commissioned services; LES: locally commissioned
- four sources of practice income

Computerised records, choice and prescribing

The current state of records in general practice

There have been considerable changes in the management of patient records as a result of the development of computerised records. The new GMS contract means that PCTs are now responsible for providing every GP practice with computerised systems for record keeping, so computers are now considered essential equipment in running general practices. The introduction of QOF payments gave even the most reluctant GPs a strong financial incentive to implement computer systems. GPs are way ahead of hospital trusts in this regard, most of whom are still using hand-held records. In the long term the NHS aims to create a national computerised patient record system called the NHS Care Record (see below).

Requirements of a record system

The traditional *functions* of clinical notes are several:

1. To improve patient care, e.g. to:
   (a) make diagnoses clearer
   (b) make management decisions clearer
   (c) make follow-up more systematic, especially in chronic illness

(d) avoid simple errors (e.g. drug interactions and sensitivities, unnecessary repetition of investigations, prescribing that is inappropriate to the patient's past history).

2. To aid communication:
   (a) between doctors (especially in large group practices and those without personal list systems)
   (b) in the primary care team
   (c) with outside agencies (medical reports, referral letters, legal correspondence, etc.).

3. As an aide mémoire:
   (a) of main events in the patient's life (physical, psychological, social) and of his family
   (b) of what was said and done at the last consultation.

4. *As a tool* in:
   (a) audit, research, epidemiology
   (b) teaching
   (c) planning of patient services.

5. *As a medicolegal record* (important in a climate of increasing litigation).

6. *As a means of maximising income*, by prompting clinicians to record QOF targets and items of service payments.

The requirements of a good record system are:

1. A complete database
2. Information recorded at the level of certainty (e.g. suspected vs confirmed diagnosis)
3. Important information indexed and highlighted
4. Clear progress notes (in order!) recording objectives.

Advantages and disadvantages of computerised records

Advantages

1. As a clinical *prompt*:
   (a) in opportunistic screening
   (b) in long-term maintenance.For example, lists can be printed with reminders for cervical smears, blood pressure checks, etc. Furthermore, computers can sort into 'degree of over-dueness' so that with limited resources a start can be made according to priority.

2. As a source of *information*:
   (a) drug formulary information
   (b) warning of drug interactions or contraindications (computerised prescribing in a study in the *New England Journal of Medicine* led to >50% reduction in serious medication errors (Bates and Gawande (2003)
   (c) a guide to the QOF targets (on-screen patient alert messages)
   (d) a word processor and printer of patient information pamphlets
   (e) legibility (a major improvement)
   (f) reference access point via the internet (to medical images, NICE [National institute for Health and Clinical Excellence] guidance, patient leaflets, etc.).

3. In record keeping, e.g.:
   (a) summary screens
   (b) age–sex registers
   (c) morbidity registers
   (d) patient lists
   (e) rapid access to patient letters (scanned and filed).
4. As an *administrative* tool, e.g.:
   (a) computer-run repeat prescribing systems
   (b) accounts and workload analysis
   (c) as a claim prompt
   (d) as a check of PCT returns
   (e) as a practice-based commissioning tool.
5. In *audit, research* and *epidemiology*.

Disadvantages
1. Capital costs are fairly high, but are now completely reimbursed by the PCT.
2. The administrative work needed to transfer patient records onto a computer is considerable (there are many patient records remaining that need summarising onto computer; this is especially difficult because many records are not orderly to begin with).
3. Staff must be trained to use the new equipment.
4. Confidentiality of records is a source of concern. Access must be keyword protected to prevent unauthorised access, and users must be registered with the Data Protection Registrar.

Lloyd George records
This was the main form of hand-held records before the introduction of computerised records. They were often poorly organised, illegible (to all but the authors), lacked space for documentation, and were bulky due to patient letters being folded and crammed in the back.

Problem-oriented medical records (POMRs)
Proposed by Lawrence Weed (1969), the basic structure can be seen in the layout of current day computerised records. There are three main ingredients in his model, which correlate to the three main sections of an electronic patient record:
1. Problem list (active and inactive, significant and minor, medical and social)
2. Background information:
   (a) fixed information, e.g. sex, date of birth, personal and family history, immunisations
   (b) changing information, e.g. marital status, job, address, screening tests
3. Progress notes made on each consultation (mnemonic – SOAP):
   (a) *s*ubjective: the patient's observations
   (b) *o*bjective: the doctor's observations and tests
   (c) *a*nalysis: the doctor's understanding of the problem
   (d) *p*lans: goals, further information needed, action, advice to patient.

Advantages and disadvantages of POMRs
Advantages
- Encourages logical thought and approach; information is recorded at the level of understanding.
- Makes records much clearer to other readers.
- Records can easily be audited and are a better research and teaching tool.
- The database is more comprehensive.
- Orderly notes allow planning of preventive care.

Disadvantage
- 'SOAP' is long-winded and inappropriate for straightforward problems.

The NHS Care Records service

The NHS is developing an individual electronic record for each NHS patient called the NHS Care Record. The aim is to make patient information readily available wherever the patient accesses NHS services, e.g. primary care, secondary care or through multidisciplinary services. The deadline for implementing the full system is 2010. Data are stored on the NHS Spine (a central database).

The Care Record (BMA 2006) will consist of two parts:
1. The summary record, which can be accessed anywhere in England by NHS staff who are directly providing care to a patient. The content is yet to be finalised but it is likely to include the recent medication history, significant and recent problems, and adverse/allergic reactions to medication.
2. The detailed record: the full electronic record, i.e. the complete GP and hospital records, detailed parts of which may be shared locally. A consultant, for example, may directly access the record to gain more information about a condition mentioned in a referral letter.

Advantages
- Paper records phased out:
  - no need to store bulky records
  - reduced administrative burden associated with caring for and accessing notes
  - improved data storage – no lost notes (hopefully)
  - environmental benefits from electronic storage
- Quick access to notes (this should reduce delay in management decisions)
- Improved legibility
- Improved audit and research capabilities
- Improved patient safety
- Improved communication between services (no more illegible discharge summaries).

Disadvantages
- A large change in the way NHS staff operate means considerable potential disruption to clinical and non-clinical staff due to:
  - reduced data entry speed as staff learn a new system

- ➤ time out for training staff
- ➤ difficulties of integrating non-computer-literate staff and techno-phobes; particularly a problem with older members of staff who haven't grown up with computer skills
- ➤ stress associated with change in working procedures
- ➤ increased risk of errors – incorrect data entry, loss of data, software failure.
- Security fears:
  Professional bodies and patient representatives have raised concerns over the electronic storage and accessibility of large amounts of personal data. Security features have been incorporated to address these concerns and allow patients choice as to how their personal data is used:
  - ➤ to protect particularly sensitive information, patients will be able to restrict information available for sharing; this may mean restricted access via 'electronic sealed envelopes' containing particularly sensitive parts of a record, or restricting access between organisations, e.g. not allowing the hospital access to the GP notes or vice versa
  - ➤ patients have the right not to have their information uploaded to the system; this should be an informed decision based on the benefits and risks of the system; it is not yet clear how consent will be given, i.e. opt in/opt out
  - ➤ the NHS Care Record will provide information on a 'need to know' principle; legitimate relationships define *who* needs to know and role-based access defines *how much* they need to know, where legitimate relationships mean that patient records can be accessed only by those directly involved in their care, i.e. the GP and any specialist to whom they are referred, and role-based access involves the elements of a record that can be accessed being dependent on role. A receptionist is likely to see minimal information, such as demographic details and the appointment schedule, whereas doctors would be able to see the full record
  - ➤ audit trails and alerts: access to records will be monitored and unusual patterns of access will raise an alert
  - ➤ smart cards: access to the NHS Care Record service will be possible only using a smart card
  - ➤ consent will be required to share the Care Record with services outside the NHS, e.g. private healthcare providers, social services.

GP2GP – transfer of electronic health records

GP2GP enables patients' electronic health records to be transferred directly between GP practices. It means that the patient record can be transferred within 24 h of registering a new patient so that the doctor has access to the full record at the first appointment. This should save both the patient and the doctor time, and reduce errors and delays through lack of accurate or incomplete information. It will also save administrative time from processing incoming patient records. At the beginning of 2007 GP2GP was active in over 500 surgeries, and is now available nationally.

Choose and book – patient choice on being referred

This system enables patients to choose which services they wish to be referred to and in many cases book with a named health professional. Appointments are made 'live' during the consultation by logging onto the choose-and-book website, www.chooseandbook.nhs.uk. If patients want more time to make a decision they can take a request letter away with them and book their appointment later. Choose and book is an enhanced service for GPs.

Disadvantages
- Increase in time of GP consultation
  - ➤ slow to log on (at present)
  - ➤ inconvenient for doctors – despite the need to print off A4 documents and prescriptions few PCTs have provided dual tray printers to cope with this.
- Cost to the practice of time required for training staff.
- Cost and potential reduction of patient satisfaction from extended consultation times.
- May raise false expectations, if choice seems more limited or attractive than at first sight (e.g. when the patient realises the distance and counts the costs of travel for appointment and follow-up).

Advantages
- Financial incentives for running the service (enhanced service payment)
- Increased patient choice of where and when to receive care
- The ability to attach electronic files to aid in diagnosis, e.g. images of changing skin lesions
- Improved auditing of patient waiting times from referral date. The government has set a target called the '18-week pathway'. Its aim is that, by December 2008, the longest that any patient would wait for non-emergency treatment would be 18 weeks from referral to treatment. A study of choose and book in Northamptonshire showed a 9-day reduction in referral times compared with standard paper referrals.

Repeat prescribing
The scale of repeat prescribing

In 2006 736 million items were prescribed by GPs, costing the NHS over £8000 million pounds. Approximately 70% of these prescriptions were issued for repeat medication. This means that on average a GP issues 23 000 scripts for repeat medication per year (a cost per doctor of £250 000 per year, or £4500 per week). The number of prescriptions issued is expected to rise by 5% each year.

Repeat prescribing without face-to-face review
Problems

1. Failure to review patients properly:
   (a) the drug may be inappropriate or the diagnosis questionable
   (b) the patient's needs may have changed
   (c) side effects, interactions and problems of concordance cannot be assessed
   (d) the *illness* for which the drug was given may require review.
2. The doctor–patient boundary may be widened.

Advantage

The main advantage is time saving to patients and doctors, especially in chronic illness where repeated consultations may be unnecessary.

Requirements of a good repeat prescribing system

1. Patients should receive scripts promptly, e.g. within 24-48·h.
2. Scripts should be accurate and error free.
3. The system should be simple and cheap.
4. It should have a built-in recall system, clear to all.
5. It should be auditable.
6. A doctor using the records should know what the patient is taking and when last supplied.
7. A doctor should be able to gauge concordance and/or abuse.

Systems of repeat prescribing

Repeat prescribing is virtually all computer based and has the following benefits:

- printed scripts (legibility)
- indicates recall frequency
- checks concordance
- carries out automatic audit
- updates the records
- minimises written errors and frees staff time
- warns of drug interactions and contraindications
- enables practices to monitor drug expenditure more closely.

Electronic prescription service (EPS)

The problem with the current computer system is that it involves large amounts of paper and administrative time and is not all that convenient to patients. The introduction of EPS will address these issues. EPS will enable prescribers – such as GPs and practice nurses – to send prescriptions electronically to a dispenser (such as a pharmacy) of the patient's choice. The GP authorises the prescription, which is uploaded to the EPS database. The dispenser then downloads and issues the prescription.

Advantages

- Reduced patient inconvenience: reduced travelling (e.g. to the surgery to request or collect prescriptions, to the pharmacy by using a dispenser near home), a potential to reduce waiting times at pharmacies (as dispensers will be able to prepare prescriptions in advance).
- Reduced administrative burden: currently all repeats have to be printed, sorted, distributed to doctors, re-filed and then issued. EPS will manage these tasks automatically saving administrative time.
- Electronic signatures: allow prescribers to sign prescriptions electronically and cancel prescriptions at any point until they are dispensed.
- Easier for dispensers to claim their reimbursements (which used to involve posting prescriptions off each month to the reimbursement agency).

In 2007 a quarter of GP surgeries in England and a third of pharmacies were running EPS – with plans to roll out nationally in the near future.

> **MEMORY BOX:** Computerised records, choice and prescribing
> NHS spine: database for the NHS Care Record
> GP2GP: direct transfer of electronic health records between GPs
> Choose and book: choice on referral, directly bookable appointments to secondary care
> Repeat prescribing: average GP prescribes £4500 a week of repeat medications
> EPS: electronic prescribing system, near patient dispensing, electronic signatures

Innovative access to primary care

The NHS Plan (DH 2000) set out changes in the way we provide access to primary care. It aims to improve access for all and launched initiatives such as NHS direct and NHS Walk In Centres. Further changes in patient access are set out in the 2006 White Paper Our Health, Our Care, Our Say (DH 2006) with the promotion of nurse consultation, e-mail advice, prescription ordering services, pharmacy initiatives, and alternative provider medical services amongst other initiatives.

What are the innovative access points to primary care and what impact have they made?

Chapman et al. (2004) deal with this.

Telephone advice
The burgeoning requirement for out-of-hours care has caused doctors to consider the role of the telephone as an alternative to home visiting. There is some evidence that telephone consultations with GPs or nurses can safely substitute for face-to-face consultations, although it is not clear that this reduces the number of face-to-face consultations over time, i.e. patients often book a further appointment later on.

Walk-in centres
Walk-in centres improve access but cater mainly for white middle-class patients with minor and self-limiting complaints. This may exacerbate access inequalities. A third of patients visit their GP after attending a walk-in centre – duplicating existing service provision. There is no conclusive evidence for a reduction in workload as a result of walk-in centres.

Nurse practitioners
Studies have shown that nurse practitioners are safe and effective, can tackle over 70% of presenting cases and provide high patient satisfaction rates. Nurse-led telephone triage has been shown to reduce the number of GP home visits and telephone consultations. However, the number of routine appointments may increase. Nurses take longer to consult, and carry out more tests, but no difference in outcome has been found. Concern remains over the ability of nurses to recognise early serious disease – and responsibility remains with the GP to provide appropriate support/supervision to ensure that the practitioner works within her or his boundaries of competency.

Pharmacy initiatives

Pharmacists are easily accessible and there is some evidence that patients can be safely managed by pharmacist advice with low rates of onward referral to GPs. Disadvantages include lack of privacy and lack of prescribing power for patients entitled to free prescriptions. A new contract for community pharmacies launched in 2005 remunerates pharmacies for providing the following:

- Repeat dispensing (GPs able to prescribe repeats for up to a year which the pharmacist dispenses)
- Public health advice, e.g. healthy eating, stopping smoking and regular exercise (aimed at reducing inequalities in access to primary care; pharmacies will be taking part in local and national health promotion campaigns)
- Medicine use reviews: for those with long-term conditions (aimed at resolving problems with medication at an early stage, so helping to reduce hospital admissions)
- Minor ailments scheme (where people exempt from prescription charges can obtain medicines, for a certain range of common conditions without going to their GP for a prescription), e.g.
  - contraception, including emergency hormonal contraceptive services
  - anticoagulant (anti-blood clotting) monitoring
  - clinics for people with long-term conditions such as diabetes
  - needle-and-syringe exchange clinic for drug misusers
  - stop smoking services
  - supervised administration of prescribed medication.

The effectiveness of these measures is unclear, although with 260 000 visits a day to pharmacies specifically for health advice, there is clear potential.

Email advice

The medical profession exhibit a polarity of views on emails, ranging from enthusiasm about the convenience that they provide, to hostility based on concerns about security and intrusion into clinicians' work patterns (Neville et al. 2004). When used for prescription orders, appointment booking and clinical enquiries, small studies have shown positive outcomes for patients and practices in terms of satisfaction and workload.

Alternative provider medical services

See The capital cost of practice premises, page 114.

MEMORY BOX: Innovative access to primary care
- Telephone advice: safe but only delays face to face contact
- Walk-in centres: no reduction in GP workload
- Nurse practitioners: safe, cost-effective and popular with patients
- Pharmacy initiatives: multiple schemes aim to improve convenience for patients
- Email advice: jury out on safety and efficacy

Practice-based commissioning

Commissioning is the process by which health needs of a local population are assessed, and appropriate services purchased to meet these needs. Practice-based commissioning (PBC) is a government policy that passes responsibility for commissioning services from PCTs to local GP practices. The PBC concept was first announced in the White Paper, The NHS Plan (DH 2000), and developed further in The Improvement Plan (DH 2004). It was first implemented in practice in 2005, and is now run by all PCTs.

Traditionally the money (i.e. the budget) and the responsibility for running these services and achieving good health outcomes were those of the PCT. Under PBC, practices take on this responsibility and are given a commissioning budget with which to provide services. The budget is an 'indicative' budget only, i.e. the PCT continues to hold the actual funds. Individual practices can commission or groups of practices can club together to form practice commissioning groups (PCGs). These allow for division of labour between practices, the ability to commission services that they might not otherwise be able to (e.g. employ a specialist nurse) and share risks.

The government believed that PBC would give local clinicians greater control over resources, freeing them up to respond better to local and individual need. In principle most GPs supported this concept. However, cost savings are clearly at the heart of PBC, with the Department of Health documents referring to how the 'cost savings', 'efficiency gains' and 'freed up resources' will be distributed. There is, however, an incentive for practices to make efficiency savings because a proportion of these savings can be used by the practice to reinvest and develop their patient services. If a practice is unable to balance their budget over a 3-year period they lose the right to an indicative budget for 3 years, although the PCT has the power to waive this rule.

Here is an example of how PBC might work (DH 2006):

- Consider whether patients really need to go back to outpatients for follow-up appointments for which there is a tariff and carry out the follow-up treatment locally at the practice instead.
- Invest resources that would otherwise be spent on outpatient tariffs on re-designing services by, for example, employing a specialist nurse or working with a physiotherapist, providing direct access to diagnostics for those patients who would previously have been referred to outpatients.
- Over time, as more resources accrue as a result of reduced outpatient referrals, invest these freed-up resources in a case manager or community matron for people with a long-term condition. Such case management has been proved to reduce the need for hospital treatment, again freeing up further resources to spend on community services.

Fundholding and PBC

A similar scheme to PBC called fundholding was stopped in 1999 – principally because it was creating a two-tier system with preferential access to health care for fundholders' patients, but also because the efficiency savings gained were outweighed by the management costs. The principle of the two schemes is the same (local GPs are given a budget to provide primary care services) but in fundholding GPs were given their own budget completely independent of their PCT, could negotiate the price of care with providers (e.g. private or NHS) and were responsible for the administration (for which they were paid). PBC differs in that the PCT administers the budget not the GP, the range of services that can be commissioned is much wider and under PBC the prices are predetermined by national tariffs. PBC is the government's attempt to take the positive aspects of fundholding (efficiency savings, flexibility to meet local need, etc.) and remove the negative aspects (the two-tier service – fundholders vs non-fundholders, the complex financial and administrative burden, the legal and ethical dilemmas, e.g. the cheapest service may not be the best one – nationally set standard tariffs tackle this).

Potential pitfalls of PBC

- It is unclear whether the management costs of PBC will be any less than those of fundholding –where costs were greater than efficiency savings.
- The government recommends that PCTs reserve a proportion of the PBC budget in case practices overspend. This effectively means that practices start relatively under -funded compared with their baseline figures.
- Perverse incentives may be created, e.g. a potential conflict between budget and clinical judgement. Practices may be tempted to under-refer or under-prescribe to minimise their financial risk. PCTs are required to monitor referral activity to guard against this.

The government sets out its aims for the future of PBC and general practice in the 2006 White Paper Our Health, Our Care, Our Say (DH 2006):

- More services to be provided in a community setting
- More services to be provided by practices
- Longer opening hours for practices
- Greater use of a wide range of providers
- More convenient services for patients
- More integration between health care and social care.

MEMORY BOX: Practice-based commissioning
- GPs directly purchasing services to meet the health needs of their patient population
- Aimed at improving services and making efficiency savings

Medical certificates

GPs form an important part of the welfare benefits system by issuing medical certificates. It is part of our contractual agreement to issue certificates (including for Disability Living Allowance or Attendance Allowance) to patients who are unable to complete their own job or usual occupation. Candidates need to be aware of the guidance from the Department for Work and Pensions (DWP). The forms that GPs most commonly issue are the Med 3, 4 and 5. The memory box below summarises the commonly used forms. Copies of the forms are included in the appendix for your reference.

General Med form requirements (Med 3, 4, 5)
- Complete in ink
- Include the patient's name, diagnosis and advice given to the patient
- Sign, date and stamp with the practice address
- Reissue only if lost, marking the second copy clearly as a duplicate.

Med 3 Rules (standard sick notes)
- Issue only if the patient is examined on the same day or the day before
- Closed certificates:
  - ➤ a return to work date is given
  - ➤ this must be within 2 weeks of the date of issue
  - ➤ no further certificate is necessary to return to work.
- Open certificates:
  - ➤ used to specify when you plan to review the patient, i.e. 2 weeks
  - ➤ the first issue can be for up to 6 months (if justifiable clinically!)
  - ➤ subsequent issues can be for any period or 'until further notice'
  - ➤ when fit for work issue a further Med 3 and circle 'You need not refrain from work'.

Note that a new Med 3 is to be issued in April 2009 that emphasises the work a patient can do as well as work they can't; it also makes it easier for GPs to identify work within limits (e.g. modified hours, lighter duties).

Med 5 Rules (special sick notes)
- Retrospective certificates can be issued if:
  - ➤ they are based on a previous examination by you
  - ➤ the patient is unable to work for the whole period that the certificate covers.
- Certificates based on a medical report can be issued if:
  - ➤ the report was issued less than 1 month previously *and*
  - ➤ the certificate does not cover forward a period of more than a month.

Med 4 Rules (personal capability assessment note)
A Med 4 form is filled in on request from the DWP and in addition to the general Med form requirements should include details of:
- limitations as a result of mental or physical incapacity caused by the diagnosis
- Current treatment and progress.

Continue to issue Med 3s until the DWP write to say they are no longer necessary for the patient to receive incapacity benefit.

Return to work

It may not be in the best interests of your patient to refrain from work. 'Work is important in providing economic independence, prosperity and personal fulfilment. It helps reduce health and social inequalities.' Patients out of work are twice as likely to suffer depression and anxiety. Those out of work for over a year are eight times more likely to experience mental health problems and have higher mortality rates. The negative effects of unemployment are reversible on re-entry to work. It is important to make patients aware of the positive health benefits of work and support patients in returning to work. GPs can access support for patients wishing to return to work or obtain alternative work through Jobcentre Plus. If you feel that the patient will need Jobcentre Plus support record this on the Med 3 form comments section. Jobcentre Plus has access to personal and disability employment advisers to support people overcome employment barriers due to ill health.

(Department of Work and Pensions 2004)

MEMORY BOX: Medical certificates

Med 3: • a standard sick note issued after seeing a patient on the same day or the day before.
  • The patient should have self certified for the first 7 days.

Med 4: • a form for personal capability Assessment requested by the Department of Work and Pensions (DWP) usually after 6 months of Med 3 forms.

Med 5: • special sick note to be used if:
  (a) a note is to be backdated OR
  (b) you want to issue a note based on a report from another doctor

Med 6: • used when the doctor does not want to include the exact diagnosis on the Med 3 form because it is not in the patient's best interests (i.e. where the patient or employer should not know the diagnosis)

RM7: • a request for the DWP to make an independent assessment of your patient's capacity to work (used if you doubt the patient's incapacity)

Welfare benefits

The areas of benefits of most interest to general practice are those benefits arising from:
1. sickness
2. handicap and disability
3. industrial injury and diseases.

Sickness

The major sickness benefits are:
1. *Statutory Sick Pay* (SSP): paid by employers to employees who have made qualifying class 1 National Insurance (NI) contributions. This covers them for 28 weeks.
2. *Incapacity Benefit.* Paid at three rates:
   (a) Short-term Incapacity Benefit at the lower rate. Paid for the first 28 weeks to those who do not qualify for SSP (e.g. the self-employed,

unemployed and non-employed) who have made qualifying class 1 or 2 NI contributions.

(b) Short-term Incapacity Benefit at the higher rate. Starts at 28 weeks, i.e. when the SSP and low rate incapacity run out. Expires at 1 year.

(c) Long-term Incapacity Benefit. Paid after a year to those below retirement age who are unfit to work.

3. *Income Support and Disability Premium*. A means tested benefit for those whose lack of NI contributions prevents them receiving incapacity benefit.

Tests for incapacity

Eligibility for all categories is decided by an adjudication officer. In the first 28 weeks GP medical certificates are accepted as evidence that the claimant is not fit for his or her usual work ('the *own occupation test*'); after 28 weeks a form Med 4 is requested from the GP and a Benefits Agency doctor may conduct 'an *all-work test*' (patients with illness that is severe and obviously incapacitating, e.g. dementia, tetraplegia, terminal illness, are exempted from the test). The personal capability assessment is intended to provide a common, more objective assessment of physical, sensory and mental capability.

DS1500 – Terminal Illness Benefits

DS1500 allows patients rapid access to claim Disability Living Allowance, Attendance Allowance or Incapacity Benefits at the higher rates.

- Issued to patients expected to die within 6 months.
- The form requires the diagnosis, treatment plan and current clinical state. You must also state whether the patient is aware of the condition or not.

Mat B1 – Maternity Certificate

Maternity certificates provide evidence of pregnancy, thereby allowing patients to claim maternity entitlements, e.g. Statutory Maternity Pay or Maternity Allowance.

- Issue if less than 20 weeks before the expected date of birth (i.e. more than 20 weeks' pregnant).

Handicap and disability

Disability Living Allowance (DLA) and Attendance Allowance (AA) are available to support the living costs of disability. It is available to patients requiring aid with personal care, supervision or personable mobility (no means testing or national insurance requirements):

1. *Attendance Allowance*: for the over 65s, paid at a lower and higher rate. Although normally available only if conditions are likely to be met for 6 months, an exception is made in the case of those with terminal illness.

2. *Disability Living Allowance*: a similar allowance for those aged 5–65. Has two components:

(a) a *care* component, e.g. help washing, dressing, using the toilet (paid at three rates)

(b) a *mobility* component, for those over 5 who are unable (or virtually unable) to walk (paid at two rates). To qualify the claimant must have been affected for at least 3 months, and be expected to need the benefit for at least 6 months more (except in terminal illness).

Industrial injury and diseases

The major benefits are:

1. *Sickness benefits*: these are SSP and Incapacity Benefit, paid as for acute illness except that qualifying contributions for Incapacity Benefit may be waived.
2. *Industrial Injuries Disablement Benefit*: paid for injuries arising during the course of work or for prescribed industrial diseases.
3. *Industrial death benefits*: a pension is paid to the spouse or children in two instalments: a short-term pension (first 26 weeks), then a permanent pension.

Health benefits

In addition to the welfare benefits, a range of health benefits are available to dependent groups such as:

- pregnant women and mothers in their first postnatal year
- children under 16 years old
- low-income groups (those on income support or family credit)
- the retired (men and women over 60).
  Benefits include:
- Free NHS prescriptions, dental treatment; hearing aids on free loan (if prescribed by a consultant); help with the cost of glasses
- Free milk and vitamins (expectant and nursing mothers, children under school age from low-income families)
- Hospital travelling expenses (means tested).

Additional prescription charge exemptions

Certain other groups are exempt from NHS prescription charges by virtue of the chronic nature of their illness. These include:

1. People with epilepsy
2. Those with continuing physical disability to the point where the patient cannot leave home without the help of another
3. Patients with fistulae
4. Those undergoing replacement/maintenance treatment, e.g. patients suffering from:
   (a) Addison's disease
   (b) hypopituitarism
   (c) myxoedema
   (d) hypoparathyroidism
   (e) myasthenia gravis
   (f) diabetes mellitus
5. War and service pensioners.

Other welfare benefits

For more information on the benefits available to those incapable of work, on low income, bereaved, carers, disabled and others go to www.direct.gov. uk and look under the Money, tax and benefits section.

PART 2 PRACTICE POINTS

The building

Types of ownership

Premises are in three major categories:

1. Owner occupied
2. Rented (from the PCT or private owners)
3. Alternative provider owned and run.

Types of building

1. Purpose built
2. Adapted (adapted premises have to be approved for medical use by the PCT).

The capital costs of practice premises

In the case of *rented* premises the capital cost (cost of buying the buildings) is borne by the owner and not the GP. Purpose-built rented premises are usually health centres and owned by either PCTs or local improvement finance trust (LIFT) companies (see below). They are built specifically to rent to GPs. Alternatively private developers may build health centres to rent with PCT agreement.

In *owner-occupied* premises the capital is raised by the partner(s), usually by loans from banks or building societies. The interest on the loan for purpose-built premises is usually covered by the cost-rent scheme (see below).

In *alternative provider-owned* premises private companies pay for the buildings and provide primary care services. They are new – the law was changed to allow private companies to do this in 2006. Alternative provider medical services (APMSs) are targeted at areas with under-provision of primary care services, due to problems with GP recruitment and retention, e.g. inner cities. PCTs are in control of APMS contracts and can award them to the independent sector (e.g. United Healthcare Europe and Mercury Healthcare), voluntary sector, not-for-profit organisations, NHS trusts, other PCTs, foundation trusts or even GPs in current practices (www. dh.gov.uk/en/Healthcare/).

The future of general practice premises

The government is funding the re-provision of GP premises, and development of one-stop primary care centres, integrated health and local authority service centres, and community hospitals. It wants to modernise GP premises by creating purpose-built surgeries with many services available at a single site, e.g. GP, pharmacy, physiotherapist.

The present inadequacy of GP premises has been highlighted:
- Only 40% of primary care premises are purpose built
- Almost half are either adapted residential buildings or converted shops
- Less than 5% of GPs' premises are co-located with pharmacy and around the same proportion are co-located with social services
- Around 80% are below the recommended size.

The modernisation is being paid for by LIFT projects. These are private finance initiatives (PFI) a way of funding major capital investments, without needing capital from the public purse. But there is a debate about polyclinics and many GPs don't like them. The BMA says that it erodes individual patient care by a named and trusted doctor.

LIFT Projects

LIFT companies are created by PCTs to run LIFT projects. A LIFT company is owned partly by the private sector and partly by the public sector. The company consists of a private sector partner, the local NHS (i.e. the PCT) and the national NHS (Partnerships for Health – which represents the Department of Health). This company is then used to build, maintain and operate primary care buildings. Contracts typically last for 30 years, during which time the building is leased by a public authority. The public interest is protected because the company is part owned by the NHS (www.dh.gov. uk/en/Procurementandproposals/).

The running costs of practice premises
In rented premises

The 1966 GP Charter undertook to provide rent and rate reimbursements to GPs. In PCT-run practices this is essentially a formality: a rent is charged and fully reimbursed, making it a book transaction only.

In other rented premises a 100% reimbursement is also available, provided that the rent charge is 'reasonable'. An employee of the Inland Revenue called the *district valuer* determines what is 'reasonable' by inspecting and comparing it with the current market rent charged on comparable properties in the same area.

In owner-occupied premises

If these are purpose built under an approved cost-rent scheme, the rent and rates are again entirely reimbursed. If the premises are adapted, the owner–doctor is compensated for the capital that they have tied up in bricks and mortar by the payment of a notional rent, i.e. although they pay no actual rent, they receive an annual payment comparable to the current market rent of similar local property (the sort of rent that they could have received if the premises were used otherwise). The value of the notional rent is set by the district valuer and reassessed every 3 years or when any change occurs. (GPs who dispute the district valuer's assessment can employ an independent valuer to argue their case, and can ultimately appeal to the Secretary of State.)

(Note that the GP's terms of service impose the responsibility of providing 'adequate' surgery premises and PCTs can withhold reimbursements if premises are substandard.)

Running costs other than rent and rates are *not* reimbursable although they are tax deductible – GPs in PCT-run health centres pay a quarterly consolidated service charge (covering use of heat, light, cleaning services, etc., in proportion to their overall use of the building), and other GPs pay their own service expenses as they arise.

The borrowing cost reimbursement scheme (cost-rent)

This scheme is controlled by the PCT and covers the cost of:
1. the building of completely new premises
2. substantial modification of existing practice premises
3. the acquisition of premises 'for substantial modification'.

The *principle* is that the partners raise the capital and the PCT meets the interest payments on the loan. Several *practical* points apply:
1. In all cases, prior PCT approval and consultation are needed as well as planning permission. The PCT has discretion to accept or reject a scheme, depending on their budget and priorities.
2. Regulations exist about allowable expenditure, e.g. acceptable building costs per square metre, architects' fees, planning consent costs.
3. The final rent reimbursed is the *cost-rent* renamed in the GMS contract 2004 as the 'borrowing cost reimbursement'. It is calculated from the capital costs of the project and the interest rate charged.
4. As the cost-rent is a scheduled percentage of the building cost, there comes a time when the notional rent exceeds it. At the next triennial review the practice can then opt to switch from cost-rent to notional rent.

In 1990 strict cash limits were imposed on the scheme, and a civil service report labelled it 'archaic and complex'. Despite this the cost-rent and notional rent schemes continue to run.

Improvement grants

These are included in the new GMS contract (see below) and available from the Department of Health provided that:
• there is prior PCT approval
• work is on facilities for patients (and not primarily on doctors' accommodation)
• the grant is to improve 'what already exists' and not to provide new premises.

Pros and cons of PCT centres and owner-occupied premises

See Table 5.2.

Table 5.2 Pros and cons of PCT centres and owner-occupied premises

	PCT centres	Owner occupied
1. Initial financing	By the PCT; the GP only invests minimally in practice equipment	By the partners; this means capital is needed early in a GP's career, and may cause problems in expensive areas with high housing prices
2. Capital growth	None for the doctors	Appreciable long-term investment (especially since the cost-rent scheme effectively grants an interest-free loan)
3. Control of premises	Limited: (a) consultation on the initial design may be limited (b) it may prove difficult to make substantial alterations (funds come from the community trust's budget and compete directly with other community services: delays in decision-making and the 'drying up' of funds are common problems) (c) maintenance and redecoration are the trust's responsibility; unless covered by prior agreement the timing can be a source of dispute between GPs and their landlord	Design is in the hands of the GP and his architect Alterations are easier to make (and can be covered by improvement grants and the cost-rent scheme) Maintenance decisions are in the hands of the principals
4. Staff employment	Staff may be shared with the PCT by joint appointment or entirely employed by the practice. If they are on the PCT payroll, the administrative burden of calculating and paying salaries is borne by the trust, but the GPs sacrifice control over their activities and may find themselves in dispute with the PCT over shared staff	The GP hires and fires his own staff and has control over their wage levels and work activities
5. Running costs	A service charge is set by the PCT; this varies considerably and GPs may find themselves in dispute over the level set	These are more directly under the control of the GPs and dependent on their management policies. They are usually higher than those of average health centres
6. Allowed use of premises	At present virtually unrestricted, except that, if private work comprises more than 10% of total income, reimbursements are reduced in proportion and stopped if 50% is private. However, as the property is not owned by the partners, it is conceivable that further conditions could be placed upon its use	As for PCT-owned centres (although security of future use is possibly greater)

PCT, primary care trust.

Branch surgeries

Many practices, especially those in rural areas, have branch surgeries; these often arise from the historical amalgamation of separate practices.

Advantages
1. The major advantage is to patients in rural areas who have shorter distances to travel, and do not have to depend on infrequent rural bus services to see doctors.
2. Home visiting to this group of patients is reduced by encouraging them to attend a surgery.
3. GPs in rural areas are able to sustain a higher list size, with consequent increase of profits.

Disadvantages
1. Facilities are often primitive compared with the main surgery.
2. There is a duplication of administrative and running expenses, which drains practice profits (unless GPs dispense from branch surgeries the net result is usually a financial loss).
3. Various practical problems are posed, e.g.:
   (a) the security of largely unattended premises with drug stocks and confidential records
   (b) how to run an appointment system and staff the premises
   (c) where to house paper clinical records.
4. They cannot be closed save by permission of the PCT. As branch surgeries are jealously defended by consumers and local communities, it often proves difficult for doctors to terminate this responsibility once they have undertaken to provide it.

Staff finances

Reimbursements

Under the old contract 70% of the cost of practice staff salary was reimbursable plus employers' national insurance, superannuation contributions and relevant training. Now most staff costs are reimbursed with the exception of staff training (now the responsibility of the practice – except for IT). This is paid in the global sum. It is up to the practice to decide how many, what type of staff and what salary to pay them.

Salaries

There is no fixed salary scale for employees of GPs. Employees' rights are protected by law and by standards laid out in the QOF. QOF rewards practices for complying with good human resources practice in staff contracts, e.g. holiday pay, induction and training guidance.

Note that the 'Agenda for Change' is the single pay scheme for the NHS aimed at equalising pay for equivalent job roles. It was introduced in 2004 for all NHS staff but excludes doctors, dentists or staff employed by GPs.

Staffing

The practice manager
The introduction of the QOF in 2004 (see page 49), with its organisational markers as well as clinical markers, means that the role of practice manager is even more important in the process of managing clinical data and organising the surgery. Practice management demands a wide range of skills to which practices will need to have access, to run at maximum efficiency. Different practices will be able to do this by a variety of means depending on their size. Some practices may have a single practice manager who encompasses most of these skills; others may have a practice manager who can access other colleagues (either in their own or other GP practices or via the PCT) to help them in the variety of areas of their work. The role encompasses staffing, finances, administration, management of premises and stock, and future planning.

The practice nurse
There are approximately 25 000 practice nurses in the UK. Most are experienced nurses who value part-time work, fixed hours and general practice-based responsibilities. Many now have family planning training.

Role
The role of the practice nurse depends in part on personal interests, confidence and experience, and also on the degree of responsibility and freedom encouraged by the GP employers. Whatever the degree of freedom allowed, the GP remains ultimately responsible for the practice nurse's decisions and must take steps to ensure that:
• the nurse is adequately trained for the job
• the boundaries of responsibility are defined and understood.
    The RCGP defines three main types of practice nurse: the practice nurse, specialist practice nurse and nurse practitioner.

Practice nurse
• Delivers nursing care (dressings, venepuncture, injections, basic observations [weight, blood pressure, urine testing], suture removal, ear syringing, taking swabs, etc.)
• Provides health promotion advice
• Carries out immunisations and smear tests
• Inducts new staff
• Has knowledge of chronic disease management, general health care, family planning and well woman care.

Specialist practice nurse
In addition to the duties carried out by a practice nurse, a specialist practice nurse is able to undertake nurse-led clinics in specialty areas. They have qualifications in specialties such as asthma, diabetes, family planning,

cervical cytology and travel health. Specialist practice nurses also undertake research and carry out audit for the practice.

Nurse practitioner

In addition to the above roles, nurse practitioners work independently similar to GPs, running their own minor illness clinics, prescribing appropriate medicines and referring on to GPs when necessary. Nurse practitioners are accountable for their own professional actions, and are lead specialists for a defined area.

Advantages of employing a practice nurse
1. The service is relatively inexpensive. Part of the salary may be reimbursable and the remainder allowable against tax. Increased income from item-of-service work undertaken in the treatment room and health promotion and disease management clinics may help to pay the difference.
2. Nurses are said to be better than GPs in following clinic protocols, and may thus achieve more by running protocol-led clinics, e.g. asthma review, COPD (chronic pulmonary obstructive disease) review, diabetes checks.
3. It saves the GP's time, leaving him or her free to do other work.
4. Patients express a high level of satisfaction with the facility and appreciate it (e.g. Murray and Paxton 1993).
5. The service can be very effective. Marsh and Dowes (1995) trained their nurse to manage minor illness, and offered an appointment with her to patients requesting same-day consultations. Eighty-nine per cent of those seen in the ensuing 6 months were dealt with by the nurse alone, and 79% did not present again through the same illness episode. It was concluded that a lot of minor illness in general practice can be managed by an appropriately trained nurse.

Disadvantages
1. Practice nurses need adequate training, which the GP may have to provide, especially when the nurses are asked to take on new responsibilities.
2. There is a problem in defining the boundaries of responsibility – a GP who delegates must live with the possibility that he or she may, at some time, be answerable for someone else's error. GPs are liable for the acts and omissions of their staff, and mishaps arising from ill-considered delegation may be punished by the General Medical Council (GMC). It is difficult to provide a fail-safe referral policy that covers all possible circumstances. GPs must also satisfy themselves that the correct decisions are being made without appearing to question their colleagues' professional competence – this is a difficult balance to achieve and the relationship hinges on it.
3. The facility may generate more work when its convenience is appreciated. In particular, patients may use the practice nurse to bypass the appointment system, causing the GP's surgery to be interrupted because it transpires that a doctor's opinion was required.

Trends

Through the 1980s an expansion was seen in the number of practice-employed nurses because they held two clear advantages over district nurses (who are employed by the PCT):

1. The GP has tighter control over their activities as the employer.
2. It circumvented the awkward problem of asking PCT-paid nurses to undertake item-of-service work, the profits of which went to the practice.

The introduction of the 1990 GP contract fuelled extra demand, as doctors were hard pressed to meet the various health promotion targets and well person assessments. In consequence between 1985 and 1991 the number of practice nursing whole-time equivalents rose sixfold. In 1998 nurse prescribing from a limited nurse formulary was rolled out across the UK, allowing more independent nursing practice. In May 2006 the formulary was discontinued and qualified nurse independent prescribers (e.g. nurse practitioners) became able to prescribe any licensed medicine for any medical condition within their competence, including some controlled drugs.

Some authorities believe that the trend should continue, and that the practice nurse's role should be expanded, offsetting current recruitment difficulties among doctors (and from the government's viewpoint driving down some of the cost pressures on health care). In future, according to some views, nurse practitioners will be more widely employed in a triage model of primary care: filtering out and treating minor illness, and referring more serious or difficult cases to their GP manager. The least that can be said is that the role of the nurse in primary care is evolving rapidly.

The district nurse

Employers

- Employed by the PCT and accountable to the nursing managers.
- The introduction of PBC enables practices to directly employ their own community nurses.
- *Attached* to nearly all practices.

Role

There is a broad potential overlap with other members of the primary health care team but the main role is of clinical nursing in the community. In addition district nurses have three additional responsibilities:

1. Care of vulnerable individuals (e.g. elderly, disabled and terminally ill people):
   (a) psychological support to patients and family
   (b) mobilisation of resources, e.g. incontinence aids, commodes, ripple beds, night nursing and bath nurses
2. Assessment, referral and liaison work:
   (a) with GP, health visitor and social worker
   (b) advice to patients on local resources and voluntary associations

3. Preventive work:
   (a) monitoring at-risk groups by home visiting;
   (b) health advice
   (c) influenza vaccinations.

Note that a new role of community matron was introduced in 2004 (DH 2004). Community matrons are largely PCT-employed, experienced, senior nurses working with patients with long-term conditions, to plan and organise their care at home (i.e. case managers; they typically manage a caseload of 50 such patients).

The health visitor

There are about 30 000 health visitors registered in the UK. There are three types: the health visitor, the health visitor specialist and the health visitor team manager.

The health visitor works with families with specific health and social needs, and plans and implements care. They also run child health clinics and provide advice and health education, as well as providing clinical supervision to students and other staff.

Health visitor specialists in addition undertake specialist service planning and work with other agencies. They promote public health and provide advice through clinics and home visits, as well as providing training and clinical supervision to health visitors and students.

Health visitor managers carry out the role of a health visitor with additional responsibilities to manage and provide clinical supervision to teams of health visitors and other community staff.

Employers
- Employed mainly by the PCT and accountable to the nursing managers
- Nearly all practices have an attached health visitor
- Health visitors work in a variety of settings – community, general practice, health centre, hospital.

See www.amicus-cphva.org and www.bma.org.uk/ap.nsf/Content/glossnurses#health%20visitor.

Role
1. Postnatal home visiting: this is a statutory duty from the day the midwife stops attending (usually day 10), and follow-up usually continues until the child attends school; the function is to educate and support the mother in basic baby care, common postnatal problems, and minor childhood illness and developmental milestones. Similar advice is offered at child health clinics.
2. Child developmental and screening work: undertaken in the home or at the child health clinic, and includes simple tests of sight, hearing and development.
3. Case work – targeted surveillance and support of at risk groups, e.g.:
   (a) single-parent families
   (b) cases of potential non-accidental injury

  (c) the handling of children with emotional and behavioural problems,
       or physical and mental handicap
  (d) care of elderly and frail people.
4. Preventive work and health education:
  (a) immunisations
  (b) health education (including antenatal/parent craft and relaxation
       classes, weight-watching groups, etc.)
  (c) visiting/screening elderly people
  (d) family planning advice
5. Advisory and liaison work:
  (a) advice on local resources, e.g. mother and toddler groups, day
       nurseries, self-help groups
  (b) advice on home safety, home helps, welfare benefits; liaison with GP
       and social worker
  (c) identifying the health needs of the local community and working
       with the community to address them, e.g. homelessness.

The social worker

Employers

Social workers are employed by local authority social services, i.e. they are
independent professionals, not answerable to PCTs or GPs. Their caseload
therefore includes public self-referrals.

Workload

The four basic areas are:
1. Individual casework, e.g.:
  (a) counselling those individuals and families with financial and per-
       sonal problems
  (b) marital and bereavement counselling
  (c) counselling children with behavioural problems and their families
  (d) follow-up and support for anyone with mentally illness.
2. Advice and allocation of resources:
  (a) home helps and meals on wheels
  (b) social service day-centre places
  (c) advice to impoverished, disabled and homeless individuals (to
       whom a wide range of support resources are available – home adap-
       tations, telephone installation grants, welfare benefits, legal housing
       rights, voluntary and self-help groups, etc.).
3. Statutory responsibilities (and work with legal implications):
  (a) supervision of children in care
  (b) supervision of adoption, fostering, childminding and day nurseries
  (c) the management of child abuse cases
  (d) the compulsory admission of mentally ill patients under the Mental
       Health Act 1983
  (e) responsibilities for disabled people under the Disabled Persons Act
       1970.
4. Liaison work, e.g. between clients and primary care, social services,
   hospitals and occupational therapists.

The management

Management and teamwork

Principles of teamwork

According to Gilmore the characteristics of teamwork are:

1. The members *share a common purpose* that binds them together and guides their actions.
2. Each member understands their own function, the contribution of other professions and their common interests.
3. The team works by pooling knowledge, skills and resources, and shares the responsibility for outcome.

Other authors also emphasise the importance in effective teamwork of:
- pooling
- delegation
- specialisation of function
- multidisciplinary discussion and peer group support.

Advantages and disadvantages

In principle the patient should gain from the coordinated action of specialists with a common plan, and effective teamwork should bring harmony, order and a group of self-supporting workers. However, there are practical problems as well:

1. Teamwork needs time and frequent meetings. This may encroach on the time needed for face-to-face patient care.
2. It requires commitment and agreement. QOF recognises the importance of team meetings and provides funding to encourage them, e.g. the palliative care QOF points for regular palliative care case meetings.
3. There is a danger that no one person will accept overall responsibility (the so-called 'collusion of anonymity' described by Balint). The best example of this is the Victoria Climbie case. Victoria was a 7 year old who came from the Ivory Coast to live with her aunt and her partner who abused and neglected her, culminating in her death from malnutrition and hypothermia. Victoria had been seen on 12 occasions by several agencies who had suspicions of abuse, including the child minder, hospital doctors, police and social workers. The Laming Report (2003) concluded that failure of individuals to share information, and take responsibility and action, led to this preventable tragedy. Detailed guidance followed on how child protection information should be shared between health professionals, the responsibilities of each professional and where the responsibility for coordinating action lies. These general principles:
   - share information
   - define roles and responsibilities
   - nominate a case coordinator
   - are equally valid to general practice teamwork (or any team). Although one team member must take responsibility for coordinating action, if one member assumes overall charge (primacy) there is a danger that personal status and pecking order will diminish the team's harmony and effectiveness.

4. There is a problem of size: large teams contribute more skills and viewpoints, but dilute and delay decision-making and make communication more difficult.
5. Primary health-care teams suffer the problems common to any group of workers – jealousies, prejudices, fears of exploitation or discrimination, peer group rivalry and competition. In particular, differences in training, status and remuneration have traditionally been a disruptive influence. Good will and a desire to get on are the most important elements of teamwork.

Certain ground rules aid the task of management:

1. The decision-making process should be clearly defined and not haphazard.
2. Important rules (and the reasons for them) should be known to all.
3. The processes of information sharing, feedback and grievance airing should be encouraged.

Practice meetings

It is all too easy for busy doctors to concentrate on clinical problems while neglecting longer-term plans. Practice meetings serve several purposes:

1. To ensure that necessary decisions are made
2. To review policies and agree standards of care
3. To improve communication and morale
4. To review budgetary provisions
5. To make contact with team members
6. To educate and inform (e.g. by holding journal clubs).

Regular meetings are especially important when the team is large or has a lot to discuss, or the working environment is frequently changing.

The following are the steps involved in organising a practice meeting:

1. To define its purpose
2. To define its agenda and participants
3. To make decisions, draw conclusions and communicate them effectively
4. To identify necessary action and those responsible for doing it, and finally to give feedback to the next meeting on the outcome.

Experienced campaigners advocate a formal agenda, such as: apologies for absence; minutes of the previous meeting; matters arising; items for discussion; any other business. Someone should act as chairperson and someone should record the minutes.

There are potential benefits from this chore:

• Groups in discussion often reach better decisions than an individual would acting alone.
• Communication is more efficient and complete, avoiding the piecemeal approach.

Increasingly GPs have to host or attend meetings that involve outside parties (e.g. in cooperatives, multifunds or purchasing consortia). Clear communication and a systematic approach assume even greater importance when the agenda is complex, the participants know one another only slightly and the decisions are difficult to make!

Patient lists

At present the majority (more than three-quarters) of GPs adopt a shared or combined list system.

Under this system, although patients' wishes are accommodated wherever possible and doctors try to follow up illness episodes themselves, patients have the freedom to choose a new doctor at every consultation and the practice has the freedom to direct patients and visits to doctors in a way that spreads the workload and speeds the throughput. Patients also benefit from being able to choose doctors of the same sex for embarrassing problems.

Although the GMS contract means that patients are no longer restricted to registering with a single doctor and have the right to choose an appointment with any doctor in the practice, some practices try to maintain a personal list system. By contrast to shared lists, the aim is for patients to stay with the same doctor as closely as the system will allow and on a long-term basis. The main advantage of this is continuity of care with a doctor who knows the patient well, the patient benefits from a consistent management plan and the doctor saves time as he or she knows the past history.

Recent changes in general practice (such as minor surgery, chronic disease clinics and the tendency within practices of partners to develop specialist interests) have made it more difficult to sustain personal lists. Practices often share out the clinical areas of QOF between the partners and run specialist clinics in these areas, e.g. diabetes, CHD (coronary heart disease), stroke. This helps meet the QOF targets and manages the clinical workload of keeping up to date in each area. As a result particular GPs in the practice may be best placed to advise on their QOF areas. This encourages in-house sharing of problem patients – a combined list approach.

Out-of-hours services

GPs are currently responsible for providing services between 8am and 6.30pm on weekdays. All other care is considered to be 'out of hours' (OOH). More frequent users of these services include women, those with one or more children under 16 in their household, and those aged between 35 and 54. Since 2005 GP surgeries have had the right to opt out of providing services out of hours, which then became the responsibility of the PCT. OOH provision was renegotiated in the 2004 GMS contract, largely due to the increasing intensity of workload in hours and increasing demand for out-of-hours visiting. The GMS contract states that 'Work/life balance will be improved through the out-of-hours changes'. However, it seems that the government is trying to reverse its contract commitment and get surgeries to open earlier, later and at weekends by quoting patient satisfaction surveys in which greater access is requested (www.bma.org.uk). This drive is probably a result of the government considerably underestimating the cost of providing an OOH service and the 'shambolic implementation' of new OOH services by PCTs (House of Commons report 2007); the work–life balance point is important.

OOH care is provided through a variety of services, including PCT teams, GP cooperatives, mutual organisations, commercial deputising services (e.g. Primecare), ambulance services and NHS Direct. Treatment options include advice over the telephone, face-to-face clinical assessments at out-of-hours clinics and home visits. These services are provided by a range of professionals, including doctors, nurses, paramedics and emergency care practitioners. All services must meet a series of national standards, known as Quality Requirements, determined by the Department of Health. The Quality Requirements cover response times, clinical audit, organisational elements, information flows and patient feedback.

Deputising services

Traditionally doctors have entertained mixed views about OOH services:

The public image of out-of-hours services is poor: some deputising services have clearly employed staff with inadequate experience. Medical disasters involving deputising services have been given prominent press coverage, causing the public to react with predictable concern.

Recurring worries were:
- lack of relationship, trust and familiarity
- concern that their past medical history was not known
- greater difficulty in contacting deputies
- deputies with a poor command of English.

Though patient concerns about the quality of out-of-hours services remain, a survey in 2000 showed patients are equally satisfied with the different forms of out of hours care (cooperative, practice based or deputising arrangements). In this paper the mode of consultation seemed more important to patients. Patients were more likely to be dissatisfied with a telephone consultation (Shipman et al. 2000).

Advantages
1. The personal freedom of doctors to enjoy a social life OOH and escape the pressures of work at antisocial times. This creates less personal and family strain in a profession already showing signs of it (higher than average rates of alcoholism, drug abuse and suicide).
2. (Arguably) a better standard of care in the 97–99% of daytime consultations as doctors are fresh, alert, motivated and refreshed by a break.
3. Doctors who start the night-shift fresh may make better decisions than tired doctors who have already worked a full day.
4. Surveys suggest that OOH doctors unfamiliar with the patient are likely to respond to a call by visiting, whereas their own GP is more likely to give telephone advice. This can be an advantage or disadvantage.
5. OOH providers can provide cover under difficult practice circumstances (e.g. for the single-hander in need of an annual holiday; prolonged sickness in a small practice).

Disadvantages
1. Patients are dissatisfied with OOH services (and this may affect their concordance).
2. There is a risk of inadequately qualified deputies.
3. There is no continuity of care – patients are all unfamiliar and there is limited or no access to their notes. It has therefore been suggested that OOH doctors:
   (a) make more errors
   (b) refer and treat inappropriately
   (c) have a tendency to visit, prescribe and refer more when patients are unknown – this involves unnecessary repetition and may also encourage patients to be less independent in the longer term; it also overuses hospital resources
   (d) because they lack personal knowledge of the patient, deputies often fail to appreciate the hidden agenda – the real reason for the call – so the problem is deferred but not resolved.
4. Opting OOH incurs some sacrifice of earnings (£6000 per GP in 2007 – but the cost of replacing their service is more than double this figure).
5. Some doctors oppose handing over care OOH on principle. The standing of general practice may be damaged if others believe, rightly or wrongly, that standards are being compromised.

GP cooperatives

The most popular alternative to deputising is to work in organised cooperatives with shared rotas. Cooperatives can be large enterprises (up to 180 doctors) with a central administration, remote answering services and special facilities such as chauffeured transport for visiting doctors, or a staffed night-time emergency centre that patients are encouraged to attend.

Cooperatives share a number of pros and cons in common with deputising services. However:
1. The membership of a cooperative is locally determined and drawn from a pool of local principals. To this extent a tighter control may exist over standards.
2. Members can offset the cost of getting someone else to do their night visiting by taking a turn in the rota themselves; better organisation and facilities may permit fewer doctors to provide the necessary cover, further defraying costs.
3. To be effective, cooperatives require a carefully thought-out organisational infrastructure – the degree of cover, the competency of its members, and the arrangements for prioritising care requests and transferring clinical details back to the patient's own doctor must all be addressed.

Many cooperatives assembled in haste lack adequate legal agreements, and GPs withdrawing from cooperatives have found themselves in dispute over their share of its assets, including development money.

NHS Direct

Created in 1998 NHS Direct provides telephone advice by using nurses supported by a computer-based clinical pathway tool. A national study in the *British Journal of General Practice* (Pickin et al. 2004) showed in its first 3 years that the scheme has reduced the number of calls to out-of-hours general practice (a figure that was rising year on year). It has not reduced the number of A&E admissions or use of the ambulance service. One of the criticisms of telephone triage is that it may not be cost-effective because the outcome in a high proportion of contacts is a delayed GP consultation (not an avoided one). However, this may be helpful in itself at times of high demand for services. NHS Direct also provides health promotion information and access to patient self-help guides to encourage self-management of minor illness.

Appointment systems

Since 2000 (The NHS Plan – DH 2004) all GPs are required to provide access to a health-care professional appointment within 24h and a GP appointment within 48h. Some surgeries achieved this target by only offering appointments 48h in advance. This was heavily criticised and in 2005 the government's 'access patient guarantee' pledged that patients should have the option of making appointments beyond 48h.

To achieve this an 'advanced access' guide was issued by the National Primary Care Development Team, along with the carrot of funding through QOF for meeting appointment targets (assessed through the patient satisfaction questionnaire). More than 99% of practices now achieve these targets (compared with 50% in 2000), aided by better understanding of patterns of demand and the use of innovative access to primary care, e.g. telephone consultation, nurse consultation, email advice, prescription ordering, pharmacy initiatives, NHS Direct and walk-in centres (Pickin et al. 2004; see also www.dh.gov.uk/en/Healthcare/). Evidence suggests that patients are seen more quickly in advanced access practices, but speed of access is less important to patients than choice of appointment (Salisbury et al. 2007). Open (unbooked, turn up on the day) surgeries have mostly been substituted for bookable surgeries to meet expected demand, with urgent 'extras' seen after surgery for times when demand is higher than predicted. The principal advantage is efficient use of time, space and resources. Some surgeries run open clinics in addition to a booking system. The patient satisfaction survey (DH 2006) indicates that patients want greater accessibility – longer opening hours and weekend access to their GP.

Running an appointment system

Practices running appointment systems need to review them periodically:
- How long do patients have to wait for non-urgent consultations?
- How often are patients denied the right to see a doctor the same day when they request it?
- Do appointments run to time?
- Are enough consultations on offer, or do surgeries always run over because of 'extras'?
- What provision is made to allow urgent cases to be seen promptly?

Length of appointment

The average GP consultation time in the UK is 11.7 minutes (2006–7), an increase of 40% since 1992–3. Why is consultation time increasing?

A systematic review of the relationship between consultation length and outcomes showed the evidence to suggest that patients seeking help from a doctor who spends more time with them are more likely to have a consultation that includes important elements of care (Wilson et al. 1992). Average consultation length may also be a marker of other doctor attributes. For example, in longer consultations doctors:

- identify more problems
- carry out more preventive procedures (Wilson and Childs 2002)
- spend more time listening and explaining: Risdale et al. (1992) have reported that doctors and patients ask more questions when more time is available, and that patients express their views more freely
- achieve higher patient satisfaction ratings.

Doctors offering longer appointment times may also:

- pay more attention to lifestyle and screening (Wilson et al. 1992)
- devote extra time to psychosocial issues and long-term health problems (Howie et al. 1991)
- feel less job stress (Wilson et al. 1991).

The benefits of longer consultations is recognised by QOF payments for appointment length:

> GP surgery consultation length should be not less than 10 minutes for routinely booked patient appointments or at least eight minutes for an open surgery system. (The General Medical Services Contract 2004, Department of Health)

This has led to an increase in average consultation time.

Consultations tend to be longer for certain types of problems, e.g. patients with mental health problems as a diagnosis or co-morbid diagnosis have longer consultations and more diagnoses (Zantnige et al. 2005).

Home visiting
Trends

Over the past 30 years there has been an increase in the proportion of surgery-based consultations and telephone consultations with a reduction in home visiting. During this period phone ownership has increased and telephone consultations with GPs have been made more widely available.

	1971	2002–3
Surgery consultations (%)	73%	86%
Telephone consultations (%)	4%	10%
Home visits (%)	22%	5%

Who to visit?

The reduction in home visiting rates may be attributable to more rigorous guidance on home visiting, better understanding of patterns of demand and the use of innovative access to primary care (discussed earlier).

Guidance to changes in home visiting were published by the DH in 1995 and laid out in the new GMS contract. This made clear that the medical not the social condition (i.e. lack of transport, child-minding problems) of the patient should determine the need for a home visit:

Under the new contract, the contractor must attend a patient outside practice premises if the patient's medical condition is such that, in the reasonable opinion of the contractor, it is necessary to do so.

A GP's decision on whether to visit a patient at home will depend on a number of factors. These include the severity and urgency of the condition, as well as the patient's disabilities and their ability to communicate over the phone. The highest number of home visits occurs in the over-75 age group (17% of all consultations in 2002–3). Older people are more vulnerable to illness, are less likely to own a car, may be less willing or able to use a phone and are more likely to be housebound than younger age groups. The average time for a home visit including travel is 25 minutes.

Advantages and disadvantages of home visiting
Advantages
1. *Public relations*: home visiting is a good public relations exercise and helps to cement rapport in the doctor–patient relationship. These benefits are intangible but real.
2. *Humanitarian and screening benefits*: it is kinder to elderly and infirmed people, and allows surveillance of 'at-risk' patients who might not otherwise attend and 'waste the doctor's time.
3. *Fuller assessment*: it allows whole-patient assessment – the chance to see the family together in the home environment may provide important social information that could not be gathered in the surgery. It also allows concordance to be gauged (drawers full of untouched pills tell a useful tale!).
4. It is the safest option:
   (a) serious conditions cannot easily be excluded by telephone
   (b) patients are poor judges of serious and trivial illness
   (c) 'failure to visit' is one of the more successful complaints that patients bring against doctors in service committee hearings.
5. It may be the only option when the patient appears medically unfit to travel.

Disadvantages
1. *Time*: the average surgery consultation lasts 11.7 min but the average home visit needs 25 min. Time spent in a car travelling is at the expense of other patients, through their taxes, the loss of surgery services that they could have had (e.g. extra clinics) and fewer of the 'efficient' surgery appointments on offer per day.
2. *Standards*: poor lighting, low beds, lack of access to the full patient record, lack of diagnostic facilities and equipment potentially lower the standard of care.
3. *Costs*: these are not readily calculated. At the simplest level there are travelling expenses, but more home visiting may actually mean that the

exchequer employs more GPs, which is clearly expensive to the NHS (which wishes to pay doctors to consult, not travel!).

4. *Inconvenience*: many patients who request home visits do so either on social grounds (lack of transport, difficulty getting an appointment, lack of baby sitter, bad weather), *or* through erroneous medical beliefs (e.g. fear that a febrile child will catch a chill en route). A smaller proportion is genuinely not fit to visit the surgery or elderly and infirm. The former has been clarified by the DH guidance on home visiting.

5. *The fostering of incorrect attitudes*: more motivation and self-reliance might follow if doctors rationed their visits to genuine emergencies.

6. *Risk of personal injury*: doctors who visit disreputable areas at night-time run some risk of personal injury. The surgery is a safer environment.

Variation between doctors

The variation between doctors is striking and not entirely explained:

- A *BMJ* study by Aylin et al. (1996) showed eightfold variability between general practice home visiting rates. which could not be explained by differences in apparent health needs of the population
- A study by Sullivan et al. (2004) attempted to explain the variability by adjusting the data for age, sex, social class and clinical case mix; however, this only partially explains the variation. Unmeasured factors such as patient demand, disability or differences in GP home visiting practice style are postulated as factors to explain the variability

Leaflets, reports and directories
Practice leaflets

Practices are required to produce a practice leaflet, which must be updated annually. Key requirements include:

- names of clinical staff and partners (including medical qualifications, date and place of first registration)
- details of how to register, ability to specify a preferred practitioner, and a description of the practice area
- the services available and PCT contact details (to obtain information about additional services that are not provided by the contractor), including home visits, checks for over-75s, etc.
- the appointment system, where one exists, and normal surgery hours
- whether the practice premises have suitable access for disabled patients
- the name and address of the nearest local walk-in centre
- the method of obtaining repeat prescriptions
- how to make complaints
- action that may be taken where a patient is violent or abusive, and a reminder of the rights and responsibilities of the patient, including keeping appointments and respect for race, gender, disability.

Some doctors have taken the opportunity to include general health information and advice on self-management of minor ailments; others have sought and obtained commercial sponsorship, including advertisements, in their leaflet.

Practice reports

Before the GMS contract practices were required to submit data annually to the PCT on their local demographics, workload, performance and audit. The information was used locally and nationally to help plan service development to meet local and national needs. This system has now been replaced by QMAS and data is collected throughout the year (see QOF, page 49).

Local directories

All PCTs must produce a PCT guide that contains a directory of all GP surgeries in the PCT to help patients decide where to register. The intention is to provide patients with the information needed to make an informed choice of doctor. The directory is revised annually and sent free to community health councils, libraries and citizens advice bureaux.

Principals are listed alphabetically with details of:
- their sex
- registered qualifications
- age (or date of first full registration)
- normal surgery hours and special clinics
- other relevant aspects of their practice (e.g. employment of other staff, assistants, trainees or deputies, accessibility).

Supplementary information can be provided on a voluntary basis, e.g. other languages spoken and doctors' special clinical interests.

The effect of practice size on practice matters

There is no ideal size for a practice but the character, facilities and organisation are strongly influenced by the number of principals. In Table 5.3 a large group practice (four or more doctors) is compared with a single-handed practice to illustrate this. The current trend is towards ever-bigger practices, with all the attendant pros and cons.

Dispensing

When can an item be dispensed by the practice?
1. When the drug/appliance is supplied and personally administered by the prescribing doctor. This includes:
   (a) emergency injections
   (b) anaesthetics
   (c) diagnostic reagents
   (d) intrauterine devices, caps and diaphragms
   (e) immunisations
   (f) certain pessaries and suture materials.(Separate regulations for oxygen.)
2. If the patient (or temporary resident) lives more than a mile away from the nearest chemist. These patients form the dispensing list. (Note that it is feasible, indeed common, to dispense to patients on the dispensing list from surgery premises less than a mile from the nearest chemist: it is the distance from the patient's *home* that matters!)

Table 5.3 The effect of practice size on practice matters

Aspect	Group practice (more than four doctors)	Single-handed practice
Patient care	1. More equipment and facilities, e.g. sats monitors, in-house spirometry 2. More services (e.g. specialist clinics) 3. From the patient's point of view, more choice of doctor	1. Personal care of patients with good rapport and consistent advice 2. From the doctor's point of view patients who know where they are and who they will see; who cannot 'shop around' and abuse the system
Doctors	1. On call less often – less personal and family strain; less use of deputising services 2. Fewer problems in covering sickness and holidays, or coping with epidemics 3. More opportunity for research, audit, teaching, study leave and sabbaticals	1. Own boss. No one else to get on with 2. Fewer problems with communications and organisation and no decision-making by committee 3. Other problems can be avoided (e.g. shared rota with another practice)
Staff	1. More likely to have attached staff, e.g.: • district nurse • health visitor • social worker, community psychiatric nurse, etc. 2. More likely to employ: • practice nurse • practice manager, caretaker, etc.	
Financial	1. Capital costs of the building are shared 2. More contributors to the pool when expensive practice equipment is bought	1. No dilution of the profit when capital appreciation occurs

Scale of payments

Dispensers receive:

1. The *basic price* of the drug or appliance (as defined in the *Drug Tariff*, and less a discount laid out in Para. 44/Schedule 1 of the Statement of Fees and Allowances)
2. An *on-cost allowance* – a percentage of the basic (pre-discount) price
3. A *container allowance* (per script)
4. A *dispensing fee* (depends on the volume of dispensing)
5. A *VAT allowance*.

Claims

All prescriptions, for dispensing and administering doctors, must be recorded and sent with a complete FP 34 to the Prescription Pricing

Authority (not later than the fifth day of the month after issue of the prescription).

Benefits

1. GPs make a profit on the basic cost of the drug by bulk purchase and also pocket the container fee and dispensing allowance, so dispensing is fairly lucrative and compensates rural practices for their lower lists and higher travel costs. (Profits on dispensing range from about 10% to 17% of the gross turnover of the dispensary.)
2. It also provides a good service to patients, who can find doctor and drugs under a single roof and do not have to make a separate visit to the chemist, although polyclinics will also provide this service. Doctors visiting rural patients, and elderly and infirm people can dispense the prescription in the same visit – a valuable service.
3. It imposes the discipline of limited list prescribing on the principals and forces them to examine carefully their prescribing habits and rationale. It also brings home the real cost of their prescribing. Although there are other mechanisms for this (see PACT, page 334).
4. It is an interesting and stimulating exercise.
5. Dispensing doctors can offer a wider range of drugs out of hours.

Costs

1. Inevitably choice will be limited. It is not possible to stock every prescribable item. Practical problems are more likely to develop for prescriptions arising through hospital directives.
2. It involves extra security precautions, as the dispensary may attract would-be burglars.
3. Other costs include:
   (a) insurance of drug stock
   (b) a capital cost to incoming partners (who must purchase a share of this stock)
   (c) a small capital risk (investment in drugs that may be discredited/ withdrawn from use)
   (d) the extra administrative burden, extra commitment of staff time and extra staff responsibilities.

Many dispensing practices employ a pharmacist. There is no legal obligation to employ a qualified dispenser. Nevertheless the legal obligations to dispense accurately, safely and in accordance with the various Drug Acts still apply and so responsibility for the service rests with the dispensing doctor.

The finances

Personal GP income

The three broad categories of a GP's income are:
1. Private medical income.
2. Practice income (income from the NHS)
3. Personal (non-medical) income.

Private medical income

Income from private medical work depends on the level of commitment to extra-practice activities, the opportunity for private work and the practice's policy towards private patients.

Sources of private income are numerous and include:
- insurance examinations and reports
- other private medical exams and certificates (fitness to start a job, HGV licence applications, fitness to dive, etc.)
- solicitors' reports; court witness
- cremation fees
- industrial appointments
- local authority appointments, e.g. police duties, developmental or family planning clinics; school medical officers
- hospital appointments (assistantships or practitioner posts)
- lecturing.

Practice income (see page 95 for more detail)

Practices get income from four main areas:
1. The global sum
2. Enhanced services
3. QOF payments
4. Additional payments (seniority, premises).

Outgoings

There are two broad categories of expense:
1. Running costs
2. Capital expenses.

Running costs

The major running costs are as follows:
1. Cost of premises (including rent, rate, repairs, insurance)
2. Staff costs (including wages, NI contributions and pension payments)
3. Service costs (including heat and lighting, stationery and postage, telephones)
4. Professional fees (including accountancy, subscriptions, bank charges, personal health and professional insurance)
5. Travel expenses (including petrol, road tax and depreciation).

1 and 2 are discussed in more detail in the sections devoted to reimbursements. Suffice it to say that they are to a large extent reimbursable, whereas 3 and 4 leave only a limited scope for economy. The running costs associated with a car (5) include such items as: petrol, oil and antifreeze; road fund licence and car insurance; servicing, MOT and replacement parts (e.g. tyres); AA/RAC membership; cleaning, etc. These items are tax deductible but only for the proportion attributable to practice use. A percentage (negotiable with the Inland Revenue) is not allowable, representing private use.

Capital expenses

Non-recurring expenditure on buying (or building) something new is classified as capital expense. Replacement items are included, but repairs are treated as running costs. Examples of capital expenses include a new computer or an ECG machine. For tax purposes 25% of the 'written down' value is allowable annually in the same manner as for GPs' cars.

Doctors' pensions

The NHS pension scheme was revised in September 2007, because the old scheme was no longer affordable. The key points of the NHS pension scheme are:

- Normal pension age increased from 60 to 65
- Minimum pension age increased from 50 to 55
- Pension contribution now dependent on salary bracket (e.g. £63 417 to £99 999 – 7.5%; £100 000 and over – 8.5%)
- Final pensionable pay based on an average of best 3 consecutive years annual pensionable pay in the last 10 years rather than final salary
- Pension accrual rates for GPs will be 1.87% of Career Average Revalued Earnings (CARE). CARE accruals will be dynamised by Retail Price Index + 1.5% per annum
- No tax-free lump sum on retiring, unlike old scheme
- Introduction of survivor benefits to nominated partners. Survivor benefits payable for life.

For a more detailed explanation of NHS pensions, see the BMA pension section.

Tax allowances

All running expenses legitimately and wholly incurred in the running of the practice are tax deductible. The special concessions related to car use and the tax position on capital expenditure are described above.

The history, development and future of general practice

The history and development of general practice

The 1966 General Practice Charter represented in its time something of a watershed in the development of modern general practice. Until the middle of the twentieth century it was normal for GPs to be single-handed, to work from their own homes, employing their wives as secretaries, and with a minimum of supporting staff; premises were often substandard, gloomy places; and there were no financial incentives for change. Lack of a clear postgraduate training structure and lack of academic prestige also left GPs the poor relations of their hospital colleagues in the glamour specialties, and recruitment to general practice was a problem. The Charter of 1966 made a great impact on this situation. Its principal ingredients were better pay, seniority, group practice and designated area allowances, financial recognition of out-of-hours services, and the reimbursement schemes for staff salaries.

In 1967 the General Practice Finance Corporation was founded as a source of loans, and hand in hand with these two changes there emerged an improvement in staffing, premises and general practice recruitment.

Several further developments helped to boost professional status:

1. Granting of the Royal status to the College of General Practitioners (1967).
2. The recommendation of a 3-year vocational training scheme by The Royal College on Medical Education (1968), later to become compulsory.
3. Direct access to laboratory facilities, helped by the Report on Organisation of Group Practices (1971).
4. The emergence of general practice as a specialty capable of original research and publication.
5. The building of purpose-built multidisciplinary health centres by PCTs and redevelopment/modernisation of GP premises (see LIFT projects, page 115)
6. The conformance of speciality training requirements with those of other Royal Colleges (by introducing compulsory membership before certification of completion of training, 2007).

Such was the impact of these changes (and the lack of a satisfactory career structure in hospital medicine) that general practice has became oversubscribed, with a glut of eager well-qualified trainees chasing a shortage of principal vacancies!

The future of general practice

The future of general practice is uncertain, and there have been a lot of stories in the press about the threats to general practice from private contractors (see APMS, page 114) and changes in the way that patients access care. There is no doubt that areas with historical poor provision of services (typically inner cities) are under threat from privatisation. Birmingham City PCT has discussed plans to franchise 76 practices in Birmingham city centre 'through trusted brand names such as Virgin, Tesco and Asda' aimed at tackling service provision in these areas (Univadis, 13/11/2007, Privatisation of general practice is under way). However, outside these localised pockets of deprivation general practice is thriving with over 300 million consultations a year (almost 90% of the work of the NHS) and a 91% satisfaction rating. With results such as these GPs are in a strong position to argue their effectiveness. Research in numerous countries, including the UK, indicates that a strong primary care system is key to reducing morbidity and mortality. The RCGP issued a statement in 2004 outlining its view of the future of GPs in the NHS (Royal College Statement Sept 2004).

Continuity of care
GPs no longer have, or need, a monopoly of provision of first contact care. Nevertheless, there are other occasions when continuity is important to patient care, to efficiency, and to trust. New models of

access must not damage the possibility of a patient choosing continuity of care with an individual GP if that is that patient's priority. There will inevitably be different forms of continuity including: continuity of information, team continuity, and continuity with an individual healthcare provider, which need to be considered when services are reformed.

Medical generalism
In a health service that offers an increasing focus on long-term medical conditions, the role of the medical generalist is more and more important. Co-morbidities are increasingly common and ever more important. Sixty-five per cent of patients aged 65 or over have two or more chronic conditions. Fragmentation of care leads to a greater potential for adverse medication interactions and complications, and for duplication of investigation and referral. As the proportion of older people in society increases, so will the proportion of patients with co-morbidities. To manage these patients safely and effectively, GPs will need to devote considerable time and effort to tailoring care to patient's complex individual needs. This might result in less skilled activities being delegated to other healthcare workers where it is appropriate to do so.

Trust
Public confidence in GPs is remarkably high, notwithstanding a small number of highly publicised scandals. Such trust is particularly important in a publicly funded service, and contributes to the ability of the NHS to maximise efficiency. For instance, the trusted doctor is in a strong position to advise that a particular therapy or investigation may not be necessary. Reforms that damage the ability to develop a doctor patient relationship built on trust are, ultimately, likely to be counterproductive, even if they seem to offer short-term advantages.

(Note for short-term advantages read cost savings.)
To quote Phil Hammond 'a medical degree is no substitute for clairvoyance', but it seems inevitable that technology changes will continue to have major impacts in patient care (see NPFIT). New developments in areas such as communication and diagnostics, and in patient support/treatment offer huge potential benefits but not without significant challenges to the way that we practice (Table 5.4).

Increased government focus on lifestyle diseases is leading to lead to new quality targets and innovative interventions for example the prescription of exercise programs and weight watcher classes for those with obesity. We are seeing further changes in working hours as the government pushes for longer opening hours and weekend opening, but at what price? Finally, like death and taxes rationing of health resources is here to stay and that includes in MRCGP exam questions.

Table 5.4 Current and imminent developments in general practice

Communication	Email access for patients/GPs
	Text messaging
	Direct access to medical images in the GP surgery
	Digital imaging in GP surgeries
	The electronic care record
Diagnostics	Computer-aided diagnostic algorithms
	Rapid access to medical evidence via the internet
	Advances in near patient testing
Patient support/ treatment	Improved internet access to quality regulated patient resources (Health
	On the Net kite marking of reliable sites)
	Computer-based cognitive–behavioural therapy
	Expert patient programs
	NHS Direct online

AKT questions

Q1
Match the services to the correct part of the GMS contract. Each option may be used once, more than once or not at all:
a   Essential service
b   Additional service
c   Directed enhanced service
d   National enhanced service
e   Local enhanced service
f   Designated service
g   Innovative service

1. Extended hours
2. Excision of a skin cyst
3. A case finding initiative for COPD patients in an area of under-reporting
4. Primary care multiple sclerosis service
5. Cervical screening
6. Contraception services

Q2
The following are sources of practice income EXCEPT? Select ONE option only:
a   Registration fees
b   Quality outcome framework payments
c   Enhanced services payments
d   Item of service payments for minor surgery
e   Seniority payment

Q3
There are four quality domains in QOF but five items are listed below. Identify the incorrect area. Select ONE option only:
a Organisational
b Clinical services
c Managerial
d Patient experience
e Additional

Q4
Identify the incorrect statement regarding 'Connecting for Health'. Select ONE option only:
a Access to the NHS 'Connecting for Health' means that all health professionals will require a smart card.
b Choose and book is a contractual obligation offering choice of service to patients.
c GP2GP enables the electronic transfer of health records between GP practices.
d The electronic prescription service allows prescribers to sign prescriptions electronically.
e The NHS Care Record will include role-based access to limit the parts of the record viewable to administration staff.

Q5
Which of the following services is NOT being offered by pharmacies under the pharmacy initiatives scheme? Select ONE option only:
a Anticoagulant monitoring
b Needle-and-syringe exchange for drug misuse
c Repeat prescriptions for up to a year
d Medicine use reviews
e Thyroid screening tests

Q6
Choose the correct definition of practice-based commissioning. Select ONE option only:
a Large GP practices or groups of practices form commissioning groups to commission services for their local community.
b Each GP practice is given a budget independent of the PCT with which to commission its own services.
c Local services are commissioned by the PCT and delivered through GP practices.
d Groups of practices join with the private sector and agree arrangements to provide local services.
e Individual GP practices join with the private sector and agree arrangements to provide local services.

Q7

Match the most appropriate medical certificates and forms to the statements. Each option may be used once, more than once or not at all:

a   Med 3
b   Med 4
c   Med 5
d   Med 6
e   RM7
f   DS1500
g   Private note

1. You are issuing sick notes to a patient but wish to request an independent assessment of their capacity to work.
2. A patient presents with a letter from the Department of Work and Pensions requesting a form for personal capability assessment.
3. You issue a note based on a report from a colleague.
4. A patient requests a sick note that his employer requires. He has been off work for 3 days with diarrhoea and vomiting.
5. You wish to issue a note without including the exact diagnosis.

Q8

Match the following benefits to the statements below. Each option may be used once, more than once or not at all:

a   Statutory sick pay
b   Incapacity benefit
c   Income support and disability premium
d   Attendance allowance
e   Disability living allowance
f   Industrial injuries disablement allowance

1. A benefit to patients with disability requiring help with personal care, supervision and mobility aged 5–65.
2. Paid at three rates dependent on the time on benefit.
3. Paid by employers to patients who have made National Insurance contributions.
4. Paid for injuries sustained during the course of work.

Q9

About standard sick notes: choose the incorrect statement. Select ONE option only:

a   Can be issued if the patient is examined on the day or the day before.
b   Closed certificates can be issued for up to 3 weeks from the date of issue.
c   No further certificate is needed if a closed note is issued.
d   Open notes should not be issued for less than 7 days
e   Open notes can be issued for over 12 months

Q10

Med form requirements. Identify the incorrect statement. Select ONE option only:

a   If requested reissue an identical copy if the initial copy has been lost. Mark the second clearly as a duplicate.

b   All Med forms should be stamped with the practice stamp.

c   Med 5 forms can be issued retrospectively if the patient is unable to work for the whole period identified.

d   Med 6 forms should include the details of limitations due to mental and physical disability and current treatment including the prognosis.

e   Open certificates require a further Med 3 issuing when the patient is fit to return to work.

Answers

Q1

1. c
2. c
3. e
4. d
5. b
6. b

Q2 d

Most item-of-service payments have been replaced by the additional and enhanced services and quality outcome framework payments.

Q3 c

Q4 b

Choose and book is an enhanced service and optional.

Q5 e

Q6 a

Q7

1. e
2. b
3. c
4. g
5. d

Q8

1. e
2. b

3. a
4. f

Q9 b
Maximum issue is for up to 2 weeks.

Q10 d
This is the requirements for a Med 4; Med 6 forms are used when you do not want to specify the exact diagnosis, so you would certainly not include details of the treatment course and prognosis.

References

Aylin P, Majeed FA, Cook DG. Home visiting by general practitioners in England and Wales. *BMJ* 1996;**313**:207–10.

Bates DW, Gawande AA. Improving safety with information technology. *N Engl J Med* 2003;**348**:2526–34.

British Medical Association. *The NHS Care Records Service in England – Connecting for Health*. London: BMA, 2006.

Chapman JL, Zechel A, Carter YH, Abbott S. Systematic review of recent innovations in service provision to improve access to primary care. *Br J Gen Pract* 2004;**54**:374-81.

Department of Health. *The NHS Plan*. London: DH, 2000.

Department of Health. *The NHS Improvement Plan*. London: DH, 2004.

Department of Health. *Our Health, Our Care, Our Say*. London: DH, 2006.

Department of Health. *Quality Outcome Framework*. London: DH, 2007. Available at: www.dh.gov.uk/en/Healthcare/Primarycare/Primarycarecontracting/QOF/index. htm.

Department of Work and Pensions. *Medical Evidence for Statutory Sick Pay, Statutory Maternity Pay and Social Security Incapacity Benefit purposes: A guide for registered medical practitioners*. London: DWP, 2004.

Department of Work and Pensions, MRCGP, MRCP, Society of Occupational Medicine. *The Health and Work Handbook*. London: DWP.

Howie JGR, Porter AMD, Heaney DJ, Hopton JL. Long to short consultation ratio: a proxy measure of quality of care for general practice. *Br J Gen Prac* 1991;**41**:48–54.

Marsh GH, Dowes ML. Establishing a minor illness service in a busy general practice. *BMJ* 1995;**310**:778–80.

Murray SA, Paxton F. Nurses or doctors: patient choice in family planning? *Health Bull* 1993;**51**:394–8.

Neville RG, Marsden W, McCowan C, et al. A survey of GP attitudes to and experiences of email consultations. *Inform Prim Care* 2004;**12**:201–6.

Pickin M, O'Cathain A, Sampson FC, Dixon S. Evaluation of Advanced Access in the National Primary Care Collaborative. *Br J Gen Pract* 2004;**54**:334–40.

Risdale L, Moragn M, Morris R. Doctors' interviewing technique and its response to different booking times. *Fam Pract* 1992;**9**:57–60.

Salisbury C, Goodall S, Montgomery AA, et al. Does Advanced Access improve access to primary health care? Questionnaire survey of patients. *Br J Gen Pract* 2007;**57**:615–21.

Sawyer L, Arber S. Changes in home visiting and night and weekend cover: the patient's view. *BMJ* 1982;**284**:1531–4.

Shipman C, Payne F, Hooper R, Dale J. Patient satisfaction with out-of-hours services; how do GP co-operatives compare with deputizing and practice-based arrangements? *J Public Health Med* 2000;**22**:149–54.

Sullivan CO, Omar RZ, Forrest CB, Majeed A. Adjusting for case mix and social class in examining variation in home visits between practices. *Fam Pract* 2004;**21**:355–63.

Weed L. *Medical Records, Medical Education and Patient Care*. Cleveland, OH: Cleveland Press of Case Western Reserve University, 1969.

Wilson A, Childs S. The relationship between consultation length, process and outcomes in general practice: a systematic review. *Br J Gen Pract* 2002;**52**: 1012–20.

Wilson A, McDonald P, Hayes L, Cooney J. Longer booking intervals in general practice: Effects on doctors' stress and arousal. *Br J Gen Pract* 1992;**41**:184–7.

Wilson A, McDonald P, Hayes L, Cooney J. Health promotion in the general practice consultation: A minute makes a difference. *BMJ* 1992;**304**:227–30.

Zantinge EM, Verhaak PFM, Kerssens JJ, Bensin JM. The workload of GPs: consultations of patients with psychological and somatic problems compared. *Br J Gen Pract* 2005;**55**:609–14.

www.bma.org.uk/ap.nsf/Content/glossnurses#health%visitor

www.cancerhelp.org.uk/help/default.asp?page=3293

www.dh.gov.uk/en/Healthcare/Primarycarecontracting/APMS/DH_4125918

www.dh.gov.uk/en/Healthcare/Primarycarecontracting/index.htm

www.dh.gov.uk/en/Procurementandproposals/Publicprivatepartnership/NHSLIFT/DH_091676

Further reading

British Medical Association. *Connecting for Health – The NHS Care Records Service in England*. Connecting for Health NHS Care Record. London: BMA, 2006.

British Medical Association. Focus on practice management, 2008. Available at: www.bma.org.uk/employmentandcontracts/index.jsp.

Department of Health. *General Medical Practitioners' Workload Survey 1992–93*. London: Department of Health, 1994: paragraph 6.8 and Table D5.

Department of Health. *Community Pharmacy Contractual Framework*. London: DH, 2005.

Department of Health. *Publications and Statistics*. London: DH. Available at: www.dh.gov.uk/en/Publicationsandstatistics/DH_093440 (accessed 2008).

Information Centre for Health and Social Care on behalf of the Office of National Statistics and the Department of Health. Trends in Consultation Rates in General Practice, 2007.

Royal College of General Practitioners. *Practice Nurses*, RCGP information sheet no. 19. London: RCGP, 2004. Available at: www.rcgp.org.uk/INFORMATION/PUBLICATIONS/INFORMATION/PDFINFO/19%20-%20AUG%2004.PDF (accessed December 2007).

Unison. *Practice-based Commissioning Factsheet*, 2005. Available at: www.unison.org.uk/acrobat/A2184.pdf.

Ytterdahl T, Fugelli P. Health and quality of life among the unemployed. *Tidsskr Nor Laegoforen* 2000;**120**:1308–11.

6 Healthy people (prevention and screening)

This chapter and following chapter relate to curriculum statement 5 (Healthy people)

Screening and health promotion are examined in the Applied Knowledge Test (AKT), and 'Comorbidity and health promotion' is one of the six clinical areas of competency assessed by the Clinical Skills Assessment (CSA). Candidates may be expected to discuss screening and health promotion with simulated patients and answer questions on these topics. Knowledge of and the ability to implement current health promotion and screening guidelines is also assessed through workplace-based assessment (WPBA; see the MRCGP syllabus). A review of key screening and health promotion principles follows with a summary of screening programmes and topical issues.

Principles

Definitions

There is some confusion over the use of the terms primary, secondary and tertiary prevention. One school of thought defines the three degrees of prevention as follows:

1. *(Primary) prevention*: removing the causal agent, e.g. sanitation measures of the nineteenth century
2. *(Secondary) prevention*: identifying pre-symptomatic disease (or disease risk factors) before significant damage is done, e.g. screening for hypertension
3. *(Tertiary) prevention*: limiting complications/disability in patients with established disease by regular surveillance, e.g. trying to prevent diabetic problems by good control, regular fundoscopy, foot care.

According to this definition *screening* is a form of secondary prevention. It can be defined as the application of sorting procedures to populations by doctor initiative, with the aim of identifying asymptomatic disease or people at particular risk from it.

Others have taken primary prevention to mean measures taken *before* an event (e.g. in trying to prevent a myocardial infarction), and secondary

Notes for the MRCGP: A curriculum based guide to the AKT, CSA and WBPA, 4th edition.
By K. Palmer and N. Boeckx. Published 2010 by Blackwell Publishing,
ISBN: 978-1-4051-5724-7.

prevention to mean those measures taken *after* an event to limit damage or prevent recurrence. This is the definition accepted by the National Institute for Health and Clinical Excellence (NICE).

Anticipatory care

Anticipatory care is an approach to medicine that concentrates attention on anticipating and precluding problems. It is in fact an effort to offer all appropriate forms of prevention (however defined) within the consultation and the organisational framework of primary care.

Methods of screening

Methods of screening follow two broad lines:

1. *Case finding (opportunistic or anticipatory care)*: this means taking the opportunity when the patient attends on another matter to screen him or her for the desired characteristic. This method is simple, involves no extra administration or expense, and reaches 75% of the practice population in 1 year and 90% in 5 years.
2. *True screening*: the active pursuit of cases by questionnaire, letter, home visit, purpose-designed clinic, etc. This involves more administrative work and the expense (partly offset by QOF and additional services payments – see page 97 – where applicable) is borne by the GP.

The major disadvantage is that patients do not always share their doctor's passion for screening and there is often a significant non-attendance rate. The advantages and disadvantages of these two approaches are compared in Table 6.1.

Requirements of a screening programme

Wilson and Jungner (1968) proposed these criteria:

1. The condition must be:
   (a) common
   (b) important
   (c) diagnosable by acceptable methods.
2. There must be a latent interval in which effective interventional treatment is possible.
3. Screening must be:
   (a) simple and cheap, if possible, and in any case cost-effective
   (b) continuous
   (c) on a group agreed by policy to be at high risk.

To this we can add the requirements that the disease is readily treatable and that screening tests are highly sensitive (few false negatives), highly specific (few false positives), safe, non-invasive, acceptable to the patient and easy to interpret. If used in mass screening programmes a test should have a high positive predictive value (see Chapter 4).

Relatively few conditions exist for which all criteria could be said to be met. It is certainly true, as screening is doctor initiated, that benefits should outweigh costs.

Table 6.1 Pros and cons of opportunistic versus formal screening

	Pros	Cons
Opportunistic screening	Simple, cheap to administer	Requires organisation, time and commitment
	Does not depend on patient compliance	Does not offer 100% coverage to the target group
	Reaches a section of the public who will not attend for preventive advice alone	The time used is not 'protected': more urgent demands may take precedence
	Can be made relevant to the circumstances of attendance	Patients seen when ill may be less receptive to health education
Formal screening approaches	'Protected' time for discussion	Requires organisation, time and commitment
	Purpose of attendance understood by all parties	Important non-attendance problem, wasting health-care resources
	Attendees are (by definition) motivated and more receptive to advice that they have personally solicited	Users are often those least in need of the service
	Comprehensive coverage of related health areas can be planned	Administrative obstacles are considerable
	Financial incentives now favour the formal health promotion clinic	

Weighing costs and benefits

Several theoretical and practical considerations have a bearing on the cost–benefit equation:

1. There is always a trade-off between sensitivity and specificity in a screening test, i.e. the looser the definition of a case, the fewer the number of borderline cases missed, but the larger the number of false positives.
2. Even tests of high specificity and sensitivity may have a low predictive value in populations where the prevalence of a condition is low (odd but true).
3. Screening tests often unearth disease at an earlier stage in its genesis; this may lead to the spurious belief that survival has been prolonged, when in truth treatment has been ineffective and the true time course is unaltered (Figure 6.1).
4. Decisions about the target population (e.g. age group) and recall frequency are often arbitrary and based on imperfect ideas of natural history.

Costs and benefits are not easy to establish.

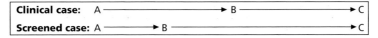

Figure 6.1 Spurious effects on survival produced by an earlier diagnosis (lead-time bias).

Benefits

1. Improvement in mortality and morbidity needs, if possible, to be confirmed by randomised trials.
2. The possible economic saving on future treatment is particularly hard to quantify.

Costs

1. Costs to patients:
   (a) unnecessary anxiety or even psychological harm
   (b) false reassurance (some of the time)
   (c) economic costs (e.g. time off work).
2. Costs to doctors: time and resource costs (test and follow-up).
3. Costs to the NHS:
   (a) costs of the test (direct and indirect)
   (b) costs of follow-up, further investigation or treatment.

Financial cost–benefit assessments have been attempted, as shown below, but these estimates remain tentative.

1. Cervical cytology: £36 000 per life-year saved.
2. Hypertension: £1700 per quality-adjusted life-year saved.

Psychological costs are well described:

1. Women with abnormal mammograms found to be normal on subsequent investigations remain significantly more anxious than those with normal results (Brett and Austoker 2001).
2. Telling patients that they have hypertension has led to absenteeism, lower self-esteem and poor marital relationships (Haynes et al. 1978).
3. There are also concerns that the communication of a negative result may be harmful. It may, for example, reinforce an unhealthy lifestyle or make participants less likely to return for repeat tests.

Marteau (1989) suggests that sensitive pre-test counselling is necessary in anticipation of these problems, and that the long-term behavioural outcomes of widespread screening initiatives need to be fully assessed. Others also see this as an ethical imperative, because in many instances the efficacy of intervention and cost-effectiveness of screening initiatives can be questioned. Informed choice is essential because, although screening programmes benefit populations, not all participants will benefit and some will be harmed by participation (Fludger et al. 2002). The General Medical Council (GMC) provides guidance on information that should be offered to those undergoing screening.

Health promotion activities and targets

Many types of screening and health promotion activity have been advocated as appropriate to primary care, despite the failure in some cases to demonstrate objective benefit:

Screening
- Hypertension screening, detection and follow-up
- Cervical cytology
- Developmental surveillance
- Well woman and well man clinics
- Visiting elderly people at home
- Mammography
- Blood fat estimation
- Faecal occult bloods
- Screening for psychiatric illness/alcohol abuse
- Well person periodic medicals
- Prostate cancer screening

Preventive interventions
- Immunisations/vaccinations
- Postmenopausal hormone replacement
- Lifestyle counselling
- Advice on smoking
- Keep-fit and aerobic programmes
- Weight-watching.

The UK National Screening Committee (NSC) created in 1996 uses research evidence, pilot programmes and economic evaluation to assess the evidence for new screening programmes against a set of internationally recognised criteria. The NSC also examines the case for continuing, modifying or withdrawing existing population screening programmes. A review of evidence by the NSC has led to a number of new screening programmes and changes to existing schedules.

New and recently introduced screening programmes

Colon cancer screening: rolled out in 2006, aiming for nationwide coverage by 2009.

Sickle cell and thalassaemia screening programme: rolled out in 2001 – linked antenatal and newborn screening.

The newborn hearing screening programme: rolled out in 2006 – identifies hearing impairment early in newborns.

Changes to existing programmes

Cervical screening: 2003 change in screening intervals in light of new evidence published in the *British Journal of Cancer* (Sasieni et al. 2003).

Obstacles to prevention

An effective programme will take account of some of the barriers to success.

Patient-related obstacles

Patients weigh costs against benefits and often perceive costs to be high. Taking smoking as an example, the costs of giving up include:

1. Sacrifice of physical pleasure – the anxiolytic pharmacological action of cigarettes
2. Sacrifice of the psychological and social benefits – smoking is:
   (a) a social activity that binds groups
   (b) a relaxation ritual
   (c) a conversation filler
   (d) a risk-taking, and hence exciting, exploit
   (e) in adolescence, a form of rebellion.

   Hence people rationalise or ignore:
   - 'It won't happen to me' (the ostrich approach).
   - 'I don't believe they know the true facts' (the sceptic's approach).
   - 'You go when it's your turn and you can't change that' (the fatalist's approach).

   Sometimes people are genuinely ignorant of relative risks ('Life's a risk – you're just as likely to be knocked over crossing the road').

Doctor-related obstacles

Costs to the doctor include:

1. Time and resources
2. Frustration (if returns are low).

There are also barriers of organisation and enthusiasm, problems with effective, clear communication (see Chapter 2), and in some areas medical debate and uncertainty that make advice-giving harder. In group practices commitment to preventive activities often varies between the partners, and this produces a source of potential friction and a check on the effectiveness of the service.

Overcoming patient-related obstacles and the cycle of change

Many areas of health promotion require a change in the individual's behaviour (e.g. lifestyle changes associated with diabetes, obesity, hypertension, etc.). Fowler, Gray and others have suggested the following plan:

1. Point out the disadvantages (seriousness and magnitude of risk)
2. Point out the benefits (social and financial as well as physical; positive as well as negative)
3. Anticipate and be prepared to discuss difficulties
4. Suggest coping strategies
5. Give simple advice and supplement it with written information (Fowler 1982; Gray & Fowler 1983).

Diclemente et al. (1991) have developed a model describing how people change. It recognises that a person's willingness to change and receptiveness to advice differs depending on where they are in a cycle of change. This model was originally based on self-help change, but research has shown

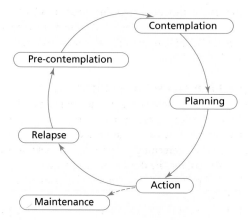

Figure 6.2 DiClemente and Prochaska's cycle of change (DiClemente and Prochaska 1991) (Blume et al. 2005; Herzog 2007).

that it is applicable to all types of change-related behaviours such as addictions through to smoking, eating and drug misuse (Blume et al. 2005; Herzog 2007). The decision to make a change is seen as a continuous process that includes several stages (Figure 6.2).

Precontemplation
The individual is unwilling to change and is happy with his lifestyle. Intervention at this stage is unlikely to lead to change but may encourage them to question their behaviour, thus moving closer to stage 2.

Contemplation (70% of smokers are at this stage)
The individual thinks about changing but does not feel ready to act. At this stage patients begin to be receptive to advice on change.

Planning
The individual is actively planning to stop. Advice on the treatment options to aid change is most beneficial at this stage.

Action
The attempt to change behaviour is made. Intensive support and encouragement are needed at this vulnerable period. As time passes the change becomes easier to maintain.

Maintenance
The individual tries to sustain the change. Continued but less intensive support and encouragement are necessary.

Relapse
Failure to maintain the desired change. The cycle starts again – or in some cases the patient makes no further effort to change.

To be effective facilitators of change GPs need to offer the appropriate intervention at each stage of the cycle. Mistimed intervention leads to wasted effort on our behalf and may alienate the patient (DiClemente et al. 1991; Blume et al. 2005).

Setting up a local screening programme

In addition to national screening programmes, practices may wish to initiate screening of local groups at high risk of disease. For example, a practice with a high proportion of African–Caribbean or south Asian individuals may institute a diabetes screening programme in view of the five times increased risk of developing the disease in these groups.

Zander (1982) has pointed out the major differences between preventive and routine care (Table 6.2).

In general terms the stages involved in setting up a screening programme are:

1. Identifying a problem that meets the Wilson criteria and that the practice agrees is a priority.
2. Auditing the records to establish the baseline performance of the practice, and then deciding whether to proceed.
3. Counting numbers – how big is the undertaking? Do you know the names of the high-risk group?
4. Defining *objectives* (e.g. screening of all African–Caribbean or south Asian individuals aged over 25 years for diabetes).
5. Defining *methods*:
   (a) opportunistic?
   (b) by patient invitation?
   (c) by patient visiting?
6. Defining the *participants* (e.g. practice nurse in hypertension screening clinics; health-care assistant in new registration clinics).
7. Participants may need training and/or equipment and need to have a protocol. They also need time to do the job.
8. Implementation of the screening.
9. Review after a trial period. Has the performance improved? Are objectives being met? Are teething problems disturbing the balance and effectiveness of the practice in other respects? Then decide whether to continue and what refinements are needed.

Table 6.2 Major differences between preventive and routine care

Routine care	Preventive care
Patient initiated, i.e. demand is unpredictable	Doctor-initiated, i.e. the demand should be predictable
Immediate-type demand	Non-urgent
Usually involving the doctor	Easily delegated to other primary health-care team members
Focused on individuals	Focused on high-risk groups
Good records are a help but audit is difficult	Good records are essential; audit is usually straightforward

Cervical screening

Key facts
- A total of 4 million smears are performed annually at a cost of £157 million a year in 2007.
- Approximately 80% of the target population (79.2% in 2007) receive screening. (If overall coverage of 80% can be achieved, the evidence suggests that a reduction in death rates of around 95% is possible.)
- Since the introduction of screening in 1988 rising mortality rates from cervical cancer have been reversed. A review in *The Lancet* estimates that cervical screening saves 5000 lives per year costing £36 000 per quality-adjusted life-year (QALY) (Peto et al. 2004). NICE approves interventions as cost-effective at a QALY of approximately £30 000. There have to be exceptional circumstances for NICE to approve interventions costing more than this (NICE 2007a). On this basis the cervical smear programme is not cost-effective but changes are unlikely in view of the considerable political investment in this programme (see Chapter 7).
- Liquid-based cytology (LBC) was introduced in 2003 following NICE guidance as a result of the lower rate of inadequate smears compared with conventional cytology. Since its introduction the percentage of inadequate samples has fallen to its lowest level (9% down to 7.2%). The reduction should have a positive impact on the quality of service and cost-effectiveness.

Background
The current campaign is based on evidence that the natural history of cervical cancer involves several pre-malignant stages (grades of dysplasia and carcinoma *in situ*) detectable by regular cervical screening several years in advance of frank carcinoma.

Certain *high-risk* groups have been described:
- low socioeconomic class
- early age of first sexual intercourse
- early age of first pregnancy
- multiple sexual partners
- frequent pregnancies
- human papillomavirus – types 16, 18 and 33.

Smoking probably doubles the risk of cervical cancer.

Women who have never been sexually active have a low risk of developing cervical cancer and may wish to decline screening.

Changes in the recall programme
The NHS Cervical Screening Programme now offers screening at different intervals depending on age. In the younger age range cervical screening intervals have been reduced from 5 to 3 years, based on evidence published in the *British Journal of Cancer* (Sasienei et al. 2003) (Tables 6.3 and 6.4). There is a benefit to 3-yearly screening versus 5-yearly screening in terms of

Table 6.3 Cervical screening intervals

Age group (years)	Frequency of screening
25	First invitation
25–49	3 yearly
50–64	5 yearly
65+	Only screen those who have not been screened since age 50 or have had recent abnormal tests

Table 6.4 Protection offered by a single negative smear

	20–39 years	40–54 years	55–69 years
3-yearly screening (%)	41	69	73
5-yearly screening (%)	30	63	73

From Sasieni et al. (2003).

detection rates apparent below the age of 40 years, but less apparent at older ages. Reducing the screening interval in older patients does not improve the detection rate, so the screening interval remains unchanged in this group.

The national NHS call-and-recall system invites women who are registered with a GP to attend for screening. It also keeps track of any follow-up investigation, and, if all is well, recalls the woman for screening in 3 or 5 years time. It is important that all women ensure that their GPs have their correct contact details and inform them if these change. Women overdue smears, who have not had a recent test, may be offered one when they attend sexual health or family planning clinics on another matter. Women should receive their first invitation for routine screening at age 25.

Limitations to cervical cytology
1. A false-negative rate of about 10% for carcinoma *in situ* (even necrotic tumours can give a negative result). LBC has shown small improvements in sensitivity and positive predictive values in the pilot programme.
2. A false-positive rate of about 5% (smears showing mild dysplasia).
3. Sampling problems: the squamocolumnar junction is not always accessible.
4. Other technical problems that upset interpretation (e.g. menstruation, pregnancy, the contraceptive pill, intrauterine devices and polyps).
5. Limitations of the *cervical smear campaign*:
   (a) guidelines have been complex, inconsistent and often lagging behind current research but are being adapted
   (b) the number of smears taken has probably been inadequate in some areas (particularly cities)
   (c) the right women have probably not been screened, in particular the high-risk groups from low social classes use the service least but need it most (the inverse care principle)

(d) organisation has often been inadequate: in some inner-city studies nearly 70% of invitation letters were inaccurately or inappropriately addressed (Beardow et al. 1989).

The future of cervical screening and HPV immunisation

Nearly all cervical cancers are attributable to human papillomavirus (HPV) infection (Garcia 2007). The most carcinogenic are HPV 16 and 18, which cause 70% of cervical cancers worldwide. Two HPV vaccines have now been licensed, a bivalent (against 16 and 18) and a quadrivalent (6, 11, 16, 18) version (Ault and Future II Study Group 2007) The bivalent version Cervarix is the one chosen for UK immunisation. Both vaccines offer high levels of protection, e.g. 98% seropositivity at 4.5-year follow-up. Studies have shown a significant reduction in the number of pre-cancerous changes in immunised individuals (Ault and Future II Study Group 2007). HPV vaccines also prevent genital warts. As HPV is most prevalent after a person has become sexually active, immunisation would need to be given before this. As 20% of adolescents are sexually active at the age of 14 years, immunisation has been implemented in all girls in year 8 (age 12–13) and is given at school. The programme commenced in autumn 2008 and there is also a 3-year catch-up programme for girls aged 13–18. The cervical screening programme will continue after the HPV vaccine has been introduced, because clinical trial data have shown that neither of the two vaccines licensed protects against all HPV types that cause cervical cancer.

Issues

- Parental concerns over the sexual implications of HPV immunisation may reduce uptake of immunisation, thereby reducing the efficacy of the HPV immunisation programme. The vaccine requires a three-dose course.
- The immunisation programme is expected to cost £100m a year (however, it is expected to potentially save 400 lives a year). Researchers have estimated a likely cost to the health service of £23 000 per QALY – less than NICE's threshold of £30 000.

Screening for bowel cancer

Key facts

In the UK 5% of the population will develop colorectal cancer leading to 16 000 deaths each year. Biennial screening for colorectal cancer using faecal occult blood (FOB) tests reduces mortality by 16% (Towler et al. 2006). The NHS bowel cancer screening programme was rolled out in 2007.

The *advantages* of FOB screening are obvious. The technique is:

- non-invasive
- cheap
- simple to administer.
  Disadvantages include:
- inconvenience
- relative insensitivity (occult blood is not uniformly distributed in faeces, and some lesions bleed intermittently)

- relative non-specificity (lesions other than cancer can generate positive tests)
- compliance (wide variation).

How good is the test in practice?
1. Two per cent of those screened will have a positive FOB and should be offered colonoscopy.
2. Of those undergoing colonoscopy:
   10% will have bowel cancer
   20% offered colonoscopy will not be suitable for the procedure or refuse
   30% will have polyps
   40% will have no abnormality.
3. If the test is negative there is still a 1 in 200 chance of a cancer and a 1 in 50 chance of an adenoma in the next 4 years.
4. Bleeding tends to occur relatively late in the tumour's natural history.

Who is eligible?
- All men and women aged 60–69 will receive 2-yearly FOBs
- Over-70s can request screening.

Risk/Benefit?
A pilot of the screening programme (2007) offered 480 000 residents screening: 56% accepted. The screening detected 552 cancers, 48% at Dukes' A grade. Of the remainder, 1% had metastasised at the time of diagnosis. The 5-year survival rate after identification and treatment is 97% for Dukes' A, 80% for Dukes' B, 30–60% for Dukes' C and 5% for Dukes' D. The positive predictive value of FOB is 10.9% for cancer and 35% for adenoma. The risks involved include perforation after colonoscopy, which occurs in 1 in 1500 cases, and death in 1 in 10 000; the psychological risks are more difficult to quantify.

Screening for prostate cancer

Prostate cancer is both the second most common cause of cancer, and cancer deaths, in men from the UK. It commonly presents in those aged over 65 and is rare under the age of 50. Only a quarter of those with prostate cancer will die because of it, as many will die of other causes due to slow disease progression. Despite this 10 000 men die annually of prostate cancer.

Screening and PSA
There have been calls for the introduction of prostate cancer screening using the prostate-specific antigen test (PSA). PSA can detect early, local-ised prostate cancer when potentially curative treatment can be offered. However, despite the ability to diagnose prostate cancer at an early stage, there is currently insufficient evidence that doing so will improve survival. Many prostate cancers are identified that would never have presented clini-cally during the man's lifetime. Treatment of these cases would undoubt-edly lead to some men (with indolent disease) suffering from impotence,

incontinence and even death, who would not have done so had screening not been introduced (NSC 2006). A recent study from the USA (Andriole et al. *N Engl J Med* 2009) of 77000 men randomised to screening or usual care found no difference in mortality between the two groups. A second European study (Schröder et al. *N Engl J Med* 2009) of 162000 men did show a reduction in mortality in the screened group. However, the screening used a tight PSA cut-off of 3, leading to over-diagnosis. In this study, to prevent one cancer death you need to screen 1410 men and treat 48 cases of prostate cancer. In light of these studies there has been no change in the guidance on PSA screening and patients should continue to be counselled about the benefits and risks of screening.

PSA facts:

- Two-thirds of men with elevated PSA do not have prostate cancer on biopsy.
- Over half of patients with a raised PSA will have a normal result if repeated 6 weeks later. Repeat testing reduces unnecessary referral for biopsy (Eastham et al. 2003).
- PSA is elevated by urinary tract infection (UTI), benign prostate hypertrophy, recent ejaculation, vigorous exercise and prostate examination (delay test by 1 week or test before digital rectal examination).
- Direct rectal examination is not recommended as a screening test for prostate cancer in *asymptomatic* men. It is recommended in patients with lower urinary tract symptoms or features of metastasis.
- PSA cannot differentiate aggressive from indolent cancers.
- PSA rises with age and age-related reference values should be used
- A borderline PSA in an asymptomatic man should be repeated in 1–3 months and referred urgently if the PSA is rising (NICE 2008a).
- A direct rectal examination and PSA (after counselling) are recommended with the following unexplained symptoms:
  - ➤ inflammatory or obstructive lower urinary tract symptoms,
  - ➤ erectile dysfunction
  - ➤ haematuria
  - ➤ bone pain, low back pain or weight loss.
- Screening is not recommended in the over-75s or in men with less than 10 years' life expectancy because treating screen-positive cancers in this group is unlikely to improve their survival.

Which treatment?

It is currently unclear which course of action – watchful waiting, radical radiotherapy or radical – is best for screen-detected prostate cancer. The PROTECT trial aims to answer this question but will not complete its report until 2021. There is a small survival advantage to radical prostatectomy versus watchful waiting in patients with localised prostate cancer presenting clinically (non-screen detected) (Holmberg et al. 2002).

To screen or not to screen?

Current evidence does not support a national screening programme because over-diagnosis and over-treatment are significant problems.

Patients requesting screening should be counselled on the risks and benefits of the PSA test.

Screening for breast cancer

The size of the problem
1. Breast cancer is *the* major form of cancer among women in the UK. It accounts for:
   (a) over 12 500 deaths per annum
   (b) 20% of all female cancer deaths. It is the most common cause of death in women aged 35–54.
2. The UK has a high breast cancer mortality rate compared with other developed countries.

Risk factors (Cancer Research UK)
- Female sex (99% diagnosed in 2004 were women)
- Previous breast cancer
- Previous endometrial or ovarian cancer
- Age (peak incidence after age of 45)
- Race: more common in white women
- Social class: breast cancer is one of the few cancers to have a higher risk in the more affluent classes
- Country of residence: higher in west, lower in east
- Family history (RR 2-12x)
- Ionising radiation to the chest: shows a linear dose–response relationship
- Alcohol
- Prolonged oestrogen exposure, i.e. increased risk with:
  - early menarche and late menopause
  - oestrogens in hormone replacement therapy (HRT) and the oral contraceptive pill (OCP)
  - obesity – increases endogenous oestrogen levels.

Note that breaks in oestrogen exposure due to childbirth and breastfeeding reduce breast cancer risk.

(www.cancerhelp.org.uk/help/default.asp?page=3293)

Prognosis
On average, two-thirds of all women with breast cancer are alive 5 years after diagnosis. However, those with early local disease fare better than those with metastatic spread.

Screening by mammography
1. Mammography involves low-level X-ray exposure on one or two planes. The amount of radiation involved is small (1 rad).
2. Women aged between 50 and 70 are routinely invited for breast screening every 3 years. The tissue of young women's breasts is dense, resulting

in practical difficulties in interpretation. Perimenopausal thinning makes the task easier, so screening is easier in older (50+) women. Magnetic resonance imaging (MRI) or ultrasonography is used for diagnosis in younger women.

3. The sensitivity of modern mammography is about 80% and the specificity 95%. (Clinical examination picks up 50–60% of abnormalities.)
4. Estimates of positive predictive value vary from 9% to 60%, with the Forrest report (1987), suggesting a 2:1 ratio of benign to malignant biopsies.

Benefits

It might be supposed, these problems not withstanding, that mammography is bound to be of benefit: after all, it detects breast lumps too small to be palpated, and 5-year survival figures are better for early disease. In fact, as Figure 6.1 illustrates, earlier diagnosis can result in longer survival times from diagnosis without altering the time course of a disease at all.

Early results appeared to show an improvement in mortality, although estimates of the benefit differed. In one of the first studies to directly assess the impact of the UK's breast cancer screening programme on mortality, it was shown that screening reduces deaths from breast cancer by 48% (Allgood et al. 2008). After adjusting for self-selection bias to account for poorer health in women who chose not to attend, researchers calculated that women who attended screening had at 35% reduction in breast cancer mortality.

Costs

1. The cost of the programme is £75 m annually (2007).
2. There is also an opportunity cost, as skilled personnel and capital funds could be deployed elsewhere.
3. A low positive predictive value implies over-diagnosis, over-investigation and over-treatment of some false positives, with all the heartache that this entails.
4. All women experience anxiety awaiting and undergoing tests, and awaiting results; some experience indignity and some may become phobic.

Breast self-examination (BSE)

There is a long-held view that BSE is a worthwhile preventive exercise, to be taught at every available opportunity. However, the evidence for this view is shaky. A Cochrane review of the evidence in 2003 (Kösters and Gøtzsche 2003) showed no reduction in breast cancer mortality but an increase in the number of invasive investigations with benign results. Furthermore guilt may be engendered in those patients with cancer who did not self-examine before diagnosis. Some doctors have suggested that it is unethical to offer a test that may harm without clearer evidence of benefit. An alternative concept of 'breast awareness' – familiarity with the normal breast throughout the monthly cycle is encouraged (DOH) with reporting of changes from abnormality rather than regular systematic self-examination.

New concepts in breast cancer

A 2008 cohort study (Perrin et al. 2008) has found a link between gestational diabetes and postmenopausal breast cancer. Women with gestational diabetes were 1.5 times more likely to develop breast cancer than women with uncomplicated pregnancies and 1.7 times more likely when diagnosed after the age of 50.

Prevention and screening in older people

In 2007 16% of the population were aged over 65 years, but the proportion of older people is increasing, and the proportion of the very elderly is increasing even more. The largest percentage growth in population in the year to mid-2006 was at ages 85 and over.

Fifty per cent of all non-psychiatric NHS beds are already occupied by the over-65s, and concern has been expressed that hospital services will not be able to cope. The solution to this dilemma may lie in better prevention and in identifying disability before it becomes severe. Better prevention could also raise the quality of life in old age and the priority areas are summarised by the National Service Framework (NSF) for Older People (Department of Health 2001).

Preventive measures (DH 2001)

Preventive measures that may help include:
- falls prevention
- mental health screening in older people
- stroke prevention
- lifestyle advice.
    The NSF also includes two key statements of principle:
- Care should be based on clinical need (age no bar to treatment).
- Independence should be promoted (intermediate care will provide supportive care in the home and help unnecessary hospital or long-term residential care).

Is screening worthwhile?

Screening studies on older people show a high prevalence of unreported problems, so it might be supposed that they would benefit from the regular attention of a screening doctor. It has been argued by some that most newly diagnosed problems in older people are trivial or irreversible, so health spin-offs are small.

Epstein et al. (1990) conducted a large-scale US study in which patients were randomly allocated between usual and intensive specialist care (geriatrician, geriatric nurse, geriatric social worker): at 3 and 12 months the health differences between the groups were marginal. Worthwhile diagnoses *can* be made (up to one in five over-75s is said to suffer some degree of depression; 6–12% have some degree of dementia, with carers stressed and unsupported).

Some spin-offs (morale, self-esteem and satisfaction) are immeasurable and come forth when it is shown that someone cares. Influenza vaccinations reduce mortality from flu by 70% in the over-65s, and halve the rate of serious associated complications and hospital admission. Today's trivial problem (e.g. uncorrected presbycusis or loose doormat) is tomorrow's major one (e.g. fractured neck of femur). Ninety per cent of the over-75s see the primary health-care team anyway over a 1-year period Targeted screening interventions have been shown to improve quality of life and reduce adverse events in the NSF areas of falls prevention, mental health, stroke prevention and lifestyle advice.

Falls prevention

Approximately 30% of over-65s living in the community have a fall each year, and an even greater proportion in care fall. Although fewer than 10% of falls result in fracture, 20% require medical attention and 14 000 die every year of osteoporotic hip fracture. Complications include significant psychological and physical disability, a threat to independence and burden on carers. The cost to the NHS and social services is large (>£900m a year). As falls are often due to multiple factors, effective prevention requires multifactorial interventions (Gillespie et al. 2009).

(DH 2001; NICE 2004; Gillespie et al. 2009)

NICE recommendations (2004)
- Case/risk identification – routinely ask elderly patients if they fall
- Fallers or at-risk patients:
  - ➢ assess gait and balance
  - ➢ refer to falls clinic for multifactorial falls risk assessment.

Falls prevention interventions with the best evidence of efficacy (Gillespie et al. 2009)
- Strength and balance training
- Home hazard intervention and follow-up
- Medication review/withdrawal (especially hypnotics, antidepressants)
- Cardiac pacing (syncope-associated falls).

Multifactorial assessment involves assessing falls history, gait, balance and mobility, muscle weakness, osteoporosis risk, functional ability, fear relating to falling, visual impairment, cognitive impairment, neurological examination, urinary incontinence, assessment of home hazards, cardiovascular examination and medication review. NICE recommends referral to a dedicated specialist falls service in view of the complexity and breadth of assessment and management, but also states that GPs need to maintain basic professional competence in falls assessment and prevention.

Osteoporosis
The size of the problem
The obvious link between osteoporosis and falls prevention means that these two areas should be assessed together. Around 70 000 people in England and Wales suffer a fractured neck of femur annually. Two-thirds

are elderly women. A tenth of women in their 60s and half in their 70s suffer an osteoporosis-related fracture. By 2010 the cost of treatment of osteoporotic fractures is estimated at £2.1bn (NICE 2008b).

Definition

The World Health Organization (WHO) defines osteoporosis in terms of the bone mineral density (BMD). The reduction in current BMD is compared with that of a woman's peak BMD (aged 25), measured as standard deviations (SD) from the mean. This is called the *T*-score:

- Normal: *T*-score no worse than −1 SD
- Osteopenia: *T*-score between −1 and −2.5 SD
- Osteoporosis: *T*-score below −2.5 SD
- Established osteoporosis: *T*-score below −2.5 SD, with one or more associated fragility fractures.

Preventive strategies

BMD remains constant in women until the menopause when it falls sharply for 5–10 years (oestrogen withdrawal bone loss), and more slowly thereafter (age-related bone loss). Preventive strategies focus on encouraging new bone formation, discouraging bone resorption and achieving a higher BMD at peak. Preventive lifestyle measures are advised for all women on treatment and those with risk factors for osteoporosis, i.e. regular weight-bearing exercise, avoidance of smoking, a calcium-rich diet, calcium and vitamin D supplementation in those deficient on testing, moderation of alcohol intake and in older patients measures to prevent falls.

Risk factors

Age-independent risk factors
- Family history of maternal hip fracture before the age of 75 years
- >4 units of alcohol/day
- Severe long-term rheumatoid arthritis.

Indicators of low BMD
- Body mass index below $22\,\text{kg/m}^2$
- Untreated premature menopause
- Inflammatory conditions,
- Hyperthyroidism or coeliac disease
- Prolonged immobility.

Primary prevention (NICE 2008b)

The definition of who to treat is not straightforward and a simplified summary is given here. The complexity of the full guidance may limit its effective implementation in clinical practice. The author prefers the National Osteoporosis Guidance Group guidance which uses an online calculator (www.sheffield.ac.uk/FRAX/index.htm) to estimate 10-year risk of a major osteoporotic fracture. Risk groups are low, medium or high. High-risk groups are treated, medium-risk groups are sent for DEXA (dual energy X-ray absorptiometry) assessment and low-risk groups are reassured and given lifestyle advice.

Who to treat?
- Women >70 with:
  - an age independent risk factor **OR**
  - an indicator of low BMD **and** *T*-score <−2.5 **OR**
  - a T score <−3.5 alone
- Women 65–70 with:
  - an independent risk factor **and** T score <−2.5
- Women <65 and postmenopausal with **all** of the following:
  - an age-independent risk factor
  - T score <−2.5
  - an indicator of low BMD.

How to treat?
- Alendronate (a bisphosphonate) is the first-line treatment (etidronate and risedronate are alternative bisphosphonates to try if alendronate is not tolerated) plus lifestyle measures.
- If bisphosphonates are not tolerated, strontium ranelate is recommended (decreases bone resorption and increases bone formation – 49% reduction in vertebral fractures in first year of use (Meunier et al. 2004).

Secondary prevention (NICE 2008c)
Who to treat?
- Women with a fragility fracture who are:
  - >75
- 65–74 with a *T*-score <−2.5
  - <65 and postmenopausal:
    - *T*-score <−3 **OR**
    - *T*-score <−2.5 and any of the risk factors listed.

How to treat?
- Alendronate (a bisphosphonate) is the first-line treatment (etidronate and risedronate are alternative bisphosphonates to try if alendronate is not tolerated) plus lifestyle measures. Bisphosphonates are effective (average risk reduction of 40% for hip fracture), but often cause upper gastrointestinal disturbance. Weekly preparations such as Alendronate help reduce the severity of symptoms. A 2007 study has now shown an annual infusion with zoldedronic acid to be effective (reduce hip fractures by 41% – Black et al. 2007).
- Raloxifene (selective oestrogen receptor modulator) and teraparatide (recombinant parathyroid hormone) are second-line options for secondary prevention in those not tolerating bisphosphonates; raloxifene is not recommended for use in primary prevention of osteoporosis.

Mental health screening in older people
Depression (Mottram et al. 2006)
Depression requiring treatment is found in 10% of those aged over 60. Depression in this group is associated with an increased mortality and is more often missed than in younger groups (fewer patients in this group

receive treatment). Older depressed patients differ in their presentation, young people showing more behavioural symptoms and older adults more somatic symptoms and fewer complaints of low mood (Serby and Yu 2003). Causal factors also differ, e.g. bereavement, poor social network, poor physical health, polypharmacy. A Cochrane review has concluded that tricyclic antidepressants (TCAs), selective serotonin re-uptake inhibitors (SSRIs) and monoamine oxidase inhibitors (MAOIs) are effective in the treatment of older patients and in patients likely to have severe physical illness. At least 6 weeks of antidepressant treatment is recommended to achieve optimal therapeutic effect. There is little evidence concerning the efficacy of low-dose TCA treatment.

Depression screening in older people (NICE 2007b)
- Patients with significant physical illnesses causing disability and other mental health problems, such as dementia, should have a two-question depression screen (see Chapter 8).
- In older adults with depression, physical state, living conditions and social isolation should be assessed.
- Antidepressants – in particular TCAs – for older adults require careful monitoring for side effects. Health-care professionals should be aware of the increased frequency of drug interactions in this group.
- Bear in mind the potential physical causes of depression and the possibility that depression can be caused by medication, e.g. many cardiovascular drugs, β blockers, calcium channel blockers, statins.

Dementia
There are approximately 700 000 cases of dementia in the UK (Alzheimer's Society 2006). It affects around 5% of the over-65s, rising to a third of the over-85s (Ott et al. 1995). The most common causes of dementia include Alzheimer's disease (about 60% of cases), vascular dementia and Lewy body dementia (about 20% of cases each). Dementia is also more common after strokes and in patients with Parkinson's disease.

Principles of dementia management (NICE 2006)
- Non-discrimination: no exclusion from services due to diagnosis or age.
- Valid consent: patients must give valid consent for interventions (if the patient lacks capacity, refer to the Mental Capacity Act 2005 guidance below).
- Help for carers: the needs of carers should be assessed (Carers Acts 2000 and 2004) and support offered. Carers of people with dementia who experience psychological distress and negative psychological impact should be offered psychological therapy, including cognitive–behavioural therapy.
- Coordination of care: care managers and care coordinators should ensure the coordinated delivery of health and social care with a combined care plan agreed by health and social services together with the patient and carers.

- Memory clinics:
  - referral of all people with a possible diagnosis of dementia
  - assessment of dementia by MRI to exclude other cerebral causes and reversible causes (e.g. normal pressure hydrocephalus).

The Mental Capacity Act 2005

The Mental Capacity Act 2005 was implemented in April 2007 and has implications for all people with dementia, their carers and those who work with them. It has five key principles:

1. Adults must be assumed to have the capacity to make decisions for themselves unless proved otherwise.
2. Individuals must be given all available support before it is concluded that they cannot make decisions for themselves.
3. Individuals must retain the right to make what might be seen as eccentric or unwise decisions.
4. Anything done for or on behalf of individuals without capacity must be in their best interests.
5. Anything done for or on behalf of individuals without capacity should restrict their rights and basic freedoms as little as possible.
   For more details see Chapter 3.

Investigations

- Mental state exam (Mini-Mental State Examination or MMSE or six-item cognitive impairment test)
- Physical examination
- Medication review to identify medication that may impair cognitive function
- Dementia screen (full blood count [FBC], urea and electrolytes [U&Es], calcium, glucose, liver function tests [LFTs], thyroid function tests [TFTs], vitamin B_{12}, folate, mid-stream urine [MSU]).

Management

- Refer those with cognitive impairment to memory clinics for imaging, and in-depth assessment of the patient and carers.
- The clinic should cater for all severities of dementia and provide a written integrated care plan for the patient including:
  - signs and symptoms
  - course and prognosis
  - treatments
  - local care and support services
  - support groups
  - sources of financial and legal advice and advocacy
  - medicolegal issues, including driving
  - local information sources, including libraries and voluntary organisations.
- A record of the care plan should be kept in the notes.

Treatment options
Non-pharmacological (accessed via memory clinic)
- Cognitive stimulation: mild-to-moderate dementia – structured group cognitive stimulation programmes.
- Interventions for agitation: aromatherapy, multisensory stimulation, therapeutic use of music and/or dancing, animal-assisted therapy (the type of animal is not specified!) and massage have been shown to be beneficial.

Pharmacological
- Acetylcholinesterase inhibitors, e.g. donepezil: for moderate Alzheimer's disease only (MMSE 10–20). Started by a specialist and stopped if MMSE <10. Meta-analysis (NICE 2007c) shows improved cognition and maintenance of functional ability compared with placebo, but differences between the two groups are small.
- Antipsychotics:
  - ➤ indicated for severe non-cognitive symptoms (psychosis and/or agitated behaviour causing significant distress)
  - ➤ avoid in mild-to-moderate symptoms due to increased risk of stroke
  - ➤ regularly review to titrate down or stop medication whenever possible.

Patients with vascular dementia should have treatment to reduce their cardiovascular risk factors, i.e. statins, hypertension management.

Well person assessments

Well person checks
These checks have the potential to offer health education to patients who are in a receptive frame of mind. They are supplementary to the patient checks required by the GP contract for those registering with their practice for the first time. Many surgeries advertise well person checks and they are usually booked as double appointments into normal nursing or health-care assistant clinics

Advantages
1. These clinics may attract patients who might not otherwise come to the surgery, who are inhibited about seeing a doctor and using up time unless ill.
2. Patients attending such clinics are in a health-conscious and receptive frame of mind.
3. It is often possible to offer more time and a more informal atmosphere.
4. A separate clinic also avoids the real pitfall of opportunistic screening, i.e. often when it is inconvenient (the surgery is running late; the patient is having a period, etc.).
5. There is a large potential for health promotion and educating towards self-help for common, minor problems (perhaps reducing demand on consulting time in the long run, and helping to relieve health-related anxieties in those with neurotic illness).

6. Income may be boosted (e.g. increased item-of-service work, helps meet Quality Outcome Framework [QOF] targets for routine data, i.e. smoking status, BMI, higher list sizes because a well-received competitive range of services is on offer).
7. Greater satisfaction for the patient and doctor, and an extended (more satisfying) role for the practice nurse.

Disadvantages
1. The obvious costs of:
   (a) time and energy
   (b) administrative effort and overheads.
2. These appointments may still reach the *most* motivated people, when the need is to reach the *least*.
3. There are dangers that it will degenerate into a sick person appointment through patient misuse.

AKT questions

Q1
With regard to screening choose the correct answer. Select ONE option only:
a   Screening for prostate cancer using the PSA meets Wilson's criteria.
b   A test is best assessed for use as a screening tool by looking at the positive and negative predictive values.
c   Specificity is a measure of the proportion of the studied population with disease currently identified by the test.
d   Screening is not associated with significant psychological and social effects.
e   Highly sensitive and specific tests have low predictive values in conditions with low prevalence.

Q2
Which of these is NOT a risk factor for cervical cancer. Select ONE option only:
a   Low socioeconomic class
b   Early age of intercourse
c   Progesterone-only contraceptive pill
d   Smoking
e   Multiple sexual partners
f   Human papillomavirus 18.

Q3
The cycle of change (Diclemente and Prochaska). Fill in the gaps with the appropriate stage description. Each option may be used once, more than once or not at all.
1. Patients are most receptive to advice on behavioural change at this stage.
2. Seventy per cent of smokers are at this stage.
3. At this stage the individual needs continued support to sustain change.

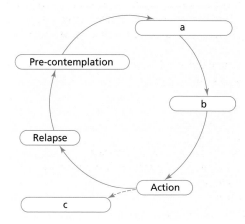

Q4

Wilson's criteria state the following EXCEPT. Select ONE option only:

a   The condition should be important.
b   Treatment should be cost-effective.
c   Screening should be performed annually.
d   Screening should be targeted at high-risk groups.
e   There should be a latent period in which effective treatment is possible.

Q5

Cervical screening. Identify the incorrect statement. Select ONE option only:

a   The false-negative rate for carcinoma *in situ* is approximately 10%.
b   The false-positive rate is around 5%.
c   The first invitation for screening is at age 25.
d   Screening is at 5-yearly intervals and ends at age 65.
e   Those with recent changes and aged >65 are invited for further screening.

Q6

Bowel cancer screening. Identify the incorrect statement. Select ONE option only:

a   Approximately 15% screened will require colonoscopy.
b   Screening is offered to all patients aged 60–69.
c   Screening is at 2-yearly intervals.
d   Screening is via faecal wipes which are returned in the post.
e   Over 70s can request to be screened.

Q7

PSA. Identify the correct statement. Select ONE option only:

a   Seventy per men of men with a raised PSA have prostate cancer.
b   Rectal examination is an appropriate screening test for prostate cancer in asymptomatic men.

c   PSA can differentiate aggressive from indolent cancers.
d   PSA is elevated by ejaculation.
e   PSA falls with age.

Q8
Breast cancer screening. Identify the correct statement. Select ONE option only:
a   Breast cancer is more common in patients with a high social class.
b   Breast cancer is the second most common cancer in women in the UK.
c   Screening commences at age 55 and ceases at age 70.
d   Breast self-examination reduces cancer mortality.
e   A third of women with breast cancer are alive at 5 years.

Q9
A Cochrane review in 2003 found that the following interventions are effective at preventing falls EXCEPT. Select ONE option only:
a   Home hazard intervention and follow-up
b   Prescription of hip protectors
c   Cardiac pacing
d   Medication review and withdrawal
e   Strength and balance training

Q10
Which of the following patients should start on a bisphosphonate for the primary prevention of osteoporosis according to the 2008 NICE guidelines? Select ONE option only:
a   A woman <65 with a T-score of above −2.5
b   A woman of <65 with untreated premature menopause
c   A woman >70 with a T-score of <−2.5 but no risk factors for osteoporosis
d   A woman 65–70 with a T-score >−2.5
e   A woman >70 with a family history of maternal hip fracture before the age of 75

Answers

Q1 e

Q2 d

Q3
1. b
2. a
3. c

Q4 c
Screening should be a continuous process.

Q5 d
Screening is 3 yearly up to the age of 50 and 5 yearly thereafter.

Q6 a

Only 2–15% would be a massive number and at this level the service could not cope due to lack of facilities and finances.

Q7 d

True – recent ejaculation can elevate the PSA. Note that only a third of those with a raised PSA will have prostate cancer.

Q8 a

Breast cancer is the number one cancer in women in the UK.

Q9 b

Hip protectors do not **prevent** falls. Medication withdrawal, especially hypnotics and antidepressants, is effective at preventing falls.

Q10 e

This guideline is complicated – see the explanation earlier in the chapter.

References

Allgood PC, Warwick J, Warren RML, Day NE, Duffy SW. A case–control study of the impact of the East Anglian breast screening programme on breast cancer mortality. *Br J Cancer* 2008;**98**:206–9.

Andriole GL, Grubb III RL, Buys SS et al., for the PLCO Project Team. Mortality results from a randomized prostate-cancer screening trial. *N Engl J Med* 2009;**360**:1310.

Ault KA and Future II Study Group. Effect of prophylactic human papillomavirus L1 virus-like-particle vaccine on risk of cervical intraepithelial neoplasia grade 2, grade 3, and adenocarcinoma in situ: a combined analysis of four randomised clinical trials. *Lancet* 2007;**369**:1861–8.

Beardow R, Oerton J, Victor C. Evaluation of the cervical cytology screening programme in an inner city health district. *BMJ* 1989;**299**:98–100.

Black DM, Delmas PD, Eastell R et al., for the HORIZON Pivotal Fracture Trial. Once-yearly zoledronic acid for treatment of postmenopausal osteoporosis. *NEJM* 2007;**356**:1809–2.2

Blume AW, Schmaling KB, Marlatt GA. Memory, executive cognitive function, and readiness to change drinking behavior. *Addict Behav* 2005;**30**:301–14.

Brett J, Austoker J. Women who are recalled for further investigation for breast screening: psychological consequences 3 years after recall and factors affecting re-attendance. *J Public Health Med* 2001;**23**:292–300.

Department of Health. *National Service Framework for Older People.* London: DH, 2001.

DiClemente CC, Prochaska JO, Fairhurst SK, Velicer WF, Velasquez MM, Rossi JS. The process of smoking cessation: an analysis of precontemplation, contemplation, and preparation stages of change. *J Consult Clin Psychol* 1991;**59**:295–304.

Eastham JA, Riedel E, Scardino PT et al., for the Polyp Prevention Trial Study Group. Variation of serum prostate-specific antigen levels; an evaluation of year-to-year fluctuations. *JAMA* 2003;**289**:2695–700.

Epstein AM, Hall JA, Fretwell M et al. Consultant geriatric assessment for ambulatory patients. *JAMA* 1990;**263**:538–44.

Fludger BS, Turner A-M, Harvey RF, Haslam N. Controlled prospective study of faecal occult blood screening for colorectal cancer in Bury, black pudding capital of the world. *BMJ* 2002;**325**:75–80.

Fowler GH. Coronary heart disease prevention: a general practice challenge. *J R Coll Gen Prac* 1988;**38**:391–2.

Forrest P. *Breast Cancer Screening*. London: HMSO, 1987.

Garcia FA. Prophylactic human papillomavirus vaccination: A breakthrough in primary cervical cancer prevention. *Obstet Gynecol Clin North Am* 2007;**34**:761–81.

Gillespie LD, Robertson MC, Gillespie WJ et al. Interventions for preventing falls in older people living in the community. *Cochrane Database Syst Rev* 2009;**2**: CD007146.

Gray M, Fowler GH. *Preventive Medicine in General Practice*. Oxford: Oxford University Press, 1983.

Haynes RB, Sackett DL, Taylor DW, Gibson ES, Johnson AI. Changes in absenteeism and psychosocial function due to hypertension screening and therapy among working men. *N Engl J Med* 1978;**299**:741–4.

Herzog TA. Are the stages of change for smokers qualitatively distinct? An analysis using an adolescent sample. *Psychol Addict Behav* 2007;**21**:120–5.

Holmberg L, Bill-Axelson A, Helgesen F et al., for the Scandinavian Prostatic Cancer Group Study Number 4. A randomized trial comparing radical prostatectomy with watchful waiting in early prostate cancer. *N Engl J Med* 2002;**347**:781–9.

Kösters JP, Gøtzsche PC. Regular self-examination or clinical examination for early detection of breast cancer. *Cochrane Database Syst Rev* 2003;**2**:CD003373.

Marteau TM. Psychological costs of screening. *BMJ* 1989;**299**:527.

Meunier PJ, Roux C, Seeman E, et al. The effects of strontium ranelate on the risk of vertebral fracture in women with post-menopausal osteoporosis. *N Engl J Med* 2004;**5**:459–68.

Mottram P, Wilson K, Strobl J. Antidepressants for depressed elderly. *Cochrane Database Syst Rev* 2006;**1**:CD003491.

National Institute for Health and Clinical Excellence. *Supporting People with Dementia and Their Carers in Health and Social Care*. London: NICE, 2006.

National Institute for Health and Clinical Excellence. *An Economic Analysis of Environmental Interventions that Promote Physical Activity*. London: NICE, 2007a.

National Institute for Health and Clinical Excellence. *Depression in Adults Guideline, Update*. London: NICE, 2007b.

National Institute for Health and Clinical Excellence. *Alzheimer's Disease: Donepezil, galantamine, rivastigmine (review) and memantine*. London: NICE, 2007c.

National Institute for Health and Clinical Excellence. *The Assessment and Prevention of Falls in Older People*. London: NICE, 2004.

National Institute for Health and Clinical Excellence. *Prostate Cancer: Diagnosis and treatment*. London: NICE, 2008a.

National Institute for Health and Clinical Excellence. *Osteoporosis – Primary prevention*. London: NICE, 2008b.

National Institute for Health and Clinical Excellence. *Osteoporosis – Secondary prevention including strontium ranelate*. London: NICE, 2008c.

National Screening Committee (NSC). *Prostate Cancer Review against UK NSC Criteria*. NSC, 2006. Available at: www.screening.nhs.uk/prostatecancer (accessed 2008).

Ott A, Breteler MMB, Harskamp F van et al. Prevalence of Alzheimer's disease and vascular dementia: association with education. The Rotterdam study. *BMJ* 1995;**310**:970–3.

Perrin MC, Terry MB, Kleinhaus K et al. Gestational diabetes and the risk of breast cancer among women in the Jerusalem Perinatal Study. *Breast Cancer Res Treat* 2008;**108**:129–35. Epub May 2007.

Peto J, Gilham C, Fletcher O, Matthews FE. The cervical cancer epidemic that screening has prevented in the UK. *Lancet* 2004;**346**(9430):249–56.

Sasieni P, Adams J, Cuzick J. Benefits of cervical screening at different ages: evidence from the UK audit of screening histories. *Br J Cancer* 2003;**89**:88–93.

Schröder FH, Hugosson J, Roobol MJ et al., and ERSPC Investigators. Screening and prostate-cancer mortality in a randomized European study. *N Engl J Med* 2009;**360**:1320–8. Epub 2009.

Serby M, Yu M. Overview: Depression in the elderly. *Mt Sinai J Med* 2003; **70**:38–44.

Towler BP, Irwig L, Glasziou P, Weller D, Kewenter J. Screening for colorectal cancer using the faecal occult blood test, Hemoccult. *Cochrane Database Syst Rev* 2006;**4**.

Wilson JMG, Jungner G. *Principles and Practice of Screening for Disease*. Geneva: World Health Organization, 1968.

Zander LI. Practising prevention: making a start. *BMJ* 1982;**284**:1241–2.

www.cancerhelp.org.uk/help/default.asp?page=3293

Further reading

Department of Health. *Breast Awareness Policy*. London: DH. Available at: www. cancerscreening.nhs.uk/breastscreen/breastawareness.html (accessed 2008).

7 Developmental milestones, immunisation and travel advice

This chapter relates to curriculum statements 5 and 16 (Healthy people and Travel advice)

This chapter presents, often in tabular form, basic factual information that may be of help in the Applied Knowledge test (AKT) and the Clinical Skills Assessment (CSA).

Developmental milestones

Some milestones have well-established predictive reliability (e.g. sitting unsupported – 90% at 8 months; using two- to three-word combinations – 90% at 24 months). Others have a wide range and may follow a particular pattern in families. There are a plethora of milestones and it is not practical to learn them all – a shortened guide to key milestones is enough for the exam (Table 7.1).

Developmental red flags (Table 7.2)

Developmental red flags are useful for identifying severe developmental problems. Although milestones indicate the normal age of achieving a certain skill, the wide range of variability means that a delay may not be significant. The developmental red flags identify significant delay by identifying the time by which 90% of children would normally have achieved specific milestones.

(Wilson Frankenburg et al. 1992)

Childhood immunisations

Types of vaccine
1. Toxoids, e.g. diphtheria, tetanus
2. Inactivated vaccines, e.g. pertussis, typhoid, anthrax and rabies
3. Live vaccines – MMR BOY (**m**easles, **m**umps, **r**ubella; **B**CG, **o**ral polio, **y**ellow fever). Note that live polio vaccine has now been replaced with killed vaccine.

Notes for the MRCGP: A curriculum based guide to the AKT, CSA and WBPA, 4th edition. By K. Palmer and N. Boeckx. Published 2010 by Blackwell Publishing, ISBN: 978-1-4051-5724-7.

Table 7.1 Shortened milestone guide

Age	Gross motor	Language and hearing	Fine motor and vision	Social
6 weeks	Holds head in a sitting position	–	Follows moving people with eyes	Smiles
3 months	Lifts head off surface	Vocalises	–	–
6 months	Sits supported	–	Hand transfer	Laughs
9 months	Crawls	Babbles (baba, mama)	9–10m pincer grip	Plays peak-a-boo
12 months	Walks	First word by 1 year	Bangs objects together.	Anxious around strangers (9–12 months)
18 months	–	–	Builds towers two to three cubes high	Self-feeds with spoon
2 years	–	Two-word sentence by 2 years	–	Drinks from a cup
3 years	–	–	Draws a circle	Plays with other children
5 years	Hops on one foot	–	Draws a triangle	Has friends

Table 7.2 Developmental red flags

Time (months)	Developmental red flag
2	Absent smile, fails to vocalise
4	Persistent fist clenching, no laugh
6	Fails to localize voice, head lag
9	Fails to sit unsupported, fails to say mama or dada non-specifically
12	Fails to stand alone for 2 seconds
15	Fails to walk alone
18	Fewer than 20 words, fails to scribble
24	Fails to kick a ball

Spacing and timing of immunisations

At birth there is some passive immunity acquired when maternal antibodies cross the placenta. At the same time the baby's own immune system is immature, so babies are not immunised at birth. (An exception is BCG (bacille Calmette–Guèrin) immunisation given when a close household member has tuberculosis.)

By 6 months passive immunity is lost and host immunity is in the ascendance. Somewhere in between these two dates the first immunisations are given, representing a compromise whereby maximum effect from immunisation is traded against the increasing vulnerability to infection as

Table 7.3 New immunisation schedule (2007)

Time	Vaccine type
2 months	5 in 1 pneumococcal
3 months	5 in 1 meningitis C
4 months	5 in 1
	Meningitis C
	Pneumococcal
12 months	*Haemophilus influenzae* type b (Hib)
	Meningitis C
13 months	MMR (measles, mumps, rubella)
	Pneumococcal
Pre-school (3–5 years)	5 in 1 (no Hib)
	MMR
12–13	HPU (girls only)
13–18	3 in 1 (tetanus diptheria, inactivated polio)

passive immunity wanes. Pertussis antibody (an IgM antibody) is too large to cross the placenta, so young un-immunised infants are particularly prone to this infection. Measles antibodies are slower to be catabolised and the longer duration of immunity allows immunisation to be deferred.

Childhood immunisation schedule

A new immunisation schedule was introduced in 2007 (Table 7.3). The main changes are the introduction of pneumococcal immunisation, meningitis C (1999) and a new five in one vaccine to replace the previous five in one. Polio has been replaced by killed vaccine because its prevalence worldwide is extremely low and killed vaccine is safer. Whole-cell pertussis vaccine has been replaced with acellular vaccine because it is as effective but with fewer side effects (fever, pain) (Bedford and Elliman 2004). The new vaccines no longer use a mercury preservative.

Components of the five in one vaccine (diphtheria, tetanus, acellular pertussis, inactivated polio and *Haemophilus influenzae* type b or Hib).

Incomplete courses

In general, live vaccines have a prolonged duration of protection because they are more antigenic, and so booster doses are less important.

Incomplete courses sometimes cause confusion. Generally speaking:

1. If only one dose is given, a further two doses with a month's gap between them will complete the course.
2. If two doses have been given, the third will still be effective if given within 12 months of the second.

Contraindications to live vaccines

1. Acute febrile illness
2. Pregnancy
3. Within 3 weeks of another live vaccine (except in emergency immunisation programmes)
4. Immunosuppression (e.g. immunodeficiency states, malignancy, cytotoxic treatment, radiotherapy, steroids).

Note that being human immunodeficiency virus (HIV) positive is not a contraindication to measles, mumps, rubella and polio (but yellow fever and BCG should not be given). There are few absolute contraindications to killed vaccine other than a reaction to previous doses. Patients with a history of anaphylactic reaction to egg should not receive influenza of yellow fever vaccines (other than under controlled conditions supervised by a specialist).

Points of importance
Most vaccines can cause local reactions and mild fever. These reactions are short lived (<24h) and should be managed with simple analgesia and reassurance.

Tetanus
A total of five doses is considered adequate to provide lifelong immunity. Rarely a hypersensitivity response occurs when injections are too frequent.

BCG
No longer routine. For high-risk individuals only (e.g. for babies with parents/grandparents from countries of increased risk). Sometimes causes local reactions, including discharging skin ulcers and subcutaneous abscess formation. Contraindicated when there is local sepsis.

Measles, mumps and rubella (MMR)
The MMR vaccine is regarded as safe (Demicheli et al. 2005) and concerns regarding a link between MMR and autism (the Dr Wakefield fiasco) have been widely discredited (as has a link between MMR and Crohn's disease – Seagroatt 2005). Localised reactions are mild and resolve within 1 week. Much damage was caused by the MMR scare. Due to reduced uptake of immunisation and the lowered levels of herd immunity, there has been a rise in the number of cases of measles. There is less evidence for the safety of single vaccines than that of the combined vaccine.

Infectivity periods
These are shown in Table 7.4.

Table 7.4 Infectivity periods

Disease	Infectivity period
Scarlet fever	10–21 days after rash onset (but only 1 day if penicillin given)
Chickenpox	A few days before the rash first appears and upto 6 days after
Measles	From onset of prodromal illness to 4 days after the rash onset
Mumps	3 days before salivary swelling to 7 days after
Whooping cough	7 days after exposure to 3 weeks after onset of symptoms (but only 7 days if antibiotics given)
Rubella	7 days before onset of rash to 4 days after

Table 7.5 Interval between disease onset and rash

Disease	Interval in days
Scarlet fever	1–2
Chickenpox	0–2
Measles	3–5
Rubella	0–2
Typhoid	7–14

Interval between disease onset and rash

These are shown in Table 7.5.

Influenza and pneumococcal immunisation

Influenza and pneumococcal immunisation should also be offered to all patients over 65 and those under 65 in an at-risk group. At-risk groups are the immunocompromised and patients with chronic disease (lung, liver, heart, renal), although some other minority groups are not listed here. In addition the influenza vaccine is offered to those in residential homes and nursing homes, and carers and NHS employees. Influenza vaccine is given annually. Pneumococcal vaccine is a single dose course.

Immunisation for foreign travel and general travel advice

Recommendations

This is an area of the MRCGP that the RCGP have said candidates are scoring poorly on. Immunisation schedules depend on the countries being visited, the degree of risk of contracting the disease and the amount of time left before travel. Ideally travellers should consult at least 8 weeks before the date of departure to ensure enough time for immunisation if required. Candidates should have a general idea of which vaccines are necessary in the different world regions, immunisation schedules and which vaccines are charged for (see Table 7.6). As recommendations change from time to time, it is important to keep abreast of the changes. An excellent online resource is www.nathnac.org (the National Travel Health Network and Centre). *MIMS* also has a good table for travel vaccines and is regularly updated.

Do I have to pay?

The following travel vaccines are available without charge under the NHS:
- typhoid
- hepatitis A
- polio.

The following are charged for as a private prescription:
- yellow fever
- meningococcal meningitis
- Japanese and tick-borne encephalitis
- hepatitis B

Table 7.6 The common travel vaccines and regional risk of infection

Disease and schedule	Regions primarily affected	Comments
Typhoid fever Single dose At least 4 weeks before travel	Developing world, particularly the Indian subcontinent	Mainly transmitted through contaminated water or food (avoidable)
Tetanus If 5 doses nil further	Worldwide	Treatment for a suspected tetanus wound may be difficult in some developing countries – in this case a further booster may be offered before travel
Hepatitis A Single dose 2 weeks before travel[a]	Worldwide	Immunisation is recommended outside western Europe, North America and Australasia
Hepatitis B 0, 1, 2 months (rapid schedule)	High-prevalence regions include sub-Saharan Africa, most of Asia and the Pacific islands Intermediate-prevalence regions include the Amazon, southern parts of central and eastern Europe, the Middle East and the Indian subcontinent Low-prevalence regions include most of western Europe and North America	The risk of hepatitis B for tourists is considered to be low. The risk increases with, for example, unprotected sexual intercourse, receiving blood transfusions in countries that do not screen donated blood, sharing needles, working in medical settings, receiving injections or body piercing
Yellow fever Single dose 10 days before travel	Sub-Saharan Africa and tropical South America (including Paraguay and certain areas of Argentina and Brazil)	An International Certificate of Vaccination or Prophylaxis (ICVP) is a condition of entry for some countries
Meningococcal meningitis Single dose 3 weeks before travel	Worldwide, but some strains (especially A) are much more common outside the UK	Saudi Arabia requires proof of immunisation with a quadrivalent vaccine (ACWY vax) for visitors arriving for the Hajj (Mecca) and Umrah pilgrimages, or for seasonal working in the Hajj areas
Poliomyelitis Single dose if required[b]	Largely eradicated, but still endemic in some areas – 98% of new cases are from Nigeria, Pakistan and India	Booster doses if travelling to endemic regions

Continued

Table 7.6 *Continued*

Disease and schedule	Regions primarily affected	Comments
Rabies Three doses days 0, 7, 21 Complete the course 7 days before travel	Endemic in most regions of the world. Exceptions include the British Isles, Scandinavia, Japan and Australasia	Treatment for a suspected rabies wound may be difficult in some developing countries
Japanese encephalitis Three doses day 0, 7, 28 Complete the course 10 days before travel	South-east Asia and the Far East	Risk is highest in rural and agricultural areas, and there may be seasonal variations
Tick borne encephalitis Three doses 0, 3, 1 2 months	Forested areas of western Europe, Scandinavia and countries of the former Soviet Union	Risk is low for short stays. Maximum immunity occurs 1 week after dose 2
Cholera Two doses 6 weeks apart Complete course 7d before travel	Endemic in developing countries, especially the Indian subcontinent, Africa, the Far East and South America	Transmitted through contaminated water or food (avoidable). An oral vaccine is now available

www.nathnac.org; National Travel Health Network and Centre 2004.

[a]Note that a second dose will provide extended immunity (20 years).

[b]No single vaccines are available so give the three in one formulation.

- rabies
- cholera.

Note that antimalarial medication is also issued as a private script. Table 7.6 gives the common travel vaccines and countries.

Malaria

Malaria is common in Africa, Asia and South America.
1. *General advice*: the standard insect bite avoidance advice is appropriate (use nets, sprays, screens). Also:
    (a) start tablets 1 week before departure and continue for at least 4 (possibly 6) weeks after return
    (b) if you omit any doses, you are taking a risk
    (c) drugs are prophylactic, not curative; furthermore protection is probably only 60–90%, so report fevers within 2 months of return. (Patient UK 2007)
2. *Drugs*: the appropriate choice is not straightforward. Recommendations change frequently, so get up-to-date information from www.nathnac. org. The highest risk areas are the Amazon Basin in South America, Africa south of the Sahara, the Indian subcontinent, Papua New Guinea, Irian Jaya and the Solomon Islands.

Table 7.7 gives information on common antimalarial regimens.

Table 7.7 Common antimalarial regimens

	Weekly cost (£) in 2008
Chloroquine + proguanil (moderate-risk areas)	0.63
Mefloquine (high-risk areas)	1.80
Doxycyline (high-risk areas)	0.60

Medical advice to travellers

Medical contraindications to flight

Physiological problems produced by air flights include:
1. Reduced atmospheric pressure: aircraft cabins are not pressurised to sea level, and cabin pressure drops with ascent until about 7000 feet (2000 m), hence gas trapped in body cavities *expands*.
2. Hypoxia: reduced atmospheric pressure means a reduced partial pressure of oxygen (Po_2). At 6000 feet (1800 m) oxyhaemoglobin is reduced by 3–4% – a small amount if you are healthy, but not if you are an unhealthy hypoxia-sensitive individual.
3. An upset in the normal circadian rhythms (jet lag).

Other problems can arise from the risk of spreading contagious disease in a confined space, and the impossibility of providing anything other than the most basic medical care during travel.

Most of the contraindications can be remembered by applying these principles in a common sense way. Table 7.8 is a simple aide mémoire.

Table 7.8 Contraindications to flying

This problem …	… may exacerbate these conditions
Expansion of gas trapped in body cavities	Asthmatic attack
	Recent middle-ear disease, middle-ear surgery, and sinusitis with catarrh
	Unresolved pneumothorax
	Recent chest surgery (within 3 weeks)
	Recent abdominal surgery (within 10 days)
	Diving (if within 12 h for aqualung divers or 24 h if diving depth is more than 100 feet or 30 m)
Hypoxia	Recent myocardial infarction (within 3–6 weeks)
	Uncontrolled cardiac failure
	Severe anaemia (e.g. haemoglobin <7 g/dl)
	Severe respiratory disease
	Recent cerebrovascular accident (within 3–6 weeks)
	Sickle cell disease
Spread of infection in a confined space	Contagious diseases in their infectivity period
Remoteness from medical care	Recent gastrointestinal haemorrhage
	Pregnancy (after 35 weeks for long flights and after 36 weeks for domestic ones)
	Acute mental illness (unless the patient is escorted and sedation is to hand)

Motion sickness

1. *Who?* One-third of the population, especially children (peak age 10 years).
2. *What?* Various symptoms, including: pallor; cold sweats; nausea and vomiting; malaise; yawning; headaches; drowsiness.
3. *Why?* Probably multifactorial, but a mismatch between motion information from the eyes and vestibular apparatus/proprioceptors is the main stimulus.
4. *Advice?*
   (a) sit children up high, so that they can see out
   (b) provide good ventilation
   (c) provide activities (e.g. games), but no reading
   (d) limit alcohol intake
   (e) if severe, lie down with eyes closed
   (f) choose the most stable part of the vehicle to sit (car – front seat; boat – the middle; plane – between the wings).
5. *Drugs?*
   (a) take preparations 1–2 h before travel (otherwise absorption may be impaired)
   (b) either an anticholinergic or antihistamine; anticholinergics are very effective, but associated with more side effects; the antihistamines offer a choice in the duration of action (e.g. cyclizine – short acting; promethazine – once-daily preparation). Tailor the time course of the drug to the duration of travel.

Jet lag

1. *What?* An upset in the circadian rhythms (e.g. sleep cycle, hunger pattern, bowel and urinary habits). Occurs if the time difference is greater than 5 h. *Less* marked when the day *lengthens* (i.e. going westwards).
2. *Advice?*
   (a) avoid unnecessary stress (e.g. arrive in good time for flight)
   (b) avoid smoking, food and alcohol
   (c) maintain a good fluid intake (non-diuretic beverages)
   (d) sleep on the plane if you can
   (e) allow an easy first 24 h to adjust after arrival. Remember that performance may be impaired for a week after travel (businessmen and -women beware!).

Food hygiene

1. *The problem*: food-borne and water-borne infections, e.g.:
   (a) contaminated drinking water may transmit *Escherichia coli*, *Shigella* spp., cholera, typhoid, hepatitis A, amoebic dysentery or giardiasis
   (b) poultry are notorious sources of *Campylobacter* and *Salmonella* spp.
   (c) shellfish may transmit typhoid
   (d) unpasteurised milk is a possible source of tuberculosis, brucellosis and Q fever.
2. *Advice?*
   (a) boil drinking water or chlorinate it (remember – all water)
   (b) avoid unpasteurised milk
   (c) do not buy food or ice-cream from street vendors
   (d) avoid salads and unpeeled fruit and vegetables
   (e) eat only food that has been recently cooked (and is hot and steaming)
   (f) be wary of seafood, especially shellfish.

Traveller's diarrhoea

1. *Where?* Worldwide, but most commonly in Africa and Asia.
2. *What?* Seventy per cent of cases are due to enterotoxic *E. coli* strains; other culprits include *Campylobacter* sp., rotavirus, *Salmonella*, *Shigella*, *Amoeba* and *Giardia* spp. Symptoms, which usually only last a few days, include:
   (a) Nausea and vomiting
   (b) colic
   (c) watery diarrhoea.
3. *Drugs?*
   (a) *Prophylactic antibiotics* have been shown to be beneficial but consideration of possible side effects and drug resistance suggests they are best reserved for elderly, infirmed people and high-risk cases.
   (b) *In treatment.* Imodium/lomotil will reduce stool frequency and abdominal pain, and Septrin/trimethoprim reduces symptoms considerably if taken early. The mainstay of treatment, however, is fluid replacement. Electrolyte mixtures are very useful.
   (c) *medical advice* may be needed in severe cases (prostration, severe vomiting, fever and blood per rectum) and for very young children.

AKT questions

Q1

Developmental milestones. Match the skills to the appropriate age group. Each option may be used once, more than once or not at all.

a 6 weeks

b 3 months

c 6 months

d 9 months

e. 12 months

f 18 months

g 2 years

1. Builds a tower two to three cubes high
2. Forms two-word sentences
3. Sits supported
4. Crawls
5. Smiles

Q2

The following immunisations form part of the UK routine childhood immunisation schedule (either as a single or as a combined vaccine) EXCEPT. Select ONE option only:

a BCG

b Diphtheria

c Polio

d Measles

e Pneumococcal

Q3

Choose the correct statement. Select ONE option only:

a Five in one vaccinates against *Haemophilus influenzae* type b, diphtheria, tetanus, polio and pneumococcal.

b Pneumococcal vaccine is given at 2, 4 and 6 months.

c MMR is associated with Crohn's disease and autism.

d Meningitis C vaccine is given at 3, 4 and 12 months.

e A history of asthma is a contraindication to the five in one vaccine.

Q4

Live vaccines. All are true EXCEPT. Select ONE option only:

a Are contraindicated in acute febrile illness

b Include yellow fever

c Have been removed from the childhood immunisation schedule and replaced by inactivated vaccine

d Should be avoided in pregnancy

e Should not be administered with 3 weeks of another live vaccine

Q5

Infective disease. Identify the incorrect statement. Select ONE option only:
a   Chickenpox is no longer infective 1 week after the onset of the rash.
b   Chickenpox in pregnancy is a risk for congenital abnormality.
c   Pregnant women uncertain of past exposure to chickenpox who are exposed to it should have antibody testing and receive immunoglobulin if antibody positive.
d   The paediatricians should be contacted so that immunoglobulin can be given to a baby whose mother develops chickenpox 7 days before or 28 days after delivery.
e   Children with chickenpox should be excluded from school for 5 days from the onset of the rash.

Q6

Which of the following travel vaccines is normally issued on an NHS script without charge. Select ONE option only:
a   Yellow fever
b   Meningitis C
c   Hepatitis B
d   Rabies
e   Hepatitis A

Q7

Choose the incorrect statement. Select ONE option only:
a   Hepatitis B is given to those working in medical settings abroad.
b   Yellow fever is given as a single dose given at least 10 days before travel
c   Rabies is endemic in most regions of the world.
d   Cholera is a single dose vaccine given at least 1 week before travel
e   Japanese encephalitis vaccine should be given to those travelling to south-east Asia and the Far East.

Q8

Which of the following is a recommended regimen for travellers to high-risk areas of malaria. Select ONE option only:
a   Chloroquine and proguanil 1 week before travel and 4 weeks after return.
b   Pyrimethamine once weekly started on the day of travel and continued 2 weeks after return.
c   Doxycycline started 2 days before travel and continued for 4 weeks after return.
d   Mefloquine 1 week before travel and continued 4 weeks after return
e   Proguanil 1 week before travel and continued 6 weeks after return.

Q9

The following are contraindications to flying EXCEPT. Select ONE option only:
a   Chest surgery 2 weeks previously
b   Myocardial infarction 2 weeks previously

c Chickenpox rash onset 2 days ago
d Pregnancy – 37 weeks
e Grommets

Q10
The following are common causes of travellers' diarrhoea EXCEPT. Select ONE option only:
a *Bacillus cereus*
b *Campylobacter* sp.
c *Entamoeba histolytica*
d *Shigella* sp.
e *Giardia* sp.

Answers

Q1
1. f
2. g
3. c
4. d
5. a

Q2 a
BCG is no longer routine as part of the UK schedule. It is still given to those considered at high risk.

Q3 d
Pneumococcal vaccine is given at 2, 4 and 13 months. No link has been shown between MMR and autism or Crohn's disease.

Q4 c
Although live polio has been removed and replaced with inactivated vaccine, the MMR vaccine is live and remains part of the schedule.

Q5 c
You should receive immunoglobulin if antibody negative indicating no immunity from past exposure– not positive. Note that when a pregnant woman contracts chickenpox near birth neonates are at risk of severe complications because they have not developed passive immunity.

Q6 e

Q7 d
Cholera vaccine is a two-dose vaccine given 6 weeks apart.

Q8 c

Q9 e

Grommets allow free movement of air to the middle ear so there is no danger of pressure differences causing pain or damage.

Q10 a

Bacillus cereus is a cause of food poisoning, typically in reheated rice. It is not associated with travellers' diarrhoea.

References

Bedford H, Elliman D. Misconceptions about the new combination vaccine: Pentavalent vaccine is better in many ways. *BMJ* 2004;**329**:411–12.

Demicheli V, Jefferson T, Rivetti A, Price D. Vaccines for measles, mumps and rubella in children. *Cochrane Database Syst Rev* 2005;**4**:CD004407.

Seagroatt V. MMR vaccine and Crohn's disease: ecological study of hospital admissions in England, 1991 to 2002. *BMJ* 2005;**330**:1120–1.

Patient UK. Malaria prophylaxis. *HPA Guidelines for Malaria Prevention*. National Travel Health Network and Centre, 2007 www.nathnac.org.

Wilson Frankenburg W, Dodds J, Archer P, Shapiro H, Bresnick B. The Denver II: A major revision and restandardization of the Denver Developmental Screening Test. *Pediatrics* 1992;**89**:91–7.

8 Chronic disease management, QOFs and urgent referral

This chapter relates to the following clinical curriculum statements:
- Care of acutely ill people (7)
- Care of people with cancer and palliative care (12)
- Care of people with mental health problems (13)
- Cardiovascular problems (15.1)
- Digestive problems (15.2)
- Metabolic problems (15.6)
- Neurological problems (15.7)
- Respiratory problems (15.8).

The current evidence for chronic disease management in major Quality Outcome Framework (QOF) areas is summarised here. QOF areas not included and summaries of other important chronic disease areas e.g. chronic kidney disease are to be found in the following chapter. This is core GP knowledge and the basis for MRCGP AKT questions and CSA cases.

Cardiovascular disease (CVD)

Coronary heart disease (CHD) is the most common cause of death in the UK. The government set a target and action plan in 2000 to cut mortality rates by 20% (National Service Framework for CHD, Department of Health, 2000). The principles are still up to date today and can be broadly divided into primary and secondary prevention strategies. CHD primary preventive involves addressing cardiovascular risk factors in the population. Secondary prevention measures are summarised later under Coronary heart disease.

CVD risk
The Joint British Societies' guideline (JBS2) is the established tool of choice for cardiovascular risk assessment. The risk assessment requires knowledge of a patient's age, sex, smoking status, systolic blood pressure, total cholesterol (TC):high-density lipoprotein (HDL) ratio, triglyceride level and the presence of left ventricular hypertrophy (LVH). JBS2 calculates risk based on a study in Framingham, USA, which analysed risk factors to create a

Notes for the MRCGP: A curriculum based guide to the AKT, CSA and WBPA, 4th edition.
By K. Palmer and N. Boeckx. Published 2010 by Blackwell Publishing,
ISBN: 978-1-4051-5724-7.

model for predicting coronary heart disease. The JBS2 score is a modified version that also includes risk of other vascular disease, e.g. stroke, transient ischaemic attack (TIA) and peripheral vascular disease.

QRISK2 is an alternative cardiovascular risk score developed for the UK using UK GP data based on 2.3 million registered UK general practice patients. It includes additional CVD risk factors (social deprivation score, type 2 diabetes, treated hypertension, rheumatoid arthritis, renal disease and atrial fibrillation). QRISK2 has a closer association between predicted and observed risk than the Framingham-based models, i.e. it seems better at predicting risk in a UK population (Hippisley-Cox et al. 2008). This score may supersede the JBS2 risk score and has been included in draft NICE (National Institute for Health and Clinical Excellence) guidance.

Primary prevention of CVD is recommended in patients with a 10-year risk of >20%. A JBS2 calculator is available online at www.patient.co.uk and currently risk tables are included in the back of the *British National Formulary* (BNF).

Hypertension
The problem
Hypertension is common affecting 30% (National Centre for Social Research 2004) of the UK adult population. It is largely asymptomatic and a significant cardiovascular risk factor. CVD is the number one cause of death in the UK. Table 8.1 gives the QOF for Hypertension.

When to start treatment (Table 8.2)
- Sustained systolic >160 or diastolic >100 or
- Sustained systolic >140, diastolic >90 with:
  - ➤ CVD risk >20% or
  - ➤ diabetes or
  - ➤ target organ damage (i.e. ECG evidence of LVH, hypertensive retinopathy, renal impairment, microalbuminuria).

Initial investigations in general practice (to look for target organ damage and assess cardiovascular risk)
- Urinalysis for protein/blood
- Glucose, U&Es/eGFR (urea and electrolytes/estimated glomerular filtration rate), cholesterol (total and HDL)
- ECG for LVH.

Treatment guidelines (NICE 2006)
Antihypertensives
A = ACE inhibitor
B = β blockers
C = calcium channel blocker
D = diuretic
Meta-analyses confirm that, in general, the main determinant of benefit from BP-lowering drugs is the achieved BP, rather than the choice of antihypertensive therapy (Blood Pressure Lowering Treatment Trialists' Collaboration [BPLTTC] 2003; NICE 2006). However, specific groups of

Table 8.1 Quality Outcome Framework (QOF) for hypertension

Indicator	Evidence
The practice can produce a *register* of patients with established hypertension	A disease register is common to all the QOF areas – without one it is not possible to undertake planned systematic care for patients
The percentage of people diagnosed with hypertension after 1 April 2009 who are given lifestyle advice in the last 15 months for: increasing physical activity, smoking cessation, alcohol consumption and healthy diet	There is grade A evidence summarised in the NICE 2006 guidance for reduction in cardiovascular risk associated with lifestyle changes (NICE, *Hypertension: Management of hypertension in adults in primary care*, 2006)
The percentage of patients with a new diagnosis of hypertension without established cardiovascular disease who have had a face-to-face *cardiovascular risk assessment* within 3 months of diagnosis	Cardiovascular risk calculation helps to provide an informed decision on the risk–benefit ratio of starting treatment. Treatment is recommended for those with a 10-year risk score above 20% (NICE 2006)
The percentage of patients with hypertension whose notes record *smoking status* at least once since diagnosis The percentage of patients with hypertension who smoke, whose notes contain a record that *smoking cessation advice* or referral to a specialist service, if available, has been offered at least once The percentage of patients with hypertension in whom there is a record of the BP in the past 9 months	Smoking is an established risk factor for cardiovascular and other diseases
The percentage of patients with hypertension in whom the last BP (measured in the last 9 months) is 150/90 or less	Hypertension Optimal Treatment trial (Hansson et al. *Lancet* 1998) Lowest CVD risk found at systolic BP of 139 and diastolic BP 83. Patients with diabetes benefited from lower values (diastolic <80)

BP, blood pressure; CVD, cardiovascular disease; QOF, Quality Outcome Framework.

Table 8.2 Treatment targets

	Optimal treatment (NICE 2006)	QOF audit standards
BP target	140/90[a]	(150/90)
Diabetic BP target	140/80[b]	(145/85)
Diabetic nephropathy/CRF	135/75[c]	

[a]HOT trial (Hansson et al. *Lancet* 1998;**351**:1755–62) found 140/85 as the optimal treatment level.
[b]Type 2 diabetes (type 1 target is still lower at 135/85).
[c]Type 2 diabetes target.

patients respond better to specific agents. The agents ABCD fall into two modes of action: ACE (angiotensin-converting enzyme) and β blockers act primarily to suppress renin levels that are already low in African–Caribbean and older patients. Calcium and diuretics promote vasodilatation and salt excretion. African–Caribbean and older patients have salt-sensitive hypertension. Calcium channel blockers and β blockers are first-line treatments for women of childbearing age. The HYVET (Hypertension in the Very Elderly Trial – Beckett et al. 2008) and BPLTTC (2008) have confirmed the benefit of treating hypertension in older people – with a number needed to treat (NNT) of 40 to prevent one death in a 2-year period in HYVET.

The stepwise approach to management of hypertension
(Proceed to the next step if target blood pressure is not achieved.)

Step 1
- Age <55: A (ACE inhibitors and ACE 2 receptor blockers (A2RBs) have a similar side-effect profile except that ACE can cause a persistent cough. ACE inhibitors are the first-line choice and A2RBs the second line if cough occurs)
- Age >55 or African–Caribbean individuals: C or D

Step 2
- A + C OR A + D

Step 3
- A + C + D

Step 4
- Other diuretics, α blockers or β blockers.

Lifestyle measures
All hypertensive and borderline hypertensive patients:
- Exercise (30 min a day)
- Weight loss (one in five of the UK population is obese)
- Smoking cessation: low salt diet
- Alcohol: <21 units a week
- Dietary modification: low saturated fat intake, high fruit and vegetable diet.

Primary prevention (CVD risk >20%)
- A statin for all.

Secondary prevention
- Add aspirin and a statin for all.

Landmark studies in hypertension
HOT (Hypertension Optimal Treatment)
Publication: Hansson et al. *Lancet* 1998;**351**:1755–62
Question posed: How much should we lower blood pressure?
Findings: 19 000 patients. Lowest CVD risk found at SBP of 139 and DBP 83. People with diabetes benefited from lower values (diastolic <80).
Key point: evidence for optimal BP targets of 140/85.

ASCOT (Anglo Scandinavian Cardiac Outcomes Trial)

Publication: Dahlöf et al. *Lancet* 2005;366:895–906

Question posed: Are newer antihypertensive combinations more effective? (Is amlodipine plus perindopril more effective than atenolol plus bendroflumethiazide?)

Findings: 19 000 patients. Reduced cardiovascular mortality in the calcium channel blocker plus ACE inhibitor group (23% reduced risk of stroke). This may be due to the lower BP achieved by the ACE inhibitor/calcium channel blocker group. Increased onset of diabetes in the β blocker/ thiazide group.

Key points:

- Higher doses of β blockers than routinely prescribed were used (100 mg), and may explain the increased incidence of diabetes without improving BP lowering.
- This study contributed to the removal of β blockers as a first-line antihypertensive agent. Thiazides remain a first-line choice – see ALLHAT study (note that β blockers remain appropriate first-line agents in specific patient groups, e.g. coronary heart disease).

ALLHAT (Antihypertensive and Lipid Lowering to Prevent Heart Attack Trial)

Publication: The ALLHAT Officers and Coordinators for the ALLHAT Collaborative Research Group *JAMA* 2002

Question posed: Which antihypertensive is most effective (ACE, calcium channel blocker, diuretic or doxazosin)?

Findings: 42 000 patients. Largest hypertension trial to date. All patients aged over 55 with a large diabetic and African–Caribbean component. BP lowering best in the thiazide diuretic group. Prevention of myocardial infarction similar in all groups except doxazosin. ACE inhibitors less effective in the African–Caribbean population than calcium channel blocker or thiazide.

Key points:

- Evidence suggests that the best choice of antihypertensive varies by race and age.
- The study investigators conclude that thiazide-type diuretics should be the initial treatment of hypertension in most patients requiring drug therapy (including those with type 2 diabetes).
- Doxazosin was associated with increased risk of death from heart failure.

BP Lowering Treatment Trial Collaboration

Publication: BPLTTC *Lancet* 2003

Question posed: Which antihypertensive is most effective (meta-analysis)?

Findings: 29 trials. ABCD agents equally effective at reducing cardiovascular events.

Key point: ABCD agents are the main antihypertensive choices and are equally efficacious. Choice is determined by side effects of the agents and efficacy in subgroups, e.g. age and race dependent (see ALLHAT).

Coronary heart disease

The secondary prevention measures and evidence base are outlined in the QOF framework and notes in Table 8.3 (SIGN 2007).

Cardiovascular disease and antiplatelets

The evidence for benefit of 75mg daily aspirin in established cardiovascular disease is very strong (Stott 1994). Until recently aspirin also had a role in the management of patients with hypertension, diabetes or a cardiovascular risk score of >20% without established heart disease. However, a meta-analysis in the *British Medical Journal* (Antithrombotic Trialists' Collaboration 2002) brought this into question. A more recent trial (the prevention of progression of arterial disease and diabetes or POPADAD – Belch et al. 2008) looking specifically at primary prevention in a high-risk group has shown no benefit for the use of aspirin in primary prevention. A Cochrane 2009 review (Lip and Felmeden 2004) looking at aspirin for primary prevention in patients with hypertension concurs that there is no benefit.

Clopidogrel is an alternative antiplatelet with a reduced risk of gastrointestinal (GI) bleeding (Hallas et al. 2006) of 1.8 for aspirin and 1.1 for clopidogrel. However, combining aspirin with a proton pump inhibitor (PPI) has shown an even lower risk of GI bleed than clopidogrel and is the recommended option for patients at increased risk of GI bleeding (Francis et al. 2005, NICE 2007).

Combinations of antiplatelets are recommended in two situations:

1. 2 years post CVA/TIA – aspirin + dipyridamole M/R (see Stroke below)
2. 1 year post-coronary stenting or acute coronary syndrome – aspirin + clopidogrel (CURE 2001).

MEMORY BOX: Antiplatelets
- Aspirin is no longer recommended for the primary prevention of cardiovascular disease
- Aspirin plus a PPI is safer than clopidogrel for patients at risk of a GI bleed
- The indications for anti-platelets in combination are post stroke and post stent

---

Lipids – who to treat and how low to go (NICE 2008a)
Who to treat
- >40 years old and a CVD 10-year risk score of >20%
- Total cholesterol:HDL ratio >6
- Those with type 1 + 2 diabetes age>40, familial hyperlipidaemias, BP >160/100, secondary prevention.

All patients requiring lipid therapy should have advice on lifestyle changes (see hypertension section for summary of lifestyle advice).

How low to go
Primary prevention
- 'Fire and forget' strategy: there is no lipid target set by NICE for primary prevention. Hence after starting the statin there is no need to check cholesterol levels. All patients on statins require LFT monitoring at 3 and

Table 8.3 Quality Outcome Framework (QOF) for coronary heart disease (CHD) secondary prevention

Indicator	Evidence
The practice can produce a register of patients with CHD	See the first point in the first QOF summary table
The percentage of patients with newly diagnosed angina (diagnosed after 1 April 2003) who are referred for exercise testing and/or specialist assessment	Confirmation of diagnosis and a prognostic indicator (Antiplatelet Trialists' Collaboration *BMJ* 1994;**308**) 75% with IHD test positive. A stronger positive result (downsloping ST) is a more significant marker of disease
The percentage of patients with CHD whose notes record smoking status in the past 15 months, except those who have never smoked, where smoking status need be recorded only once since diagnosis The percentage of patients with coronary heart disease who smoke, whose notes contain a record that smoking cessation advice or referral to a specialist service, where available, has been offered within the last 15 months	Cook et al. *Lancet* 1986;**ii**: 1376–80 Cigarette smoking approximately doubles the risk of morbidity and mortality from IHD compared with those who have never smoked. Risk is dependent upon duration and intensity of smoking history
The percentage of patients with CHD whose notes have a record of BP in the previous 15 months The percentage of patients with CHD in whom the last BP reading (measured in the last 15 months) is 150/90 or less	*Heart* 2005;(suppl 5):v1–52 (review primary and secondary prevention) Lowest CVD risk in normotensive patients Hypertension Optimal Treatment Trial (Hansson et al. *Lancet* 1998) (Primary prevention) Lowest CVD risk found at SBP 139 and DBP 83. Patients with diabetes benefited from lower values (DBP <80)
The percentage of patients with CHD whose notes have a record of total cholesterol in the previous 15 months The percentage of patients with CHD whose last measured total cholesterol (measured in last 15 months) is 5 mmol/l or less	4S study 1994 *Lancet* Simvastatin reduced mortality in the treatment group by 30% CARE study *N Engl J Med* 1996 Pravastatin prevents coronary events in patients with average cholesterol levels
The percentage of patients with CHD with a record in the last 15 months that aspirin, an alternative anti-platelet therapy, or an anticoagulant is being taken (unless a contraindication or side effects are recorded)	Antiplatelet Trialists' Collaboration *BMJ* 1994;**308** (meta-analyses) Reduction in CV events and all cause mortality in patients with established CVD risk
The percentage of patients with CHD who are currently treated with a β blocker (unless a contraindication or side effects are recorded)	ISIS-1: *Lancet* 1986;**ii**:57–66; CAPRICORN: Dargie *Lancet* 2001;**357**:1385–90 Improved survival on β blocker in patients with established CHD

Table 8.3 *Continued*

Indicator	Evidence
The percentage of patients with a history of myocardial infarction (diagnosed after 1 April 2003) who are currently treated with an ACE inhibitor (or α_2 antagonists)	SAVE trial: *N Engl J Med* 1992 – secondary prevention HOPE study: *N Engl J Med* 2000 – primary prevention Reduced CV events on ACE inhibitor
The percentage of patients with CHD who have a record of influenza immunisation in the preceding 1 September to 31 March	Influenza infection is associated with poorer outcomes in patients with chronic disease Department of Health. *The Green Book*, 2009

ACE, angiotensin-converting enzyme; CVD, cardiovascular disease; DBP, diastolic blood pressure; IHD, ischaemic heart disease; SBP, systolic blood pressure.

12 months. If normal further LFT monitoring is not required. Stop the statin if the alanine transaminase (ALT) rises to >3 × the upper limit of the reference range.

Secondary prevention
- Aim for a total cholesterol of 4 mmol/l (and a low-density lipoprotein [LDL]-cholesterol of <2 mmol/l, or a 25% reduction in total cholesterol and 30% reduction in LDL-cholesterol, whichever results in the lowest number) (Joint British Societies 2005; NICE 2008a).
- Simvastatin 40 mg is first-line treatment. Increase dose to 80 mg if target is not achieved. If still not achieving target consider swapping to atorvastatin or rosuvastatin or adding other lipid-lowering agents, e.g. ezetimibe, fibrates, nicotinic acid (which raises HDL-cholesterol and reduces triglycerides), and omega-3 fish oil supplements (reduce triglycerides).

How low to go
- Aim for a total cholesterol of 4 mmol/l (and a LDL-cholesterol of <2 mmol/l, or a 25% reduction in total cholesterol and 30% reduction in LDL-cholesterol, whichever results in the lowest number (Joint British Societies 2005).

Landmark studies in hyperlipidaemia
HPS (Heart Protection Study)
Publication: Collins et al. 2002
Question posed: Statins for primary prevention of CHD?
Findings: 20 000 patients. Cholesterol lowering in patients with risk factors but no established CHD showed significant risk reduction in all groups.
Key points:
- Largest primary prevention study of cholesterol lowering
- Risk of myocardial infarction (MI) and stroke reduced by a third.

WOSCOPS (West Of Scotland Coronary Prevention Study)
Publication: Shepherd et al. 1995
Question posed: Statins for primary prevention of CHD?
Findings: 7000 patients. Cholesterol lowering in patients with total cholesterol >6 as primary prevention reduced CHD events.
Key points:
- Reduction in coronary events by 30%
- Reduction in mortality by 20%.

4S (Scandinavian Simvastatin Survival Study)
Publication: Scandinavian Simvastatin Survival Study Group 1994
Question posed: Statins for secondary prevention of CHD?
Findings: 4444 patients. Cholesterol lowering in patients with established CHD and moderate hyperlipidaemia showed significant risk reduction in all groups.
Key points:
- Secondary prevention study of cholesterol lowering
- Reduced mortality by 30%.

REVERSAL (Reversing Atherosclerosis with Aggressive Lipid Lowering)
Publication: Nicholls et al. 2005
Question posed: How low should we go?
Findings: 502 patients. Aggressive lipid lowering significantly slowed the progression of atheroma compared with moderate lipid lowering.
Key point: the lower the better (see also the PROVE IT study: Cannon et al. *N Engl J Med* 2004;**350**:1495–504).

Heart failure
In the UK 900 000 people have heart failure, and it is estimated that an equal number of pre-symptomatic individuals are undiagnosed). Ischaemic heart disease (IHD) is the most common cause. Survival rates are poor, being similar to those of colon cancer (approximately 40% die within the first year of diagnosis – London Heart Failure study 2002 – see www.heartstats.org/datapage.asp?id=752). An average GP will manage around 30 cases with 10 new cases a year (NICE 2003). Table 8.4 shows the relationship between CHD and left ventricular dysfunction.

Assessment of heart failure
Heart failure is characterised by breathlessness, fatigue and signs of fluid retention. Echocardiography is the single most effective tool in the diagnosis of heart failure, but the appropriate use of earlier investigations (electrocardiograph [ECG] and/or B-type natriuretic peptide [BNP] testing) increases the likelihood that patients referred for echocardiography actually have heart failure, and reduces unnecessary referrals (National Prescribing Centre 2008; SIGN 2007).

Table 8.4 Coronary heart disease (CHD) and left ventricular (LV) dysfunction

Left ventricular dysfunction	Evidence
The practice can produce a register of patients with CHD and LV dysfunction	See the first point in the first QOF summary table
The percentage of patients with a diagnosis of CHD and LV dysfunction (diagnosed after 1 April 2003) which has been confirmed by an echocardiogram	Confirmation of diagnosis and investigation of aetiology (SIGN, *Heart Disease Guidelines* 2007)
The percentage of patients with a diagnosis of CHD and LV dysfunction who are currently treated with ACE inhibitors (or α_2 antagonists)	ACE MI Collaborative Group (Flather et al. *Lancet* 2000;**355** – meta-analyses) Reduction in CV mortality rate by >20%
The percentage of patients with a diagnosis of heart failure treated with an ACE inhibitor, who are additionally treated with a β blocker licensed for heart failure (bisoprolol, carvedilol, nebivolol)	COMET (Remme et al. *J Am Coll Cardiol* 2007;**362**); CIBIS-II (*Lancet* 1999;**352**); COPERNICUS (Eichhorn and Bristow. *Curr Control Trials Cardiovasc Med* 2001;**2**) The benefit of β blockers on mortality is not equal between different agents. COMET compared carvedilol and metoprolol – carvedilol had a superior outcome. Prescribing should therefore be limited to those with proven efficacy

CV, cardiovascular; QOF, Quality Outcome Framework.

First-line investigations:
- ECG for LVH
- BNP (if available in your area)
- Refer for echocardiography if either abnormal.

A BNP has a high negative predictive value (96%) when used to investigate patients with a history suggestive of heart failure. A negative result therefore makes the diagnosis of heart failure unlikely (Baughman 2002). Note that it is important to be aware that predictive values differ depending on the prevalence of disease in the population tested, e.g. the prevalence of heart failure is greater in symptomatic patients than in the practice population as a whole, so the negative predictive value, if applied to the practice population, will be much lower. A positive BNP can also provide information about severity of heart failure. A study in 2007 showed that high levels of BNP correlate with increased risk of death and cardiovascular events (März et al. 2007).

Managing heart failure
Treatment in primary care involves addressing lifestyle factors (see Stroke) and using drugs directed at treating heart failure (CHF), with the aim of relieving symptoms, improving quality of life, and reducing morbidity and mortality.

Associated issues that may arise from and/or further aggravate CHF also need to be addressed, e.g. use of non-steroidal anti-inflammatory drugs (NSAIDs).

Which drugs, what benefit, where's the evidence! (National Prescribing Centre 2008)

- ACE inhibitors should be considered in all patients with any degree of CHF, unless specifically contraindicated, because there is consistent evidence that they improve symptoms and life expectancy. ACE inhibitors reduce CV mortality by >20% (Flather et al. 2000).
- β Blockers licensed for use in CHF should also be considered in all patients with any degree of CHF as soon as their condition is stable, unless specifically contraindicated. They have been shown to improve mortality and reduce hospitalisations (Brophy et al. Beta-blockers in congestive heart failure. *Ann Intern Med* 2001;**134**:550–60).
- Diuretics are likely to be required by most patients to control congestive symptoms and fluid retention. There are no large or long-term controlled trials of these in CHF, but clinical experience supports their use. Loop diuretics are generally preferred to thiazide diuretics.
- Treatment options in those who remain symptomatic at this stage include adding in either an aldosterone antagonist (i.e. spironolactone) or an angiotensin-2 receptor antagonist (A2RA) (e.g. candesartan) to the above drugs. There are no data from randomised controlled trials (RCTs) comparing these two approaches.
    - ➤ evidence for spironolactone is mainly derived from a randomised controlled trial (RCT) of patients with symptoms on moderate exertion (New York Heart Association – NYHA III or greater – Table 8.5). The addition of spironolactone reduced both hospitalisations and mortality (Pitt et al. RALES study *N Engl J Med* 1999;**341**:709–17). It was associated with side effects, such as gynaecomastia, and increases in potassium levels, but did not increase overall drug discontinuations.
    - ➤ evidence for A2RAs is weaker in that they reduced hospitalisations but did not reduce mortality.
- Digoxin is recommended as an add-on treatment for patients in sinus rhythm who remain symptomatic despite optimised treatment. However, supporting evidence is limited to its use in patients receiving only ACE inhibitors and diuretics, and there are no direct comparisons with other approaches.

New agents

In the EPHESIS study (Pitt et al. 2003), eplerenone was shown to improve survival by 15% compared with placebo when added to existing medical therapy within 3–14 days of an acute MI in patients with evidence of heart failure. There is no evidence for eplerenone in CHF, but the Scottish Intercollegiate Guidelines Network (SIGN 2007) guideline considers eplerenone as an alternative in patients who experience the side effect of gynaecomastia with spironolactone because it is a more selective aldosterone antagonist and is less likely to cause sexual side effects.

Table 8.5 New York Heart Association classification of heart failure

Class	Definition
1	Symptoms on exercise only
2	Symptoms with ordinary daily activity
3	Symptoms with minimal activity
4	Symptomatic at rest, confined to bed or chair

Treatment with ACE inhibitors, β blockers and diuretics should be optimised in terms of initial doses and titration up to the doses used in clinical trials, where tolerated.

The NYHA classification is a widely used functional assessment of heart failure. The classes directly correspond to prognosis with mortality in the highest class at approximately 50% annual mortality.

Stroke

Stroke is defined by the World Health Organization (WHO) as rapidly developing clinical signs of focal (or global in case of coma) disturbance of cerebral function lasting more than 24 hours (in TIA features resolve in <24 h). It is the third most common cause of death in the UK, accounting for over 56 000 deaths in England and Wales in 1999 (11% of all deaths). Most people survive a first stroke, often with significant morbidity. Consequently it is the leading cause of disability in the UK. More than 900 000 people in England are living with the effects of stroke, with half of these being dependent on other people for help with everyday activities. More than a third of survivors will experience a recurrent stroke within 5 years (NICE 2008b).

Over last 10 years there has been improvement in mortality largely as a result of changes in acute management and secondary prevention. The National Stroke Strategy (DH 2007) was developed to help implement recent evidence for improved management of strokes, e.g. screening and risk assessment tools for imminent stroke, rapid access imaging and thrombolysis. A NICE guideline for stroke management was published in 2008 (NICE 2008b).

Guidance summary
Acute management
- Stroke: assessment using a validated tool – 'FAST score' (see below) and immediate referral for next slot imaging and thrombolysis.
- TIA: risk assessment using a validated tool – 'ABCD' (see below). Review within 24 h if score >4 and 1 week for all others.

Antiplatelets
- All patients should receive dipyridamole plus aspirin for 2 years after an ischaemic stroke or TIA, and aspirin alone thereafter. (The ESPS-2 study

[Diener et al. 1996] found a lower incidence of recurrent stroke with aspirin/MR dipyridamole [9.5%] compared with aspirin alone [12.5%].)
- Aspirin should be given in high dose (300 mg daily) for the first 2 weeks (NICE 2008b).

Anticoagulants
- All patients with atrial fibrillation should be anticoagulated after 2 weeks of high-dose aspirin (300mg) (Cochrane review 2004 – in patients with AF anticoagulation reduces the odds of recurrent events by roughly 50% – Saxena and Koudstaal 2004).

Lifestyle interventions (Table 8.6)
- Smoking cessation
- Blood pressure control
- Hyperlipidaemia: target – lower total cholesterol by 25% or LDL-cholesterol by 30% or to reach <4.0 mmol/l or <2.0 mmol/l, respectively, whichever is the greater
- Exercise
- Diet (salt/alcohol reduction)
- Flu immunisation
- Carotid endarterectomy: stenosis of >70% should be assessed within 1 week of presentation of symptoms and receive surgery within 2 weeks.

How has the acute management of stroke changed?
Stroke is now managed as an urgent event requiring rapid diagnosis and immediate treatment, along similar lines to an acute MI. A Cochrane review in 2003 (Wardlaw et al. 2003) of six RCTs has shown that thrombolysis with alteplase in acute ischaemic stroke significantly improves mortality and disability at 3 months in selected patients treated within 3 hours of onset of symptoms. Thrombolysis in acute stroke is associated with an increased risk of haemorrhage (up to 6% of patients) and is therefore a treatment not without hazard (Hill and Buchan 2005).

How can we improve the rapid diagnosis of stroke in primary care?
The FAST study (Mohd et al. 2004) demonstrated that use of a validated tool in primary care to identify the symptoms and signs of suspected stroke and TIA increases diagnostic accuracy and speed of access to secondary care. The FAST (face, arm and speech test) assessment has a high positive predictive value (78%) for accurate diagnosis of stroke and TIA. In suspected stoke/TIA victims there is good interobserver agreement of the neurological findings between stroke physicians and primary care workers. It is recommended by NICE and also designed to aid recognition of stroke by the general public.

Table 8.6 Quality Outcome Framework (QOF) for stroke

Indicator	Evidence
The practice can produce a register of patients with stroke or TIA	See the first point in Table 8.3
The percentage of new patients with presumptive stroke (presenting after 1 April 2003) who have been referred for confirmation of the diagnosis by CT or MRI	NICE (Stroke guidelines 2008b) To ensure appropriate secondary prevention (and manage those patients with an alternative diagnosis, e.g. metastasis)
The percentage of patients with TIA or stroke who have a record of smoking status in the last 15 months The percentage of patients with a history of TIA or stroke who smoke and whose notes contain a record that smoking cessation advice or referral to a specialist service, if available, has been offered in the last 15 months	Smoking is an established risk factor for cardiovascular and other diseases
The percentage of patients with TIA or stroke who have a record of blood pressure in the notes in the preceding 15 months The percentage of patients with a history of TIA or stroke in whom the last blood pressure reading (measured in last 15 months) was 150/90 or less	PROGRESS trial (*Lancet* 2001;**358**) and HOPE trial (Yusuf et al. *N Engl J Med* 2000 – secondary prevention) BP lowering reduces stoke risk. Ideal target 140/85 or 130/80 in people with diabetes. Use ACE inhibitor + thiazide
The percentage of patients with TIA or stroke who have a record of total cholesterol in the last 15 months The percentage of patients with TIA or stroke whose last measured total cholesterol (measured in last 15 months) was 5 mmol/l or less	LIPID trial (*N Engl J Med* 1998 – secondary prevention) Meta-analysis (Briel et al. *Am J Med* 2004) Lipid lowering reduces stroke risk. All patients with total cholesterol >3.5 require statin
The percentage of patients with a stroke shown to be non-haemorrhagic, or a history of TIA who have been prescribed aspirin (unless a contraindication or side effects are recorded)	SALT trial (*Lancet* 1991;**338**) Meta-analysis (Antithrombotic Trialists' Collaboration *BMJ* 2002;**324** – secondary prevention); 28% risk reduction of stroke vs placebo
The percentage of patients with TIA or stroke who have had influenza immunisation in the preceding 1 September to 31 March	Influenza infection is associated with poorer outcomes in patients with chronic disease (DH *The Green Book* 2009)

FAST assessment

Face: can the person smile? Has their mouth or an eye drooped?
Arm: can the person raise both arms?
Speech: can the person speak clearly and understand what you say?
The presence of any of these features warrants urgent admission.

Predicting risk of a stroke after a TIA?

The ABCD score aims to identify individuals at high risk of stroke and who may require emergency intervention. It was derived from the OXVASC study (Coull et al. 2004) where a series of clinical features in people with TIA were related to subsequent stroke risk:

- **Age** [<60 years = 0, ≥60 = 1]
- **BP** [SBP ≤ 140 mmHg and/or DBP < 90 mmHg = 0; SBP > 140 mmHg and/or DBP > 90 mmHg = 1]
- **Clinical features** (unilateral weakness = 2, speech disturbance without weakness = 1, other symptom = 0)
- **Duration of symptoms** [<10 min = 0, 10–59 min = 1, ≥60 min = 2]).

More specifically an ABCD score of 5–6 is associated with an eightfold greater 30-day risk of stroke. Furthermore, an ABCD score of 5–6 was also independently significantly associated with the 7-day risk of stroke (Tsivgoulis et al. 2006).

NICE (2008) recommends that people with a suspected TIA who are at high risk of stroke (e.g. score of 4 or above) should receive:

- immediate initiation of aspirin (EXPRESS: Rothwell et al. 2007)
- specialist assessment within 24 h of onset of symptoms (EXPRESS – see above).

Those with ABCD risk factors <4 should be assessed by a stroke clinic within 7 days of the event.

Chronic management of stroke

For the chronic management of stroke see Table 8.6.

Diabetes care

The problem

The prevalence of diabetes in the population is 3.7% (Diabetes UK 2007) of which >85% is type 2 diabetes. However, the prevalence of undiagnosed disease is thought to be equally high (National Screening Committee 2006). Diabetes (type 2) is particularly prevalent among patients of south Asian, Chinese and African–Caribbean origin living in the UK, with rates up to six times higher in south Asian communities and three to five times higher in African–Caribbean communities than among the white population. To put this is perspective, a quarter of south Asians over the age of 60 have diabetes.

The public health burden of diabetes is large. It is associated with a substantial burden of premature mortality, morbidity, suffering and financial cost, both through its macrovascular and microvascular complications. It is the leading cause of visual impairment, renal impairment and amputation in the UK and a major risk factor for heart disease and stroke.

Diagnosis and classification

Diagnosis of diabetes is based on the WHO criteria:

- Symptomatic patients (i.e. polyuria, polydipsia and unexplained weight loss) PLUS:
  - ➤ a random venous plasma glucose concentration ≥11.1 mmol/l *or*
  - ➤ a fasting plasma glucose concentration ≥7.0 mmol/l (whole blood ≥6.1 mmol/l) *or*
  - ➤ 2-hour plasma glucose concentration ≥11.1 mmol/l 2 hours after 75 g anhydrous glucose in an oral glucose tolerance test (OGTT)
- Asymptomatic patients (two samples required): diagnosis should not be based on a single glucose determination but requires confirmation by venous plasma glucose testing. At least one additional glucose test result on another day with a value in the diabetic range is essential, either fasting, from a random sample or from the 2-hour post glucose load. If the fasting or random values are not diagnostic the 2-hour value should be used (WHO 2006; National Prescribing Centre 2004).

Note that glycated haemoglobin (HbA1c) is not used for diagnosis of diabetes, just as a tool for monitoring because there can be considerable variance in the HbA1c values between individuals for the same plasma glucose – in one trial as much as 5%. This is because HbA1c is affected by the length of red blood cell survival, which can in turn be affected by many factors (GP notebook 2008: www.gpnotebook.co.uk; Kilpatrick et al. 1998).

There are two important aspects to diabetic care:

1. *Case finding* or screening
2. The *follow-up* of known people with diabetes.

These are considered separately.

Screening for new patients of diabetes
Population screening

The case for a national population diabetes screening programme has been assessed by the NSC, which concluded that whole population screening did not meet their screening criteria in two areas:

1. *Cost-effective primary prevention interventions had not been implemented as far as practicable*, e.g. interventions aimed at changing risk factors such as obesity, physical inactivity and diet, which may be effective in lowering the population mean blood glucose and reducing the proportion of individuals with disease.
2. *Cost-effective treatment for patients identified through early detection has not been established*. Although there is good evidence for multifactorial risk reduction in patients with clinically recognised disease, there is currently a lack of evidence for benefit in patients identified through screening. A 5-year prospective trial of screen-detected diabetes – the ADDITION Study (Anglo-Danish-Dutch Study of Intensive Treatment in People With Screen Detected Diabetes in Primary Care) – aims to answer this question (to be published). Early results show intensive multifactorial treatment of screen-detected patients in general practice

is feasible and associated with significant and clinically important reductions in CVD risk factors – results of a 5-year follow-up of cardiovascular events is awaited. Screening is likely to be reviewed in light of this evidence.

The argument in favour of population screening is that there may be benefits to screening specifically for diabetes and treating the cluster of metabolic abnormalities with which it is associated, rather than screening for and treating each component individually. For example, recognition of the presence of diabetes may increase calculated CVD risk above the threshold for intervention with lipid-lowering drugs, and may influence prescribing decisions about anti-hypertensive medication. However, as the prevalence of undiagnosed diabetes is thought to be equal to that of diagnosed diabetes, uncovering and managing these patients would be costly to the health service.

Targeted screening

The National Screening Committee (NSC) supports targeted screening. Intervention in subgroups at high risk of developing diabetes has been shown to be feasible and effective at reducing the incidence of diabetes (National Screening Committee 2006a). A pragmatic system for detecting new cases of type 2 diabetes and impaired fasting glycaemia in primary care (Greaves et al. 2004) concluded that screening of patients with a body mass index (BMI) ≥27 and age >50 by fasting glucose identified a substantial prevalence of undetected type 2 diabetes and impaired fasting glucose. In addition there is evidence to support targeted screening of patients presenting with the following risk factors:

- Age (>40 in white people, >25 in south Asian, Chinese and African–Caribbean individuals)
- First-degree relative with type 2 diabetes (concordance rate for type 2 diabetes in monozygotic twins is about 90% – much higher than for type 1)
- Waist measurement
  - ➤ women >31.5 inches
  - ➤ Asian men >35 inches
  - ➤ white and African–Caribbean men >37 inches.
- Established cardiovascular disease (hypertension, myocardial infarction, stroke)
- Impaired glucose tolerance or impaired fasting hypoglycaemia
- Gestational diabetes
- BMI >27.

Follow-up care

The standards for ongoing care of diabetes are laid out in the Quality Outcome Framework. The indicators and evidence base are summarised in Table 8.7.

Diabetic management options

(Where lifestyle interventions alone have failed to control hyperglycaemia.)

Table 8.7 Quality Outcome Framework (QOF) for diabetes

Indicator	Evidence base
The practice can produce a *register* of all patients with diabetes mellitus	See the first point in Table 8.3
The percentage of patients with diabetes whose notes *record BMI* in the previous 15 months	Weight control in overweight individuals with diabetes is associated with improved glycaemic control (Astrup and Finer 2000) BMI is an independent predictor of cardiovascular risk[a]
The percentage of patients with diabetes in whom there is a *record of smoking status*, in the previous 15 months, except those who have never smoked where smoking status need be recorded only once since diagnosis The percentage of patients with diabetes who smoke and whose notes contain a record that *smoking cessation advice* or referral to a specialist service, where available, has been offered in the last 15 months	Smoking is an established risk factor for cardiovascular and other diseases
The percentage of patients with diabetes who have a *record of HbA1c* or equivalent in the previous 15 months The percentage of patients with diabetes in whom the last *HbA1c is 8 or less* (or equivalent test/reference range depending on local laboratory in the last 15 months) The percentage of patients with diabetes in whom the last *HbA1c is 7 or less* (or equivalent test/reference range depending on local laboratory in the last 15 months) The percentage of patients with diabetes in whom the last *HbA1c is 9 or less* (or equivalent test/reference range depending on local laboratory in the last 15 months)	**HbA1c (%)** **Mean blood glucose (mmol/l)** **7** **9.5** **10** **15.5** HbA1c is a validated marker of long-term control. Lower values are associated with a reduction in complications* Diabetes Control and Complications Trial *N Engl J Med* 2000
The percentage of patients with diabetes who have a *record of retinal screening* in the previous 15 months The percentage of patents with diabetes with a *record of the presence or absence of peripheral pulses* in the previous 15 months The percentage of patients with diabetes with a *record of neuropathy testing* in the previous 15 months The percentage of patients with diabetes in whom there is a *record of microalbuminuria testing* in the previous 15 months (exception reporting for patients with proteinuria)	Screening for microvascular disease, early detection and intervention is associated with improved outcomes (see NICE 2002 for detailed guidance) *Continued*

Table 8.7 *Continued*

Indicator	Evidence base
The percentage of patients with diabetes in whom there is *a record of serum creatinine testing* in the previous 15 months The percentage of patients with diabetes in whom there is *a record of the blood pressure* in the past 15 months	Tight BP control reduces macrovascular complications and mortality. The lower the BP the lower the risk UKPDS (1998)
The percentage of patients with diabetes in whom the *last blood pressure was 145/85 or less*	Treatment with ACE inhibitors for 4.5 years in patients with type 2 diabetes and microalbuminuria has been shown to reduce cardiovascular events by 25% in both those with normal serum creatinine levels and those with mild renal insufficiency: HOPE (Heart Outcomes Prevention Evaluation) Study (2000) In patients with type 1 diabetes, ACE inhibitor therapy for 3 years was associated with a 50% reduction in a combined end-point of death, dialysis and transplantation that was independent of BP
The percentage of patients with diabetes with a diagnosis of proteinuria or microalbuminuria who are treated with ACE inhibitors (or ARB) The percentage of patients with diabetes who have a *record of total cholesterol* in the previous 15 months The percentage of patients with diabetes whose last measured *total cholesterol was 5 mmol or less* within the previous 15 months	MRFIT (Multiple Risk Factor Intervention Trial) *Arch Intern Med* 1992 (primary prevention) 1. Continuous relationship between risk of CHD and cholesterol down to at least 3.0 mmol/L 2. Therapy is perhaps more important in higher-risk groups, e.g. people with diabetes
The percentage of patients with diabetes who have had influenza immunisation in the preceding 1 September to 31 March	Influenza infection is associated with poorer outcomes in patients with chronic disease (DH 2006)

[a]Although BMI is a useful measure, it does not take into account the difference between excess fat and muscle, nor does it identify where the fat lies on the body. For example, excess fat abdominally (centripetal obesity) has more serious health consequences. Waist:hip ratio has been shown to be a more accurate predictor of cardiovascular risk (the Dallas Heart Study 2007) (waist circumference alone is also more accurate than BMI but less accurate than waist:hip ratio). Measuring waist circumference is a practical way to assess body fat and health risks. This evidence may lead to an alteration in this QOF indicator.

*Though early right control of glurose (HbA1c <7%) reduces complications and mortaling there is a paradoxical increase in mortality of 22Y. in patients 15 years after diagnosis. (NEJM 2008; The Advance Collaborative Group 2008; Diabetes Care 2001.)

Metformin (biguanide)

- **Action:** increases insulin sensitivity and inhibits gluconeogenesis.
- **Indication:** first-line choice in overweight (BMI >25) individuals with type 2 diabetes (80% are overweight at diagnosis). Joint first-line choice in non-overweight individuals with diabetes.
- **Contraindication:** renal impairment, i.e. GFR <30 ml/min per 1.73 m^2 – due to risk of lactic acidosis.
- **Evidence**: grade A evidence (Bolen et al. *Ann Intern Med* 2007;**147**: 428–30).
- **General information:** not associated with weight gain, unlike other individuals with hypoglycaemia.

Insulin secretagogues (sulphonylureas and meglitinides)

- **Action:** insulin secretagogues – increase insulin secretion from the pancreas.
- **Indication:** second-line treatment – should be used in combination with metformin when not controlled on monotherapy alone. Can be used as an alternative to metformin where it is not tolerated or if BMI <25.
- **Evidence:** grade A evidence (Bolen et al. *Ann Intern Med* 2007;**147**: 428–30).
- **General information:** first choice drug – generic sulphonylurea, e.g. glibenclamide. Meglitinides are rapid-onset secretagogues and may help achieve tight control in patients with irregular eating habits.

Thiazolidinediones (glitazones)

- **Action:** increases insulin sensitivity.
- **Indication:** third-line treatment – in those who cannot tolerate second-line treatment or have poor control despite it. Expensive, slow acting and out of favour.
- **Contraindication:** insulin therapy (injected). Heart failure – rosiglitazone is associated with an increased risk of heart failure; avoid in patients with established ischaemic heart disease or peripheral vascular disease (worrying in a diabetic population!) (Home et al. 2007; European Medicines Agency 2008).
- **General information:** slow onset of action. If replacing a hypoglycaemic agent with a glitazone there may be a short-term worsening of control.

Insulin

- **Action:** synthetic insulin.
- **Indication:** insulin should be offered to people with diabetes with inadequate blood glucose control on optimised glucose-lowering drugs.
- **General information:** when transferring a person from a combination of metformin and another oral agent to insulin therapy, continue with metformin; when transferring a person from a combination of sulphonylurea plus another oral agent (metformin not tolerated or contraindicated) to insulin therapy, continue the sulphonylurea.

Aspirin
- **Indication:** NICE (2008a) recommends that aspirin 75 mg should be given to people with type 2 diabetes if they have:
  - ➤ manifest CVD (i.e. secondary prevention)
  - ➤ or *no overt CVD but a 10-year coronary event risk >20% (i.e. primary prevention), provided that SBP is reduced and maintained to 145 mmHg or below* – this last guidance point seems out of date in light of the POPADAD trial 2008 (Belch et al. 2008), showing no evidence for aspirin in primary prevention of CVD and probably should be ignored. I have included it to make you aware of it because it is still part of current guidelines.
- Note that Diabetes UK advocates aspirin use in all people with diabetes aged over 50, all south Asian and African–Caribbean individuals with diabetes and those with a CVD risk factor other than diabetes, e.g. diabetes for >10 years, smokers, family history of CVD; once again this should also be ignored in view of the above.

Statins
- **Action:** cholesterol lowering via HMG-CoA (hydroxymethylglutaryl coenzyme A) reductase inhibition.
- **Indication:** all individuals with diabetes aged over 40 (and under 40s if risk profile poor, e.g. end-organ damage, total cholesterol >6). Targets – reduce total cholesterol by 25% and LDL by 30% or total cholesterol <4 and LDL <2, whichever is the lower target. The QOF audit standard is total cholesterol <5 and LDL <3.
- **Evidence:** Heart Protection Study (HPS) (Collins et al. 2002) – statins reduce the risk of macrovascular complications in patients with diabetes by a third regardless of cholesterol level. REVERSAL (Nicholls et al. 2005) and PROVE-IT (Cannon et al. 2004) both provide evidence of reduced CVD risk the lower the levels of cholesterol (in patients with coronary artery disease).
- **General information:** LFTs should be carried out before and within 4–6 weeks of starting statin therapy, and thereafter at intervals of 6 months to 1 year – earlier if clinical features of hepatotoxicity; also, at the first review at 4–6 weeks, enquire about adverse effects such as itching, rash, myalgia, arthralgia and insomnia

Self-management programmes – DAFNE and DESMOND
NICE guidance supports two evidence-based patient support programmes:
1. DAFNE – Dose Adjustment For Normal Eating (DAFNE Study Group 2002). This programme teaches patients with type 1 diabetes to adjust insulin around their eating patterns rather than the reverse. At 1-year follow-up both HbA1c and quality-of-life indicators were improved.
2. DESMOND – Diabetes Education and Self Management for Ongoing and Newly Diagnosed (Davies et al. 2008). This programme teaches people with type 2 diabetes to identify their risk factors and respond to them by setting their own goals. At 12 months outcomes show improvement in weight loss and smoking cessation but no improvement in HbA1c or other indicators.

Self-monitoring – effective or cost-effective?
Probably neither. A Cochrane review (Welschen et al. 2005) of monitoring in type 2 diabetes found no conclusive evidence of an improvement in glycaemic control. Also an RCT in the *British Medical Journal* in April 2008 (O'Kane et al. 2008) demonstrated a 6% higher score for depression in self-monitoring patients. Self-monitoring is costly – the cost of monitoring being greater than the cost of oral hypoglycaemic therapy. NICE has recommended that monitoring should be limited to when there is a clear need or objective agreed with the patient. Examples of a clear need would include monitoring during times of illness, or change in diabetic regimen.

Impaired glucose tolerance (IGT) and impaired fasting glucose (IFG)
IGT and IFG are states of impaired glucose regulation below the diabetic threshold:
- IGT fasting plasma glucose <7.0 mmol/l and OGTT 2-hour value ≥7.8 mmol/l but <11.1 mmol/l. This is a common condition affecting 17% of those aged 40–65 in the UK.
- IFG is defined as a fasting plasma glucose ≥6.1 mmol/l but <7.0 mmol/l

A recent trial confirms that all states of glucose regulation impairment confer increased mortality (Australian Diabetes, Obesity and Lifestyle Study 2007). Risk of death from diabetes is increased by more than half, and by a third in those with IFG and IGT in comparison to controls with normal glucose tolerance.

The risk of subsequent conversion to diabetes from IGT and IGG is about 4.7% and 2% per year respectively in white people and higher in some ethnic minority groups. Annual review is recommended (Joint British Societies 2005) to assess glucose regulation and CVD risk.

The metabolic syndrome
The underlying cause of the metabolic syndrome is not fully understood but both insulin resistance and central obesity are considered significant factors. According to the new International Diabetes Federation, the criteria for diagnosis of the metabolic syndrome are: central obesity (defined as waist circumference women >31.5 inches, Asian men >35 inches, white and black men >37 inches) plus any two of the following four factors:
1. Triglyceride level: ≥1.7 mmol/l
2. HDL-cholesterol: <1.03 mmol/l) in males and <1.29 mmol/l in females
3. SBP ≥130 or DBP ≥85 mmHg
4. Fasting plasma glucose ≥5.6 mmol/l.

Metabolic syndrome is common, affecting 40% of adults aged over 60. It is associated with a five times increased risk of developing type 2 diabetes and increased cardiovascular risk.

Management of metabolic syndrome consists of essentially assessing and managing cardiovascular risk factors:
- lifestyle interventions (weight reduction, exercise and smoking cessation)

- lipid regulation
- blood pressure lowering.

See International Diabetes Federation and the Diabetes UK websites: www.idf.org and www.diabetes.org.uk and Stern et al. (2004)

Diabetes primary care focus

The focus of care for diabetes has moved from secondary to primary care. Secondary care management is now limited to complications of diabetes and cases with complex morbidity.

Respiratory disease (COPD/asthma)

Chronic obstructive pulmonary disease (COPD)

Chronic obstructive pulmonary disease (COPD) is a common condition affecting at least 900 000 in the UK and as many suspected but undiagnosed (Halpin 2004). Mortality is difficult to estimate because many die with the disease rather than of it. Five-year survival rate from diagnosis is 78% in men and 72% in women with mild disease, but falls to 30% in men and 24% in women with severe disease. The most common cause is smoking; other causes include occupational exposure to fumes/dust/irritants and rarer causes such as hereditary disease and genetic causes (α_1-antitrypsin deficiency) (Table 8.8).

Diagnosis

COPD is characterised by airflow obstruction. The airflow obstruction is usually progressive, not fully reversible and does not change markedly over several months: FEV_1/FVC <0.7 after bronchodilator and FEV_1 <80%, where FEV_1 is forced expiratory volume in 1 second and FVC is forced vital capacity (Table 8.9). Table 8.10 shows the differential features of COPD and asthma.

Chronic COPD management – the stepwise approach (Halpin 2004)

Established management (Figure 8.1)

Smoking cessation

Getting patients with COPD to stop smoking is one of the single most important interventions. This slows the rate of decline in FEV_1, with consequent benefits in terms of progression of symptoms and survival (Halpin 2004).

Long-term oxygen therapy

Long-term oxygen therapy (LTOT) improves survival in patients with COPD who have either a PaO_2 < 7.3 kPa when stable or a PaO_2 ≥ 7.3 and <8 kPa when stable and one of: secondary polycythaemia, nocturnal hypoxaemia, peripheral oedema or pulmonary hypertension. To get the benefits

Table 8.8 Quality Outcome Framework (QOF) for chronic obstructive pulmonary disease (COPD)

Indicator	Evidence
The practice can produce a register of patients with COPD	See the first point in Table 8.3
The percentage of patients in whom diagnosis has been confirmed by spirometry including reversibility testing for newly diagnosed patients with effect from 1 April 2003 The percentage of all patients with COPD in whom diagnosis has been confirmed by spirometry including reversibility testing	SIGN/BTS 2008
The percentage of patients with COPD in whom there is a record of smoking status in the previous 15 months, except those who have never smoked where smoking status need be recorded only once since diagnosis The percentage of patients with COPD who smoke, whose notes contain a record that smoking cessation advice or referral to a specialist service, where available, has been offered in the past 15 months	See text (Halpin 2004)
The percentage of patients with COPD with a record of FEV_1 in the previous 27 months The percentage of patients with COPD who have had a review including an assessment of breathlessness using the MRC dyspnoea score (see Table 8.9) in the preceding 15 months	Disease monitoring
The percentage of patients with COPD who have had influenza immunisation in the preceding 1 September to 31 March	Influenza infection is associated with poorer outcomes in patients with chronic disease (DH *Immunisation Green Book* 2006)

FEV_1, forced expiratory volume in 1 second.

Table 8.9 Severity of asthma and predicted forced expiratory volume in 1 s (FEV_1)

Severity	Predicted FEV_1 (%)
Mild	50–80
Moderate	30–50
Severe	<30

of LTOT patients should breathe supplemental oxygen for at least 15 h/day. Greater benefits are seen in patients receiving oxygen for 20 h/day.

Inhaled steroids
Inhaled steroids are associated with a reduction in exacerbations and mortality. Greater benefits are seen in those with severe COPD (Sin et al. 2005).

Table 8.10 Clinical features differentiating COPD (chronic obstructive pulmonary disease)

	COPD	Asthma
Smoker or ex-smoker	Nearly all	Possibly
Symptoms under age 35	Rare	Common
Chronic productive cough	Common	Uncommon
Breathlessness	Persistent and progressive	Variable
Night-time waking with breathlessness and/or wheeze	Uncommon	Common
Significant diurnal or day-to-day variability of symptoms	Uncommon	Common

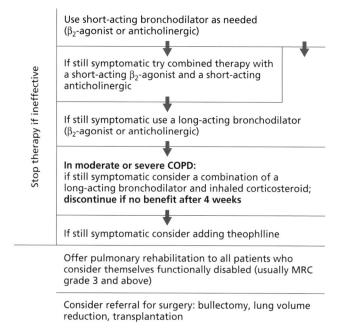

Figure 8.1 The stepwise approach to chronic COPD (chronic obstructive pulmonary disease) management.

Changes in the management of COPD
Pulmonary rehabilitation

A meta-analysis of exercise programmes for pulmonary rehabilitation 2003 (Salman 2003) demonstrates significant health improvement in quality-of-life scores, exercise capacity and shortness-of-breath indicators. There is a trend towards a reduction of days spent in hospital after pulmonary rehabilitation. The magnitude of the effects of pulmonary rehabilitation on exercise capacity, dyspnoea and health-related quality of life are significantly greater than the effects of bronchodilator drugs (Halpin 2004). NICE recommend that all patients with COPD who consider themselves func-

Table 8.11 MRC dyspnoea scale

Scale	Symptoms
1	Not troubled by breathlessness except on strenuous exercise
2	Short of breath when hurrying or walking up a slight hill
3	Has to stop for breath when walking at own pace
4	Stops for breath after about 100 m or after a few minutes on the level
5	Too breathless to leave the house, or breathless when dressing or undressing

tionally disabled to be referred for pulmonary rehabilitation. It should also be offered to all those with an MRC dyspnoea score of <3 (Table 8.11).

Mucolytics

A Cochrane review (Poole and Black 2006) of mucolytics showed no improvement in mortality but a reduction in exacerbations and hospitalisation compared with placebo. They also reduced the number of days on antibiotics. These results have been questioned in view of more recent evidence (Decramer et al. 2005), which did not replicate these findings. Nevertheless NICE recommend their usage in patients with a productive cough, although they should be stopped if there is no symptomatic improvement.

Hospital at home

Over the last few years there has been considerable interest in hospital-based rapid assessment units and early discharge schemes for patients with exacerbations of COPD – largely as a result of cost efficiency. Rapid assessment units aim to identify those patients who can safely be managed at home with additional nursing and medical input rather than being admitted. Early discharge schemes aim to facilitate the early discharge of patients admitted with an exacerbation of COPD (Halpin 2004). Home treatment may include additional equipment (e.g. a nebuliser and compressor or an oxygen concentrator), nursing supervision from visiting respiratory nurse specialists and increased social service input. Patients remain under the care of the hospital consultant. A systematic review (Ram et al. 2004) showed no significant difference in mortality or readmission between hospital and hospital at home management, i.e. they are safe.

Long-acting bronchodilators

The benefit of long-acting β agonists (LABAs) is not definitive. In a Cochrane review (Appleton et al. 2006) the largest of the trials demonstrated that LABAs reduce symptom scores: day time $P = 0.01$; night time $P = 0.001$). There were three subsequent RCTs. Using standard therapeutic doses only one trial found that symptom scores were reduced ($P < 0.001$). A meta-analysis (Salpeter et al. 2006) on LABA therapy in people with asthma showed an increase in mortality in patients on LABA monotherapy although safe in combination LABAs should not be used without concomitant steroid therapy. Long-acting anticholinergics are less contentious and studies have consistently found improvements in lung function and symptoms (Halpin 2004). NICE recommend a trial of a long-acting bronchodilator in patients with two or more exacerbations a year. If the patient fails to respond the agent should be stopped.

Asthma

There are 5.2 million asthma sufferers in the UK (Asthma UK 2004) and 12.7 million working days are lost each year through asthma (Table 8.12). Although the mortality rate is low (1400 deaths in 2002) the morbidity burden is significant. The cost to the NHS is approximately £900m but the total cost to the UK is thought to be £2.3bn per year.

Table 8.12 Quality Outcome Framework (QOF) for asthma

Indicator	Evidence
The practice can produce a register of patients with asthma, excluding patients with asthma who have been prescribed no asthma-related drugs in the last 12 months	See the first point in Table 8.3
The percentage of patients aged 8 and over diagnosed as having asthma from 1 April 2003 where the diagnosis has been confirmed by spirometry or peak flow measurement	SIGN/BTS 2008
The percentage of patients with asthma between the ages of 14 and 19 in whom there is a record of smoking status in the previous 15 months The percentage of patients aged 20 and over with asthma whose notes record smoking status in the past 15 months, except those who have never smoked where smoking status need be recorded only once since diagnosis The percentage of patients with asthma who smoke, and whose notes contain a record that smoking cessation advice or referral to a specialist service, where available, has been offered within the last 15 months	Eisner et al. (1998) Smoking cessation is associated with reduction in asthma severity scores Clough et al. (1999) Infants whose mothers smoke are four times more likely to develop wheezing illnesses in the first year of life
The percentage of patients with asthma who have had an asthma review in the last 15 months	Disease monitoring and step-down treatment where possible to reduce steroid load (SIGN/BTS 2008)
The percentage of patients aged 16 and over with asthma who have had influenza immunisation in the preceding 1 September to 31 March	Influenza infection is associated with poorer outcomes in patients with chronic disease DH (2006)

Diagnosis
Symptomatic adults
Confirm diagnosis with:
- Peak flow variability>20% (on more than 3 days in a 2-week period)
- Increase of FEV_1 >15% and minimum 200 ml):
  - after salbutamol 400 mcg by metered dose Inhaler *OR*
  - after a 14-day trial of prednisolone 30 mg/day.

Symptomatic children
Key features – wheeze on auscultation, dry cough, breathlessness, noisy breathing:
- Assessment of response to trials of treatment and ongoing assessment
- Repeated assessment and questioning of the diagnosis if management is ineffective
- Record of criteria on which the diagnosis has been made.

SIGN/BTS guidance (2008) on the stepwise management of asthma (Figure 8.2)
Key points
- Beclometasone CFC inhalers are being replaced with non-CFC propellants (HFA). They should be prescribed by brand name because they are not dose equivalent. The brand QVAR should be given at half the dose and the brand Clenil is dose equivalent to the CFC beclometasone inhalers. The normal starting dose should be 400 mcg/day or dose equivalent.
- Spacers are at least as good as a nebuliser in treating mild-to-moderate asthma exacerbations. In children 0–5 MDI (metered dose inhaler) via spacer is the preferred method of delivery. A facemask must be used until the child can breathe through the spacer mouthpiece.
- There is no evidence of benefit of sodium cromoglicate in children aged <5.
- LABAs should be added to only patients already on corticosteroids (see COPD), i.e. step 3.
- Patients on long-term steroid tablets (>3/12 a year) or frequent courses (3–4 a year) are at risk of systemic side effects (hypertension, diabetes, osteoporosis, growth retardation in children) and require monitoring.

Asthma action plans
Written asthma action plans have been shown to decrease hospitalisation for and deaths from asthma (Abramson et al. 2001; Gibson et al. 2002). Action plans should include clear instructions about the use of bronchodilators, seeking urgent medical attention in the event of worsening symptoms, how to judge severity based on personal peak flow readings and when to start a course of oral steroid. NICE previously recommended increasing the dose of inhaled steroid as part of an action plan – this has been withdrawn as recent studies failed to show improvement in control of symptoms (Harrison et al. 2004). A recent trial (Boushey et al. 2005) showed that an asthma action plan for mild persistent asthma, of short courses of inhaled or oral steroid taken only when symptoms worsen, is as effective

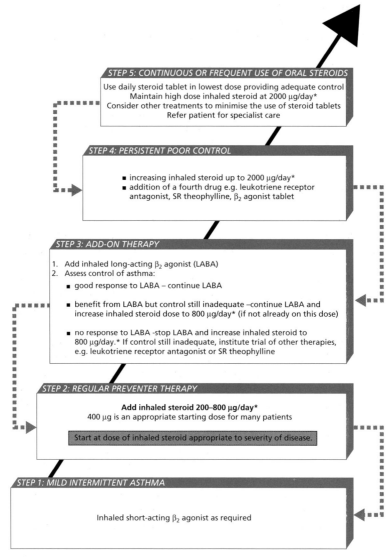

STEP 5: CONTINUOUS OR FREQUENT USE OF ORAL STEROIDS
Use daily steroid tablet in lowest dose providing adequate control
Maintain high dose inhaled steroid at 2000 μg/day*
Consider other treatments to minimise the use of steroid tablets
Refer patient for specialist care

STEP 4: PERSISTENT POOR CONTROL
■ increasing inhaled steroid up to 2000 μg/day*
■ addition of a fourth drug e.g. leukotriene receptor antagonist, SR theophylline, β₂ agonist tablet

STEP 3: ADD-ON THERAPY
1. Add inhaled long-acting β₂ agonist (LABA)
2. Assess control of asthma:
   ■ good response to LABA – continue LABA
   ■ benefit from LABA but control still inadequate –continue LABA and increase inhaled steroid dose to 800 μg/day* (if not already on this dose)
   ■ no response to LABA -stop LABA and increase inhaled steroid to 800 μg/day.* If control still inadequate, institute trial of other therapies, e.g. leukotriene receptor antagonist or SR theophylline

STEP 2: REGULAR PREVENTER THERAPY
Add inhaled steroid 200–800 μg/day*
400 μg is an appropriate starting dose for many patients
Start at dose of inhaled steroid appropriate to severity of disease.

STEP 1: MILD INTERMITTENT ASTHMA
Inhaled short-acting β₂ agonist as required

* BDP or equivalent

Figure 8.2 NICE guidance (2007) on the stepwise management of asthma.

as regular therapy. A good asthma action plan template is available at www. patient.co.uk.

Asthma monitoring
Failure to achieve control should lead to a step up in therapy. Indicators of poor control include symptomatic and objective measures.
• Symptomatic measures:
  ➤ using inhaled β₂ agonists three times a week or more

> symptomatic three times a week or more
> waking one night a week or more.
- Objective measures: PEFR measurements compared to personal best values:
  > >80% symptoms well controlled
  > 50–80% step up treatment
  > <50% – acute asthma exacerbation management.

The British Thoracic Society (BTS) recommends that all people with asthma on inhaled steroids be reviewed 3 monthly if stable, with the target of reducing the steroid dose by 25–50%.

Mental health

(For the revised mental health act see Chapter 7.)

Mental health problems are common – one in four adults experiences a diagnosable mental health problem in any one year (National Statistics: www.statistics.gov.uk/hub/health-social-care/specialist-health-services/mental-health-services/index.html). Poor mental health is associated with increased mortality and adverse lifestyle risk factors (obesity, smoking, lack of exercise) (National Primary Care Research and Development Centre [NPCRDC] 2005). Mental health disorders are a leading cause of disability, and depression alone is thought to have cost the UK annually over £9bn pounds (Sainsbury Centre for Mental Health 2003). Despite the importance of mental health, complexities of definition mean that there are relatively few markers of quality of care that can be meaningfully measured. The first QOF indicator provides a good example of this (Table 8.13). What constitutes a 'severe long-term mental health problem'? There is no universally agreed definition so some PCTs include only schizophrenia and bipolar disorder whereas others include people with depression, long-term anxiety, anorexia and obsessive–compulsive disorder. Also, patients only need be included on the register if they agree to follow-up; refusal may, however, indicate a lack of insight into the illness and consequently these patients may be the most in need of long-term support.

Common mental health problems are often managed entirely within primary care. However, most patients with long-term severe mental health problems will be cared for by specialist secondary services. In these cases the GP retains responsibility for the physical health, review of medication and coordination of care between primary and secondary services. These points are covered by the annual mental health review in the QOF.

A mental health review should include the following eight points (NPCRDC 2005):

1. Review of medication (including a discussion of concordance issues and over-the-counter medication use), including a documented agreement of the responsibilities for monitoring and prescribing treatment for those with specialist care
2. Physical health review (annual BP, glucose, lipids)

Table 8.13 Quality Outcome Framework (QOF) for mental health

Indicator	Evidence
The practice can produce a register of people with **severe long-term mental health** problems who require and have **agreed to regular follow-up**	See the first point in Table 8.3
The percentage of patients with severe long-term mental health problems with a review recorded in the preceding 15 months. This review includes a check on the accuracy of prescribed medication, a review of physical health and a review of coordination arrangements with secondary care	Glasziou et al. (2005) Monitoring aims to establish the response to treatment, detect the need to adjust treatment and detect adverse effects
The percentage of patients on lithium therapy with a record of lithium levels checked within the previous 6 months The percentage of patients on lithium therapy with a record of serum creatinine and TSH in the preceding 15 months The percentage of patients on lithium therapy with a record of lithium levels in the therapeutic range within the previous 6 months	*BNF* (2008) Lithium has a narrow therapeutic index and is associated with renal impairment and thyroid dysfunction

TSH, thyroid-stimulating hormone.

3. Review of treatment options, in particular whether to offer counselling/cognitive–behavioural therapy (CBT)
4. Crisis plan and warning signs discussed – written plan recorded and shared
5. Health promotion – especially smoking, weight management, exercise prescriptions
6. Assessment of social support needs
7. Provision of leaflets about voluntary organisations and community user groups
8. Information about accessing advocacy services.

All patients cared for by specialist secondary services will have a care plan approach (CPA), which covers many of the aspects in the mental health review. The CPA was introduced by the government in 1991, and updated in 1999 to improve coordination of care for patients with mental health problems/issues. It is important to refer to this when carrying out the annual review.

Depression

Depression is the most common mental health disorder in primary care with an estimated population prevalence of 10%. The impact on physical health puts severe forms of depression on a par with all the major chronic and disabling physical illnesses such as diabetes, arthritis and hypertension (Cassano and Fava 2002). Social and family relationships are frequently negatively affected, and parental depression may lead to neglect of and significant disturbances in children (Ramachandani and Stein 2003).

Mortality is higher in the depressed, from both impaired physical health and suicide. Two-thirds of suicides occur in depressed patients. Ninety per cent of depressed patients are managed in primary care although half of those presenting with mild depression go undiagnosed (Kisely et al. 1995).

Who is depressed?

It can be difficult to differentiate mild depression from a reduction in mood due to normal life events. GPs vary markedly in their ability to recognise depressive illnesses, with some recognising virtually all the patients found to be depressed at independent research interview, and others recognising very few (Goldberg and Huxley 1992; Üstün and Sartorius 1995). Persistence, severity, the presence of other symptoms, and the degree of functional and social impairment form the basis of that distinction. Case-finding tools such as depression questionnaires (PHQ9, HAD score, 2 question tool) improve the recognition of depression (Pignone et al. 2002). NICE recommends their use in primary care with high-risk groups, e.g. those with a past history of depression, significant physical illnesses causing disability or other mental health problems such as dementia. But a meta-analysis of 12 studies found no evidence for an improvement in the outcome of such cases (Gilbody et al. 2005). Despite this, monitoring of a depression score is included in the anxiety and depression QOF and is required within 1 month of diagnosis and again at 6–12 weeks

Two-question depression screening tool (Arroll et al. 2003)

'During the last month, have you often been bothered by feeling down, depressed or hopeless?'

'During the last month, have you often been bothered by having little interest or pleasure in doing things?'

Positive response to both questions is 97% sensitive and 67% specific for depression.

Treatment options for depressive illness (NICE 2004) (Figure 8.3)

Who is responsible for care?	What is the focus?	What do they do?
Step 5: Inpatient care, crisis teams	Risk to life, severe self-neglect	Medication, combined treatments, ECT
Step 4: Mental health specialists, including crisis teams	Treatment-resistant, recurrent, atypical and psychotic depression, and those at significant risk	Medication, complex psychological interventions, combined treatments
Step 3: Primary care team, primary care mental health worker	Moderate or severe depression	Medication, psychological interventions, social support
Step 2: Primary care team, primary care mental health worker	Mild depression	Watchful waiting, guided self-help, computerised CBT, exercise, brief psychological interventions
Step 1: GP, practice nurse	Recognition	Assessment

Figure 8.3 Stepwise treatment of depressive illness (NICE 2004).

Summary points

- Watchful waiting is recommended for mild depression; arrange further assessment – normally within 2 weeks. The following treatment options should be discussed:
  - ➤ sleep hygiene (avoid stimulants, e.g. caffeine, nicotine, use bedroom only for sleeping, quiet period 30 min before bed, avoid sleeping in daytime, write worries down on to-do list before bed time) and anxiety management
  - ➤ exercise (3 sessions per week of moderate duration, i.e. 45 min to 1 h for between 10 and 12 weeks)
  - ➤ guided self-help provision of appropriate written materials and limited support over 6–9 weeks
  - ➤ computerised CBT (NICE-recommended programs include 'Beating the Blues' and 'FearFighter' – available via your PCT)
  - ➤ psychological interventions (problem-solving therapy, brief CBT and counselling) of 6–8 sessions over 10–12 weeks
- Selective serotonin reuptake inhibitors (SSRIs) are the first-line antidepressants (better tolerated, fewer side effects than tricyclic antidepressants). Stop gradually (over a 4-week period) due to risk of withdrawal symptoms/recurrence of low mood. Effects are no greater than placebo in mild depression (Kirsch et al. 2008).
- Patients who have had two or more depressive episodes in the recent past, and who have experienced significant functional impairment during the episodes, should be advised to continue antidepressants for 2 years.
- CBT should be considered for patients with recurrent depression who have relapsed despite antidepressant treatment, or who express a preference for psychological interventions. A combination of CBT and antidepressants is recommended for severe depression.
- Suicide risk should be assessed at each appointment and documented. If patients fail to attend appointments they should be followed up. Two-thirds of suicide cases visit the GP in the month before suicide.

Postnatal mood disorders

This can take one of three forms:

1. Postpartum blues: transient low mood in the first week postpartum lasting hours to days.
2. Postnatal depression: depressive symptoms within the first 6 months postpartum.
3. Puerperal psychosis: psychotic illness usually with onset within first week postpartum (inpatient care required).

Postpartum blues is common (50% or more pregnancies) and self-limiting, requiring supportive measures only. Postnatal depression is less common (1 in 10 pregnancies) and good social (mother and baby groups, health visitor) and psychological support is as important as medication. There is evidence that SSRIs are effective in this group of patients. The Edinburgh Postnatal Depression Score (see patient.co.uk – online calculator) is a validated screening tool for detecting postnatal depression. It is not recommended for use as a routine screening tool (National Screening Committee 2006b) but should be used in patients with symptoms of postnatal depression. Puerperal psychosis is rare and requires specialist management.

Schizophrenia

There is up to a 1% lifetime risk of schizophrenia. Schizophrenia has significant adverse social and psychological effects and requires specialist management. Regular review of management in primary care is an important principle of treatment. Urgent referral of suspected cases is recommended.

Management principles for primary care (NICE 2009)

- Approach with empathy
- Urgent referral to specialist services for comprehensive assessment of suspected cases
- Partnership approach among patient, carers and multidisciplinary team
- Request informed consent before treatment
- Provide clear information (including written care plan)
- Consult advance directives when deciding treatment plans
- GPs should start antipsychotics only if they are experienced in treating and managing schizophrenia
- When starting an antipsychotic, NICE (2009) recommend:
  - oral treatment
  - a discussion of risks – the different choices and the relative potential of individual antipsychotics to cause extrapyramidal side effects (such as akathisia), metabolic side effects (such as weight gain) and other side effects (including unpleasant subjective experiences)
- Offer CBT (there is good evidence for improvement in mental state and similar efficacy to standard treatments – NICE 2002)
- Monitor physical health (weight, BP, smoking status, side effects of medication, especially extrapyramidal and endocrine side effects – glucose, prolactin)

Acute relapses should be managed by the crisis management or assertive outreach teams. Crisis teams are effective at reducing inpatient admissions (Johnson et al. 2005). Prevention of relapse through recognition of early symptoms should be included as part of the CPA (see above).

Doctors and mental health

This section is a summary of an excellent article on mental health problems in doctors from *Pulse* 2008 (C Williams).

The prevalence of common mental disorders in doctors is higher than in the general population. Compared with the general population doctors have an increased suicide rate. Moreover general practice as a specialty has a significantly increased suicide rate compared with general medicine. A survey of GPs in 2001 found that 21% reported work-related stress to be 'excessive and unmanageable'. It's not only the GP who suffers – their families do too. One study revealed that wives of GPs were four times more likely to commit suicide than other women.

Stressors include patient demands, complaints, managerial interference and target-driven requirements. Most GPs will have at least one complaint made against them during their professional life. The stress of receiving a complaint is well known in spite of help from the defence organisations.

One study found that many of the main stressors are caused or perpetuated by the GP's own policies: starting surgeries late, overbooking patients, making insufficient allowances for extra emergency patients and allowing inappropriate telephone interruptions. Partner and practice arrangements are very important. Another survey suggested that 'practices which had equitable and inclusive partner and practice relationships, managed workloads better than practices that were a collection of disparate individuals'.

Research has shown that doctors tend to be perfectionists and highly self-critical. With this background doctors are often unwilling to discuss their problems or to seek help appropriately. Instead they use a colleague for informal advice. And they self-medicate. They fear that seeking support will be viewed as a sign of weakness, or that their careers will be damaged by colleagues being aware of their emotional problems and by the stigma of mental illness. So where can the stressed GP get help? A confidential and anonymous help line 'Doctors support line' is available to provide confidential advice and support (tel: 0870 765 0001; email: deirdre@doctorssupport.org).

Urgent referral criteria (NICE 2005)

Primary care professionals are gatekeepers to specialist care and experts in the early diagnosis of medical problems. As such GPs need to be aware of the typical presenting features of cancers and take timely action using the appropriate referral pathways. Urgent referral means referral to be seen within 2 weeks (under the national 2 week wait target). Immediate referral means acute admission within a few hours or less. An urgent X-ray report should be available within 5 days.

Supporting patients with suspected cancer
Patients being referred with suspected cancer may require support while waiting for their appointment. NICE recommend offering the following information and support.

Basic information for patients
- Where patients are being referred to
- How long they will have to wait for the appointment
- How to obtain further information about the type of cancer suspected or help before the specialist appointment
- Who they will be seen by
- What to expect from the service that the patient will be attending

- What type of tests will be carried out, and what will happen during diagnostic procedures
- How long it will take to get a diagnosis or test results
- Whether they can take someone with them to the appointment
- Other sources of support, including those for minority groups.

Support
- Break bad news sensitively (see Chapter 9, Case 9, page 276, Communication and coordination)
- Share options when decision-making
- Inform patients that they are being referred to a cancer service but reassure (where appropriate) that many will turn out not to have cancer
- Invite the patient to contact you again
- Consider the need for support of the family members
- Take into account personal circumstances (age, family, work, isolation, health issues).

Make sure that you cover these points in a CSA case (and of course as part of your normal practice).

Criteria
Gynaecological cancer
Refer urgently …
- Suspicious findings on speculum examination
- Postmenopausal bleeding when:
  - not on hormone replacement therapy (HRT)
  - persisting for 6 weeks after HRT stopped
  - taking tamoxifen
- Unexplained vulval lumps/ulceration
- Persistent intermenstrual bleeding and negative pelvic examination.

Patients with palpable abdominal or pelvic masses that you suspect as gynaecological in origin should have urgent ultrasonography, or urgent referral if this is not available.

Breast cancer
Refer urgently …
Summarised in Case 1 in Chapter 9.

Upper GI cancer
Refer urgently…
- Dysphagia
- Unexplained upper abdominal pain with weight loss
- Upper abdominal masses without dyspepsia
- Obstructive jaundice.

Also consider referring urgently:
- Persistent vomiting and weight loss in the absence of dyspepsia
- Unexplained weight loss or iron deficiency
- Unexplained worsening of dyspepsia and:
  - Barrett's oesophagus
  - known dysplasia or atrophic gastritis
  - peptic ulcer surgery over 20 years ago.

Urgent endoscopy criteria
- Any patient with dyspepsia and:
  - ➤ chronic GI bleeding
  - ➤ dysphagia
  - ➤ progressive unintentional weight loss
  - ➤ persistent vomiting
  - ➤ iron deficiency anaemia
  - ➤ epigastric mass
  - ➤ suspicious barium meal result
- Patients >55 with recent onset of:
  - ➤ unexplained dyspepsia (i.e. not taking NSAIDs, aspirin)
  - ➤ persistent dyspepsia symptoms (>6 weeks).

Lower GI cancer
Refer urgently …
- Age >40 with rectal bleeding and loose stools or increased stool frequency for >6 weeks
- Age >60 with rectal bleeding for >6 weeks.
- Age >60 with loose stools or increased stool frequency for >6 weeks.
- Any patient with:
  - ➤ a right lower abdominal mass consistent with large bowel cancer
  - ➤ a rectal mass
  - ➤ unexplained iron deficiency anaemia:
    - ✦ men Hb <11 g/dl
    - ✦ women Hb <10 g/dl

Lung Cancer
Refer immediately …
- Superior vena caval obstruction (swelling of face/neck with fixed elevation of the jugular venous pressure)
- Stridor.

Refer urgently …
- Persistent haemoptysis (in smokers or ex-smokers >40)
- Chest radiograph suspicious of lung cancer (including pleural effusion and slowly resolving consolidation, especially in symptomatic patients with a history of asbestos exposure)
- A normal chest radiograph where there is a high suspicion of lung cancer.

Urgent chest radiograph …
- Haemoptysis
- Unexplained and persistent (3 weeks):
  - ➤ chest/shoulder pain
  - ➤ dyspnoea
  - ➤ weight loss
  - ➤ chest signs
  - ➤ hoarseness

- finger clubbing
- cervical or supraclavicular lymphadenopathy
- cough
- features suggestive of metastasis from a lung cancer.

Urological cancer
Refer urgently …
Prostate
- Hard irregular prostate
- Normal prostate with a rising or high age specific PSA (in an asymptomatic patient with a borderline PSA, repeat the test in 1–3 months and refer on if PSA level is rising).

Bladder/Renal
- Painless macroscopic haematuria
- Age >40 with recurrent or persistent UTI associated with haematuria
- Age >50 with unexplained microscopic haematuria
- Urinary tract masses found on imaging.

Testicular
- Swelling or masses in the body of the testis.

Penile
- Progressive ulceration or mass in the glans or prepuce (can occur in shaft also).

Haematological cancer
Refer immediately …
- Blood counts/films reported as acute leukaemia
- Spinal cord compression or renal failure where myeloma is suspected.

Refer urgently …
- Persistent unexplained splenomegaly (suggestive of chronic myeloid leukaemia).

Skin cancer
Refer urgently …
- Lesions suggestive of melanoma (seven-point check list for melanoma)
- Lesions suggestive of squamous cell carcinoma, i.e. non-healing, keratinising or crusted lesions >1 cm (a scab that keeps dropping off and reforming). Commonly found on the face, scalp or back of the hand.
Note that basal cell carcinoma – the most common type of skin cancer – is slow growing and does not require urgent referral.

Major features of lesions (score 2 points for each):
- Change in size
- Irregular shape
- Irregular colour.

Minor features of lesions (score 1 point for each):
- Largest diameter 7 mm or more
- Inflammation
- Oozing
- Change in sensation.

For low-suspicion lesions monitor over 8 weeks using the seven-point checklist. Make measurements with a ruler or photograph and marker scale. Note that you can now send images as attachments to choose and book referrals including urgent referrals. A score of >3 is suspicious and requires urgent referral. A single point may be adequate if you strongly suspect cancer.

Head and neck cancer
Refer urgently ...
- An unexplained lump in the neck, of recent onset, or a previously undiagnosed lump that has changed over a period of 3–6 weeks
- An unexplained persistent swelling in the parotid or submandibular gland
- An unexplained persistent sore or painful throat
- Unilateral unexplained pain in the head and neck area for more than 4 weeks, associated with otalgia (ear ache) but normal otoscopy
- Unexplained ulceration of the oral mucosa or mass persisting for more than 3 weeks
- Unexplained red and white patches (including suspected lichen planus) of the oral mucosa that are painful, swollen or bleeding.

For patients with persistent symptoms or signs related to the oral cavity, in whom a definitive diagnosis of a benign lesion cannot be made, refer or follow up until the symptoms and signs disappear. If the symptoms and signs have not disappeared after 6 weeks, make an urgent referral.

Note that patients with a hoarse voice persisting for 3 weeks require an urgent chest radiograph and referral to the lung team if positive findings, to the ear, nose and throat (ENT) team if negative.

Thyroid cancer
Refer urgently ...
Patients with a thyroid swelling associated with:
- a solitary nodule increasing in size
- a history of neck irradiation
- a family history of an endocrine tumour
- unexplained hoarseness or voice changes
- cervical lymphadenopathy
- very young (pre-pubertal) patient
- patient aged 65 years and older.

Brain and CNS cancer
Refer urgently ...
- Symptoms related to the central nervous system (CNS), where a brain tumour is suspected including:

- ➤ progressive neurological deficit
- ➤ new-onset seizures
- ➤ headaches
- ➤ mental changes
- ➤ cranial nerve palsy
- ➤ unilateral sensorineural deafness.
- Headaches of recent onset accompanied by features suggestive of raised intracranial pressure, e.g.:
  - ➤ vomiting
  - ➤ drowsiness
  - ➤ posture-related headache
  - ➤ pulse-synchronous tinnitus

  or by other focal or non-focal neurological symptoms, e.g. blackout, change in personality or memory.
- A new, qualitatively different, unexplained headache that becomes progressively severe.
- Suspected recent-onset seizures (refer to neurologist).

Consider urgent referral (to an appropriate specialist) in patients with rapid progression of:

- subacute focal neurological deficit
- unexplained cognitive impairment, behavioural disturbance or slowness
- personality changes confirmed by a witness and for which there is no reasonable explanation even in the absence of the other symptoms and signs of a brain tumour.

Note that headaches are an uncommon initial presenting feature of brain tumour – focal neurological deficits and fits are far more suspicious.

Cancer in children
Refer immediately ...
- Unexplained petechiae or hepatosplenomegaly (suggestive of leukaemia)
- Hepatosplenomegaly or mediastinal masses on chest radiograph (suggestive of lymphoma)
- Features suggestive of brain tumours:
  - ➤ a reduced level of consciousness
  - ➤ headache and vomiting that cause early morning waking (suggesting raised intracranial pressure)
  - ➤ new-onset seizures
  - ➤ cranial nerve abnormalities
  - ➤ visual disturbances
  - ➤ gait abnormalities
  - ➤ motor or sensory signs
  - ➤ unexplained deteriorating school performance or developmental milestones
  - ➤ unexplained behavioural and/or mood changes.

Refer urgently ...
- Any child who presents several (three or more) times with the same problem but with no clear diagnosis.

- Features suggestive of lymphoma such as:
  - non-tender, firm or hard lymph nodes
  - lymph nodes >2 cm in size
  - lymph nodes progressively enlarging
  - other features of general ill-health, fever or weight loss
  - axillary node involvement (in the absence of local infection or dermatitis)
  - supraclavicular node involvement.
- Features suggestive of retinoblastoma (usually presents under the age of 2):
  - a white pupillary reflex (leukocoria); pay attention to parents reporting an odd appearance in their child's eye
  - a new squint or change in visual acuity if cancer is suspected (refer non-urgently if cancer is not suspected)
  - a family history of retinoblastoma and visual problems (screening should be offered soon after birth).
- Features suggestive of sarcoma: an unexplained mass at almost any site that has one or more of the following:
  - deep to the fascia
  - non-tender
  - progressively enlarging
  - associated with a regional lymph node that is enlarging
  - >2 cm in diameter in size.
- Features suggestive of a brain tumour
  - a persistent headache where you cannot carry out an adequate neurological examination in primary care
  - under 2 years old with:
    - abnormal increase in head size
    - arrest or regression of motor development
    - altered behaviour
    - abnormal eye movements
    - lack of visual following
    - poor feeding/failure to thrive.
    - squint, urgency dependent on other factors.
- Features suggestive of neuroblastoma
  - proptosis
  - unexplained back pain
  - leg weakness
  - unexplained urinary retention.

AKT questions

Q1
Match the following blood pressures to the patient descriptions
a   150/90
b   140/80
c   140/90
d   135/75

e   140/85
f   135/85

1. The target blood pressure according to NICE for a 40-year-old man with established hypertension.
2. What was the optimal blood pressure target identified by the primary prevention trial HOT (Hypertension Optimal Treatment) at which cardiovascular risk was found to be lowest.
3. The target blood pressure according to NICE for someone with type 2 diabetes and microalbuminuria.
4. The audit standard blood pressure according to QOF for a 56-year-old woman with established hypertension.
5. The target blood pressure according to NICE for someone with type 1 diabetes.
6. The target blood pressure according to NICE for someone with type 2 diabetes.

Q2
A 62-year-old man has a cardiovascular risk assessment predicting a 10-year CVD risk of 36%. His risk factors include poorly controlled essential hypertension (160/94), smoking and a family history of heart disease. His total cholesterol is 5.6, HDL 1.4, triglyceride 4.5, fasting glucose 4.8. His current medication is bendroflumethiazide 2.5 mg. In addition to lifestyle modification, according to NICE guidance, what agents should be added today to further reduce his CVD risk? Choose one answer only.
a   Simvastatin, ramipril, aspirin
b   Simvastatin, ramipril
c   Simvastatin, aspirin
d   Ramipril, aspirin
e   Simvastatin, ramipril, clopidogrel

Q3
A 59-year-old woman presents to morning surgery with a 40-minute history of slurred speech that occurred yesterday evening. She has had no previous episodes and no significant past medical history. Her BP is 154/80 and she is now symptom free. Which is the most appropriate course of action?
a   Immediate initiation of aspirin and specialist assessment with 24 hours of onset of the symptoms
b   Immediate admission to hospital
c   Outpatient referral to a stroke clinic
d   Urgent referral for review in a stroke clinic within 7 days
e   Start aspirin and review in surgery in 2 weeks

Q4
Which of the following statements is correct? Choose one answer only.
a   Metformin is unsafe for use in patients with a GFR <50.

b   Rosiglitazone is associated with an increased risk of heart failure.

c   Aspirin is safe for use in a patients with diabetes and an SBP of 160.

d   Liver function tests should be carried out 6 months after starting a statin.

e   South Asians have a reduced risk of diabetes compared with the white population.

Q5

Match the studies to the findings.

a   Heart Protection Study (HPS)

b   West of Scotland Coronary Prevention Study (WOSCOPS)

c   Anglo Scandinavian Cardiac Outcome Trial (ASCOT)

d   Hypertension Optimal Treatment Trial (HOT)

e   Blood pressure-lowering treatment trial collaboration

f   Antihypertensive and Lipid Lowering Treatment to Prevent Heart Attack Trial (ALLHAT)

1.   This trial that compared the four main antihypertensive groups and found similar efficacy between all four agents.

2.   A trial of 19 000 patients comparing combination treatment of a calcium channel blocker and ACE inhibitor versus a β blocker and diuretic group.

3.   A primary prevention study for coronary heart disease using statins in patients with risk factors for cardiovascular disease. It showed risk reduction in all groups.

4.   This study investigated the blood pressure at which cardiovascular risk was lowest.

Q6

The following are risk factors for type 2 diabetes mellitus EXCEPT:

a   South Asian origin

b   BMI >25

c   Established CVD

d   Waist measurement in white people >37 inches

e   Gestational diabetes

Q7

Match the following values for predicted FEV_1 with the correct statements:

a FEV_1 60–90%

b FEV_1 50–80%

c FEV_1 40–60%

d FEV_1 30–50%

e FEV_1 <30%

f FEV_1 <50%

1.   Severe COPD

2.   Moderate COPD

3.   Mild COPD

Q8

Match the missing steps numbered in the diagram below showing the stepwise management of asthma to the treatment choices.

Treatment choices

a   Add salmeterol 25 mcg two puffs twice daily

b   Add inhaled steroid beclometasone Clenil at 100 mcg a day

c   Add inhaled steroid beclometasone Clenil at 400 mcg/day

d   Add inhaled steroid beclometasone Clenil at 800 mcg/day and stop salmeterol if there has been no response from its addition

e   Add inhaled steroid beclometasone Clenil up to 16 000 mcg/day and stop salmeterol if there has been no response from its addition

f   Add oral steroids in the lowest dose providing adequate control

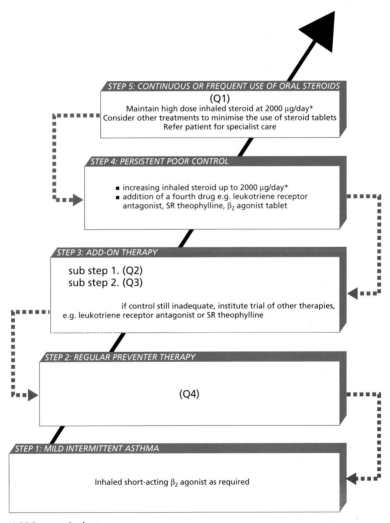

* BDP or equivalent

Q9

The following groups are eligible for the annual flu vaccination EXCEPT:

a   All patients with COPD
b   People with diabetes under the age of 60
c   Patients with chronic renal failure
d   Patients with chronic liver disease
e   Staff in nursing homes
f   All those over 60
g   Immunocompromised patients
h   Children with cystic fibrosis over the age of 6 months

Q10

There is evidence of a reduction in mortality from the following agents used to mange heart failure EXCEPT:

a   Ramipril
b   Spironolactone
c   Furosemide
d   Bisoprolol
e   Eplerenone

Answers

Q1

1. c
2. e
3. d
4. a
5. f
6. b

Q2 b

NICE guidance recommends a blood pressure target of 140/90 for patients without diabetes. As this patient is already on a diuretic, the next antihypertensive according to NICE treatment guidelines should be an ACE inhibitor. NICE recommends that patients with a CVD risk >20% should receive primary prevention with a statin using a fire-and-forget strategy. Aspirin is no longer recommended for use in primary prevention of CVD and should not be given to patients with uncontrolled blood pressure (<150/90). Hence it should not be started on this occasion.

Q3 d

This woman's ABCD stroke score is 3. NICE (2008b) recommend that people with a suspected TIA and a score of <4 should be assessed by a stroke clinic within 7 days of the event. A score of >4 warrants immediate initiation of aspirin and assessment within 24 hours.

Q4 b

Metformin is unsafe in those with a GFR <30 ml/min per 1.73 m² (risk of metabolic acidosis). Aspirin is unsafe in those with uncontrolled hypertension. NICE recommend an SBP of <145 in those with diabetes (and <150 in those without). LFTs should be monitored within 4–6 weeks of starting a statin, and thereafter at intervals of 6 months to 1 year – earlier if clinical features of hepatotoxicity. South Asians in the UK have a six times higher rates of diabetes than the background population.

Q5

1. e
2. c
3. a
4. d

Q6 b

BMI >27 confers risk of type 2 diabetes.

Q7

1. e
2. d
3. b

Q8

1. f
2. a
3. d
4. c

Q9 f

Flu vaccination is recommended to those groups most at risk of significant morbidity and mortality following an influenza outbreak. This includes those over the age of 65.

Q10 c

No trials have shown survival benefit from the use of diuretics. However, they remain an integral part of treatment. It is unlikely THAT an ethics committee will ever sanction a trial of these agents, which in practice have clear benefit.

References

Abramson MJ, Bailey MJ, Couper FJ et al. Victorian Asthma Mortality Study Group. Are asthma medications and management related to deaths from asthma? *Am J Respir Crit Care Med* 2001;**163**:12–18.

The Action to Control Cardiovascular Risk in Diabetes Study Group. Effects of intensive glucose lowering in type 2 diabetes. *N Engl J Med* 2008;**358**(24):2545–59.

The ADVANCE Collaborative Group. Intensive blood glucose control and vascular outcomes in patients with type 2 diabetes. *N Engl J Med* 2008;**358**:2560–72.

The ALLHAT Officers and Coordinators for the ALLHAT Collaborative Research Group. Major outcomes in high-risk hypertensive patients randomized to angiotensin-converting enzyme inhibitor or calcium channel blocker vs diuretic: The Antihypertensive and Lipid-Lowering Treatment to Prevent Heart Attack Trial (ALLHAT). *JAMA* 2002;**288**:2981–97.

Appleton S, Poole P, Smith B et al. Long-acting beta2-agonists for poorly reversible chronic obstructive pulmonary disease. *Cochrane Database Syst Rev* 2006;**3**: CD001104.

Antiplatelet Trialists' Collaboration. Collaborative overview of randomised trials of antiplatelet therapy – III: Reduction in venous thrombosis and pulmonary embolism by antiplatelet prophylaxis among surgical and medical patients. *BMJ* 1994;**308**:235–46.

Antithrombotic Trialists' Collaboration. Collaborative meta-analysis of randomised trials of antiplatelet therapy for prevention of death, myocardial infarction, and stroke in high risk patients. *BMJ* 2002;**324**:71–86.

Arroll B, Khin N, Kerse N. Screening for depression in primary care with two verbally asked questions: cross sectional study. *BMJ* 2003;**327**:1144–6.

Asthma UK. *Where do we stand?* London: Asthma UK. Available at: www.asthma.org.uk/document.rm?id=92.

Astrup A., Finer N. Redefining type 2 diabetes: 'diabesity' or 'obesity dependent diabetes mellitus'? *Obesity Rev* 2000;**1**(2):57–9.

Australian Diabetes, Obesity, and Lifestyle Study. Risk of cardiovascular and all-cause mortality in individuals with diabetes mellitus, impaired fasting glucose, and impaired glucose tolerance: the Australian Diabetes, Obesity, and Lifestyle Study (AusDiab). *Circulation* 2007;**116**:151–7.

Baughman KL. B-type natriuretic peptide – a window to the heart. *N Engl J Med* 2002;**347**:158.

Beckett NS, Peters R, Fletcher AE et al., HYVET Study Group. Treatment of hypertension in patients 80 years of age or older. *N Engl J Med* 2008;**358**:1887–98.

Belch J, MacCuish A, Campbell I et al. The prevention of progression of arterial disease and diabetes (POPADAD) trial: factorial randomised placebo controlled trial of aspirin and antioxidants in patients with diabetes and asymptomatic peripheral arterial disease. *BMJ* 2008;**337**:a1840.

Blood Pressure Lowering Treatment Trialists' Collaboration. Effects of different blood-pressure-lowering regimens on major cardiovascular events: results of prospectively-designed overviews of randomised trials. *Lancet* 2003;**362**:1211–24.

Blood Pressure Lowering Treatment Trialists' Collaboration. Effects of different regimens to lower blood pressure on major cardiovascular events in older and younger adults: meta-analysis of randomised trials. *BMJ* 2008;**336**:1121–3.

Bolen S, Feldman L, Vassy J et al. Systematic review: comparative effectiveness and safety of oral medications for type 2 diabetes mellitus. *Ann Intern Med* 2007;**147**:428–30.

Boushey HA, Sorkness CA, King TS et al. National Heart, Lung, and Blood Institute's Asthma Clinical Research Network. Daily versus as-needed corticosteroids for mild persistent asthma. *N Engl J Med* 2005;**352**:1519–28.

Briel M, Studer M, Glass TR, Bucher HC. Effects of statins on stroke prevention in patients with and without coronary heart disease: A meta-analysis of randomized controlled trials. *Am J Med* 2004;**117**:596–606.

Brophy JM, Joseph L, Rouleau JL. Beta-blockers in congestive heart failure. *Ann Intern Med* 2001;**134**:550–60.

Cannon CP, Braunwald E, McCabe CH et al., Pravastatin or Atorvastatin Evaluation and Infection Therapy-Thrombolysis in Myocardial Infarction 22 Investigators.

Intensive versus moderate lipid lowering with statins after acute coronary syndromes. *N Engl J Med* 2004;**350**:1495–504.

Cassano P, Fava M. Depression and public health: An overview. *J Psychosom Res* 2002;**53**:849–57.

CIBIS-II investigators and Committee. The Cardiac Insufficiency Bisoprolol Study II (CIBIS-II). *Lancet* 1999;**352**:9–13.

Clopidogrel in Unstable Angina to Prevent Recurrent Events Trial Investigators (CURE). Effects of clopidogrel in addition to aspirin in patients with acute coronary syndromes without ST-segment elevation. *N Engl J Med* 2001;**345**:494–502.

Clough JB, Keeping KA, Edwards LC, Freeman WM, Warner JA, and Warner JO. Can we predict which wheezy infants will continue to wheeze? *Am J Respir Crit Care Med* 1999;**160**:1473–80.

Collins R, Peto R, Armitage J. The MRC/BHF Heart Protection Study: preliminary results. *Int J Clin Pract* 2002;**56**:53–6.

Cook DG, Pocock SJ, Shaper AG, Kussick SJ. Giving up smoking and the risk of heart attacks: a report from the British Regional Heart Study. *Lancet* 1986;**ii**: 1376–80.

Coull AJ, Lovett JK, Rothwell PM, on behalf of the Oxford Vascular Study. Early risk of stroke after a TIA or minor stroke in a population-based incidence study. *BMJ* 2004;**328**:326–8.

Dahlöf B, Sever PS, Poulter NR et al., for the ASCOT Investigators. Prevention of cardiovascular events with an antihypertensive regimen of amlodipine adding perindopril as required versus atenolol adding bendroflumethiazide as required, in the Anglo-Scandinavian Cardiac Outcomes Trial-Blood Pressure Lowering Arm (ASCOT-BPLA): a multicentre randomised controlled trial. *Lancet* 2005;**366**: 895–906.

The Dallas Heart Study. The association of differing measures of overweight and obesity with prevalent atherosclerosis. *J Am Coll Cardiol* 2007;**50**:752–9.

DAFNE Study Group. Training in flexible, intensive insulin management to enable dietary freedom in people with type 1 diabetes: dose adjustment for normal eating (DAFNE) randomised controlled trial. *BMJ* 2002;**325**:746.

Dargie HJ. Effect of carvedilol on outcome after myocardial infarction in patients with left-ventricular dysfunction: the CAPRICORN randomised trial. *Lancet* 2001;**357**:1385–90.

Davies MJ, Heller S, Skinner TC et al., on behalf of the Diabetes Education and Self Management for Ongoing and Newly Diagnosed Collaborative. Effectiveness of the diabetes education and self management for ongoing and newly diagnosed (DESMOND) programme for people with newly diagnosed type 2 diabetes: cluster randomised controlled trial. *BMJ* 2008;**336**:491–5.

Decramer M, Rutten-van Mölken M, Dekhuijzen PNR et al. Effects of *N*-acetyl-cysteine on outcomes in COPD. The Bronchitis Randomized on NAC Cost–Utility Study (BRONCUS). *Lancet* 2005;**365**:1552–60.

The Diabetes Control and Complications Trial/Epidemiology of Diabetes Interventions and Complications Research Group. *N Engl J Med* 2000;**342**:381–9.

Diabetes UK. *Quality Prevalence Indicator Data (QPID)*, 2007. Available at: www.diabetes.org.uk/Professionals/Information_resources/Reports/Diabetes-prevalence-2007.

Diener HC, Cunha L, Forbes C, Sivenius J, Smets P, Lowenthal A. Dipyridamole and acetylsalicylic acid in the secondary prevention of stroke: European Stroke Prevention Study 2. *J Neurol Sci* 1996;**143**:1–13.

Department of Health. *Coronary Heart Disease: National Service Framework for coronary heart disease – modern standards and service models*. London: DH, 2000.

Department of Health. *National Stroke Strategy*. London: DH, 2007.

Department of Health. *The Green Book*. London: DH, 2009.

Duckworth WC, McCarren M, Abraira C. Glucose control and cardiovascular complications: the VA diabetes trial. *Diabetes Care* 2001;**24**(51):942–5.

Eichhorn EJ, Bristow MR. The Carvedilol Prospective Randomized Cumulative Survival (COPERNICUS) trial. *Curr Control Trials Cardiovasc Med* 2001;**2**(1):20–3.

Eisner MD, Yelin EH, Henke J, Shiboski SC, Blanc PD. Environmental tobacco smoke and adult asthma: the impact of changing exposure status on health outcomes. *Am J Respir Crit Care Med* 1998;**158**:170–5.

European Medicines Agency. Press statement 24 January 2008: New warnings and contraindications for rosiglitazone. *N Engl J Med* 2008;**357**:28–38. Available at: www.emea.europa.eu/humandocs/PDFs/EPAR/avaglim/4223208en.pdf.

Flather M, Yusuf S, Køber L et al. Long-term ACE-inhibitor therapy in patients with heart failure or left-ventricular dysfunction: a systematic overview of data from individual patients. *Lancet* 2000;**355**:1575–81.

Francis KL, Chan MD, Jessica YL et al. Clopidogrel versus aspirin and esomeprazole to prevent recurrent ulcer bleeding. *N Engl J Med* 2005;**352**:238–45.

Gibson PG, Powell H, Coughlan J et al. Self-management education and regular practitioner review for adults with asthma. *Cochrane Database Syst Rev* 2002;**3**: CD001117.

Gilbody S, House AO, Sheldon TA. Screening and case finding instruments for depression. *Cochrane Database Syst Rev* 2005;**4**:CD002792.

Glasziou P, Irwig L, Mant D. Monitoring in chronic disease: a rational approach. *BMJ* 2005;**330**:644–8.

Goldberg DP, Huxley PJ. *Common Mental Disorders: A bio-social model*. London: Tavistock/Routledge, 1992.

Greaves CJ, Stead JW, Hattersley AT, Ewings P, Brown P, Evans PH. A simple pragmatic system for detecting new cases of type 2 diabetes and impaired fasting glycaemia in primary care. *Fam Pract* 2004;**21**:57–62.

Hallas J, Dall M, Andries A et al. Use of single and combined antithrombotic therapy and risk of serious upper gastrointestinal bleeding: population based case-control study. *BMJ* 2006;**333**:726.

Halpin D. NICE guidance for COPD. *Thorax* 2004;**59**:181–2.

Hansson L, Zanchetti A, Carruthers SG et al. Effects of intensive blood-pressure lowering and low-dose aspirin in patients with hypertension: principal results of the hypertension optimal treatment (HOT) randomised trial. *Lancet* 1998;**351**: 1755–62.

Harrison DM, Oborne J, Newton S, Tattersfield AE. Doubling the dose of inhaled corticosteroid to prevent asthma exacerbations: randomised controlled trial. *Lancet* 2004;**363**:271–5

The Heart Outcomes Prevention Evaluation Study Investigators: Yusuf S, Sleight P, Pogue J, Bosch J, Davies R, Dagenais G. Effects of an angiotensin-converting-enzyme inhibitor, ramipril, on cardiovascular events in high-risk patients. *N Engl J Med* 2000;**342**:145–53.

Hill MD, Buchan AM. Thrombolysis for acute ischemic stroke: results of the Canadian Alteplase for Stroke Effectiveness Study (CASES) Investigators. *Can Med Assoc J* 2005;**172**:1307–12.

Hippisley-Cox J, Coupland C, Vinogradova Y et al. Predicting cardiovascular risk in England and Wales: prospective derivation and validation of QRISK2. *BMJ* 2008;**336**:1475–82.

Home PD, Pocock SJ, Beck-Nielsen H et al., for the RECORD Study Group. Rosiglitazone evaluated for cardiovascular outcomes – an interim analysis. *N Engl J Med* 2007;**357**:28–38.

Heart Outcomes Prevention Evaluation. Scholarly articles for HOPE (Heart Outcomes Prevention Evaluation) Study. *Lancet* 2000;**355**:253–9.

International Study of Infarct Survival Collaborative Group. Randomised trial of intravenous atenolol among 16027 cases of suspected acute myocardial infarction: ISIS-1. *Lancet* 1986;**ii**:5–66.

Johnson S, Nolan F, Pilling S et al. Randomised controlled trial of acute mental health care by a crisis resolution team: the north Islington crisis study. *BMJ* 2005;**331**:599.

Joint British Societies (British Cardiac Society, British Hypertension Society, Diabetes UK, HEART UK, Primary Care Cardiovascular Society, Stroke Association). JBS2: Joint British Societies' guidelines on prevention of cardiovascular disease in clinical practice. *Heart* 2005;**91**(suppl 5):v1–52.

Kilpatrick ES, Maylor PW, Keevil BG. Biological variation of glycated hemoglobin. Implications for diabetes screening and monitoring. *Diabetes Care* 1998;**21**: 261–4.

Kirsch I, Deacon BJ, Huedo-Medina TB, Scoboria A, Moore TJ, Johnson BT. Initial severity and antidepressant benefits: a meta-analysis of data submitted to the Food and Drug Administration. *PLoS Medicine* 2008;Feb.

Kisely S, Gater R, Goldberg DP. Results from the Manchester Centre. In: Üstün TB, Sartorius N (eds), *Mental Illness in General Health Care: An International Study*. Chichester: Wiley, 1995: 175–91.

Lip GYH, Felmeden DC. Antiplatelet agents and anticoagulants for hypertension. *Cochrane Database Syst Rev* 2004;**3**:CD003186.

The Long-Term Intervention with Pravastatin in Ischaemic Disease (LIPID) Study Group. Prevention of cardiovascular events and death with pravastatin in patients with coronary heart disease and a broad range of initial cholesterol levels. *N Engl J Med* 1998; **339**:1349–57.

Marz W, Beate T, Seelharst U, et al. N-Terminal Pro-B-Type Natriuretic peptide predicts and cardiovascular mortality in individuals with or without stable coronary artery disease: The Ludwigshafen Risk and Cardiovascular Health Study. *Clin Chem* 2007;**53**:1075–83.

Mohd Nor A, McAllister C, Louw SJ et al. Agreement Between ambulance paramedic- and physician-recorded neurological signs with face arm speech test (FAST) in acute stroke patients. *Stroke* 2004;**35**:1355–9.

National Centre for Social Research. *Health Survey for England 2003*. Commissioned by Department of Health. London: National Centre for Social Research, Department of Epidemiology and Public Health at the Royal Free and University College Medical School, 2004.

National Institute for Clinical Excellence. *Diabetes Guidance*. London: NICE, 2002a.

National Institute for Clinical Excellence. *Schizophrenia: Core interventions in the treatment and management of schizophrenia in primary and secondary care*. London: NICE, 2002b.

National Institute for Clinical Excellence. *Management of Chronic Heart Failure in Adults in Primary and Secondary Care*. London: NICE, 2003.

National Institute for Clinical Excellence. *Depression: Management of depression in primary and secondary care*. London: NICE, 2004.

National Institute for Health and Clinical Excellence. *Referral Guidelines for Suspected Cancer*. London: NICE, 2005.

National Institute for Health and Clinical Excellence. *Hypertension: Management of hypertension in adults in primary care*. London: NICE, 2006.

National Institute for Health and Clinical Excellence. *Secondary prevention in primary and secondary care for patients falling a myocardial infarction*. London: NICE, 2007.

National Institute for Health and Clinical Excellence. *Cardiovascular Risk Assessment and the Modification of Blood Lipids for the Primary and Secondary Prevention of Cardiovascular Disease*. London: NICE, 2008a.

National Institute for Health and Clinical Excellence. *Stroke: NICE guideline.* London: NICE, 2008b.

National Institute for Health and Clinical Excellence. *Core Interventions in the Treatment and Management of Schizophrenia in Primary and Secondary Care.* London: NICE, 2009.

National Prescribing Centre. *Type 2 Diabetes (part 1): The management of blood glucose.* MeReC Briefing no. 25. London: NPC, 2004.

National Prescribing Centre. Chronic heart failure: overview of diagnosis and drug treatment in primary care. *MeReC Bull* 2008;**18**(3):1–9.

National Primary Care Research and Development Centre. *QOF Evidence-based Reports Mental Health.* London: NPCRDC, 2005. Available at: www.npcrdc.ac.uk/QOF_Evidencebased_reports.htm.

National Screening Committee. The UK NSC policy on diabetes screening in adults: Policy Position Statement, 2006a.

National Screening Committee. Depression. The UK NSC policy on depression screening in adults, July 2006b. Available at: www.screening.nhs.uk/depression.

Nicholls SJ, Tuzcu EM, Schoenhagen P et al. Effect of atorvastatin (80 mg/day) versus pravastatin (40 mg/day) on arterial remodeling at coronary branch points (from the REVERSAL study). *Am J Cardiol* 2005;**96**:1636–9.

O'Kane MJ, Bunting B, Copeland M, Coates VE, on behalf of the ESMON study group. Efficacy of self monitoring of blood glucose in patients with newly diagnosed type 2 diabetes (ESMON study): randomised controlled trial. *BMJ* 2008;**336**:1174–7.

Pfeffer MA, Braunwald E, Moyé LA et al. The Survival And Ventricular Enlargement study. Effect of captopril on mortality and morbidity in patients with left ventricular dysfunction after myocardial infarction. *N Engl J Med* 1992;**327**:669–77.

Pignone MP, Gaynes BN, Rushton JL et al. Screening for depression in adults: A summary of the evidence for the US Preventive Services Task Force. *Ann Intern Med* 2002;**136**:765–76.

Pitt B, Zannad F, Remme WJ et al., for the Randomized Aldactone Evaluation Study Investigators. The effect of spironolactone on morbidity and mortality in patients with severe heart failure: 'the RALES study'. *N Engl J Med* 1999;**341**:709–17.

Pitt B, Zannad F, Remme WJ et al., for the Eplerenone Post-Acute Myocardial Infarction Heart Failure Efficacy and Survival Study Investigators. Eplerenone, a selective aldosterone blocker, in patients with left ventricular dysfunction after myocardial infarction. *N Engl J Med* 2003;**348**:1309–21.

Poole P, Black PN. Mucolytic agents for chronic bronchitis or chronic obstructive pulmonary disease. *Cochrane Database Syst Rev* 2006;**3**:CD001287.

Ram FSF, Wedzicha JA, Wright J, Greenstone M. Hospital at home for patients with acute exacerbations of chronic obstructive pulmonary disease: systematic review of evidence. *BMJ* 2004;**329**:315.

Ramachandani P, Stein A. The impact of parental psychiatric disorder on children. *BMJ* 2003;**327**:242–3.

Remme WJ, Torp-Pedersen C, Cleland JG et al. Carvedilol protects better against vascular events than metoprolol in heart failure: results from COMET. *J Am Coll Cardiol* 2007;**49**:963–71.

Rothwell PM, Giles MF, Marquardt L et al., on behalf of the Early use of Existing Preventive Strategies for Stroke (EXPRESS) study. Effect of urgent treatment of transient ischaemic attack and minor stroke on early recurrent stroke (EXPRESS study): a prospective population-based sequential comparison. *Lancet* 2007;**370**: 1432–42.

Royal Pharmaceutical Society of Great Britain and the BMA. *British National Formulary.* London: RPS Publishing, 2008.

Sacks FM, Pfeffer MA, Moye LA et al., for The Cholesterol and for Recurrent Events Trial Investigators. The effect of pravastatin on coronary events after myocardial infarction in patients with average cholesterol levels (The CARE Study). *N Engl J Med* 1996;**335**:1001–9.

Sainsbury Centre For Mental Health. *The Economic and Social Costs of Mental Illness: Policy Paper 3*. London: Sainsbury Centre For Mental Health, 2003.

Salman GF. Rehabilitation for patients with chronic obstructive pulmonary disease. Meta-analysis of randomized controlled trials. *J Gen Intern Med* 2003;**18**: 213–21.

Salpeter SR, Buckley NS, Ormiston TM, Salpeter EE. Meta-analysis: effect of long-acting ß-agonists on severe asthma exacerbations and asthma-related deaths. *Ann Intern Med* 2006;**144**:904–12.

The Salt Collaborative Group. Swedish Aspirin Low-dose Trial (SALT) of 75 mg aspirin as secondary prophylaxis after cerebrovascular ischaemic events. *Lancet* 1991;**338**:1345–9.

Saxena R, Koudstaal PJ. Anticoagulants for preventing stroke in patients with non-rheumatic atrial fibrillation and a history of stroke or transient ischaemic attack. *Cochrane Database Syst Rev* 2004;**2**:CD000185.

Scandinavian Simvastatin Survival Study Group. Randomised trial of cholesterol lowering in 4444 patients with coronary heart disease: the Scandinavian Simvastatin Survival Study (4S). *Lancet* 1994;**344**:1383–9.

Scottish Intercollegiate Guidelines Network. *Heart Disease Guidelines*. Edinburgh: SIGN, 2007.

Scottish Intercollegiate Guidelines Network, British Thoracic Society. *British Guideline on the Management of Asthma*. Edinburgh: SIGN, 2008.

Shepherd J, Cobbe SM, Ford I et al., for The West of Scotland Coronary Prevention Study Group. Prevention of coronary heart disease with pravastatin in men with hypercholesterolemia. *N Engl J Med* 1995;**333**:1301–7.

Sin DD, Wu L, Anderson JA et al. Inhaled corticosteroids and mortality in chronic obstructive pulmonary disease. *Thorax* 2005;**60**:992–7.

Stern MP, Williams K, González-Villalpando C, Hunt KJ, Haffner SM. Does the metabolic syndrome improve identification of individuals at risk of type 2 diabetes and/or cardiovascular disease? *Diabetes Care* 2004;**27**:2676–81.

Stott N. Screening for cardiovascular risk in general practice. *BMJ* 1994;**308**: 285–6.

Tsivgoulis G, Spengos K, Manta P et al. Validation of the ABCD score in identifying individuals at high early risk of stroke after a transient ischemic attack: a hospital-based case series study. *Stroke* 2006;**37**:2892–7.

UK Prospective Diabetes Study Group. Tight blood pressure control and risk of macrovascular and microvascular complications in type 2 diabetes: UKPDS 38. *BMJ* 1998;**317**:703–13.

Üstün TB, Sartorius N, eds. *Mental Illness in General Health Care: An International Study*. Chichester: Wiley, 1995.

Wardlaw JM, del Zoppo GJ, Yamaguchi T, Berge E. Thrombolysis for acute ischaemic stroke. *Cochrane Database Syst Rev* 2003;**3**:CD000213.

Welschen LMC, Bloemendal E, Nijpels G et al. Self-monitoring of blood glucose in patients with type 2 diabetes mellitus who are not using insulin. *Cochrane Database Syst Rev* 2005;**2**:CD005060.

Williams C. GP stress: seeking help when you can no longer cope. *Pulse* 2008;10 Apr.

World Health Organization. *Definition and Diagnosis of Diabetes and Intermediate Hyperglycaemia*. Geneva: WHO, 2006.

9 The Clinical Skills Assessment

This chapter relates to curriculum statements 6–16 (Table 9.1)
The cases list 22 common topics covering the range of the clinical syllabus.

What is the CSA?

The Clinical Skills Assessment (CSA) is 'an assessment of a doctor's ability to integrate and apply clinical, professional, communication and practical skills appropriate for general practice' (RCGP 2007). On the day of the exam you will sit in a consulting room and see 13 'patients' (role played by an actor). You have 10 minutes per consultation. A few minutes before the start of the exam you will receive the patient order and brief details on each of the patients. Once the exam starts, you will be expected to explore the presenting complaint and work through history and examination as you would in a normal surgery, giving explanations and options as you go to arrive at an agreed management plan. Your consultation approach, investigations and management plan should be in line with good medical practice and current evidence/guidelines. An examiner will observe the consultation. There will be a 2-minute gap between consultations. One of the 13 consultations is a practice case for new exam material and will not count in your final mark. You need to achieve a pass in approximately 8 out of 12 cases to achieve an overall pass.

How are the cases selected?
Cases are selected to provide a range of presentations (e.g. acute illness, chronic illness, undifferentiated illness, psychological and social, preventive and lifestyle) across the disease spectrum. Cases may include a telephone consultation and home visit. For each of these the candidates are taken to a separate room.

Notes for the MRCGP: A curriculum based guide to the AKT, CSA and WBPA, 4th edition.
By K. Palmer and N. Boeckx. Published 2010 by Blackwell Publishing,
ISBN: 978-1-4051-5724-7.

Table 9.1 Clinical curriculum statements

Case no.	Page	Case title	Curriculum statement	Curriculum statement no.
1	245	Familial breast cancer	Genetics in primary care	6
2	248	Antibiotics in general practice	Care of acutely ill people	7
3	253	Child abuse	Care of children and young people	8
4	256	Grief	Care of older adults	9
5	259	Emergency contraception	Women's health	10.1
6	264	HRT		
7	268	Erectile dysfunction	Men's health	10.2
8	271	Vaginal discharge	Sexual health	11
9	274	Death, dying and palliative care	Care of people with cancer and palliative care	12
10	281	Tired all the time	Care of people with mental health problems	13
11	284	Cardiovascular and learning disability	Care of people with learning disabilities	14
			Cardiovascular problems	15.1
12	287	Dyspepsia	Digestive problems	15.2
13	290	Alcohol abuse	Drug and alcohol problems	15.3
14	296	Drug abuse		
15	299	Acute sinusitis	ENT and facial problems	15.4
16	301	Red eye	Eye problems	15.5
17	304	Obesity	Metabolic problems	15.6
18	307	Advising the person with epilepsy	Neurological problems	15.7
19	311	Smoking cessation	Respiratory problems	15.8
20	313	Low back pain	Rheumatology, musculoskeletal and trauma	15.9
21	317	Acne vulgaris	Skin problems	15.10
22	320	Chronic kidney disease	Renal	16

How is the CSA marked?

The assessor will be marking you against the three domains of assessment:

1. Data gathering
2. Clinical management
3. Interpersonal skills.

There is also a mark for the overall impression, called the global mark. The examiners have a pre-set marking sheet specific to the case. For each

domain the mark sheet lists positive and negative descriptors, e.g. acute exacerbation of asthma:
- Positive descriptor: clarifies the problem taking a focused asthma history
- Negative descriptor: disorganised history taking focusing on non-important issues.

There is no guidance for examiners on the proportion of negative/positive indicators attained that constitutes a clear pass, marginal pass, marginal fail or clear fail. To pass a case you must be deemed competent in each of the domains. The domains have equal weighting.

RCGP summary of assessment criteria for CSA

- **Data gathering, technical and assessment skills**: gathering and using data for clinical judgement, choice of examination, investigations and their interpretation. Demonstrating proficiency in performing physical examinations and using diagnostic and therapeutic instruments.
- **Clinical management skills**: recognition and management of common medical conditions in primary care. Demonstrating a structured and flexible approach to decision-making, and the ability to deal with multiple complaints and co-morbidity, and promote a positive approach to health.
- **Interpersonal skills**: demonstrating the use of recognised communication techniques to gain understanding of the patient's illness experience and develop a shared approach to managing problems. Practicing ethically with respect for equality and diversity issues, in line with the accepted codes of professional conduct.

Preparing for the CSA

You will not be able to practise for every conceivable eventuality because the range of potential cases is vast. Some basic principles apply to CSA consultations:
- To achieve the best marks in the CSA your consultation should be systematic, comprehensive and well time managed.
- Approach the cases as though you were a GP in a well-equipped surgery with all investigations available and access to a full range of secondary care services.
- Admit lack of knowledge – offer to phone a friend (i.e. discuss with a colleague in the surgery, check guidelines, discuss with a consultant) and arrange a follow-up consultation. Knowledge of your limitations is essential (GMC *Good Medical Practice* 2006). Making things up is a fast way to fail.
- Try to listen without interrupting for the first 2 minutes. Most patients will talk for less than this (Langewitz et al. *BMJ* 2002;**325**:682–3) and will reveal the main history points during this time. Then ask the salient questions. This will demonstrate good interpersonal skills and can help improve time management.

The exam is looking for competency – you are not expected to manage a case from diagnosis to cure in 10 minutes. Being comprehensive means covering the important consultation points at the current stage of illness. If you take a relevant history and examination, request investigations where appropriate starting with the simple, and show safe practice and empathy, you should pass. The needs consultation model may provide a useful structure on which to develop a concise, systematic and comprehensive approach to the CSA dilemmas. Videoing consultations will allow you to review and assess your strengths and weaknesses. Use the cases in this chapter to practise role-playing and score each other against the CSA marking schedule provided at the end of each section. Practise your examination routines to make them slick – a partner or large teddy bear is a good guinea pig!

CSA and the MRCGP curriculum

The three domains (data gathering, clinical management, interpersonal skills) cover the following curriculum areas:
- Primary care management: recognition and management of common medical conditions in primary care.
- Problem-solving skills: gathering and using data for clinical judgement, choice of examination, investigations and their interpretation. Demonstration of a structured and flexible approach to decision-making.
- Comprehensive approach: demonstration of proficiency in the management of co-morbidity and risk.
- Person-centred care: communication with patients and the use of recognised consultation techniques to promote a shared approach to managing problems.
- Attitudinal aspects: practising ethically with respect for equality and diversity, within accepted professional codes of conduct.

Useful questions to use in the CSA

Three areas of the consultation are often missed. By asking three questions you can address these problem spots:
1. Putting the condition in social context: 'How is … affecting your daily activities or work?'
2. Exploring the patient's health understanding: 'What do you think the problem might be?'
3. Confirming the patient's understanding: 'Sometimes I don't explain myself well. Can I check your understanding by getting you to explain the problem and the plan we have agreed?'

Equipment list for the CSA (RCGP 2008)

Candidates should bring the following in their doctor's bag:
- *BNF*
- Stethoscope
- Ophthalmoscope
- Auroscope
- Thermometer
- Patella hammer
- Sphygmomanometer (aneroid or electronic)

- Tape measure
- Peak flow meter and disposable mouthpieces (note that these must be EU standard).

Tips from CSA examiners, trainers and candidates on passing the CSA

1. Make sure that your equipment works and bring spare batteries (candidates have failed cases because of inadequate equipment).
2. Any technical jargon used should be accompanied by an explanation.
3. Candidates often hunt imagined hidden agendas – use the trigger phrase 'Is there anything you are particularly worried about' to force the role player to disclose any hidden agenda.
4. Take the exam seriously – one candidate has been referred to the GMC following their exam performance.
5. The role-player will redirect you if you start down the wrong path. Listen to the responses carefully and don't persist if warned off, e.g.
   Candidate: Do you think stress at home or work might be a factor?
   RP: No, I'm happy at home and work, everything's fine.
6. Not completing the consultation in 10 minutes does not mean that you have failed the case. If you have covered the main points, you may still score well.
7. Sharing your concerns with the patient can be a useful consultation tool, e.g. vaginal discharge:
   Candidate: 'One of my concerns is that vaginal discharge can be caused by sexually transmitted infections. Are you concerned about this?' (Followed by risk assessment for STI)
8. You are expected to fill investigation forms in (so examiners can assess the use of appropriate investigations). Complete the forms starting with the tests first, and leave the patient details until last, in case you run out of time.
9. Ten minutes goes very fast – time management is critical.
10. You are videoed from start to finish in your consultation room – don't forget! Act professionally until you leave the building. There have been embarrassing recordings of some candidates.
11. Housekeeping – once you have finished a consultation start preparing yourself mentally for the next. Don't dwell on imagined failings or successes.
12. Read through the first half of the cases sheet provided in the few minutes before the start of the exam, and the second half in the tea break. You can scribble notes on the sheets to help prepare yourself, e.g. list red flags or important management options.
13. Always introduce yourself and stand to greet the patient (helps demonstrate accordance with Attitudinal aspects curriculum area).
                    (Trainer's Workshop 2008 at West Midlands Deanery)

Case 1

Candidate information

Name: Michelle Fielding
Age: 28
Social and family history: librarian, one sister age 30, BMI 27
Past medical history: termination of pregnancy age 21
Drug history: Microgynon

A 28-year-old librarian presents to the surgery regarding a lump in her breast noticed by her partner.

Role-player information

Michelle is a 28-year-old librarian who lives with her partner, Ian. Ian's aunt is being investigated for a breast lump and is waiting the results post-surgery. Consequently Ian was very concerned on finding a lump in Michelle's breast. The lump has been present for 7 days with no change in size. Michelle has not noted any nipple discharge or skin changes, and no swelling of the glands under her arm. She can move the lump in the breast. It is pea-sized. She has had no children, and other than her mother, who had breast cancer aged 58, no other family members have had breast cancer. Michelle is a non-smoker. She had not noticed the lump before being alerted by her partner. She is worried about her risk of breast cancer. Her concerns are that she may be at increased risk of breast cancer because her mother has had the disease. She is also concerned that she will need chemotherapy and lose her hair. She has heard about screening for breast cancer and expects an urgent referral for a mammogram. Michelle wants to know what, if anything, she can do to reduce her risk of breast cancer. If her risk of breast cancer is well explained, Michelle will agree a shared management plan to review her breast lump. Michelle is on day 17 of the OCP.

Examination card

Mobile area of increased nodularity lateral to the areola present in the left breast. Mild tenderness on palpation. No skin changes or lymphadenopathy. Right breast normal. No nipple discharge and otherwise normal on inspection.

Topic summary: Breast lumps

This summary outlines the assessment of breast lumps in patients both with and without a family history of breast cancer.

The scale of the problem

Breast cancer is the most common malignancy in women. One woman in eleven will suffer from breast cancer at some point in their life. It is rare before the age of 30 years with the highest proportion of breast cancers diagnosed between the ages of 50 and 64 (Office for National Statistics 2007).

Family history (NICE 2006a)

The risk of breast cancer doubles if a first-degree relative (mother or sister) is affected compared with a woman with no family history of the disease. If two or more relatives are affected the risk increases further. Around 10%

are said to be due to genetic disposition, about 5% being caused by dominant genes. The most important gene is said to be the *BRCA-1* gene. Carriers have a lifetime risk nearing 80% of developing breast cancer and an increased risk of developing ovarian cancer.

Familial breast cancer risk assessment

Women at or **near population risk** of developing breast cancer (i.e. a 10-year risk of <3% for women aged 40–49 years and a lifetime risk of <17%) are cared for in primary care. Women at **raised risk** of developing breast cancer (i.e. a 10-year risk of 3–8% for women aged 40–49 years or a lifetime risk of 17% or greater but <30%) are generally cared for in secondary care. Women at **high risk** of developing breast cancer (i.e. a 10-year risk of >8% for women aged 40–49 years or a lifetime risk of 30% or greater) are cared for in tertiary care. High risk also includes a 20% or greater chance of a faulty *BRCA-1*, *BRCA-2* or *TP-53* gene in the family.

Familial breast cancer referral criteria
Near population risk (no referral)
- Single relative affected after the age of 40.

Women who may be at increased risk (refer on their 40th birthday)

Female breast cancers only:
- One first-degree relative diagnosed before age 40
- One first-degree relative and one second-degree relative diagnosed after average age 50
- Two first-degree relatives diagnosed after average age 50.

Women who may be at high risk (refer on)

Female breast cancers only:
- One first-degree relative and one second-degree relative diagnosed before average age 50
- Two first-degree relatives diagnosed before average age 50
- Three or more first- or second-degree relatives diagnosed at any age.

Male breast cancer:
- One first-degree male relative diagnosed at any age.

Bilateral breast cancer:
- One first-degree relative where first primary diagnosed before age 50.

Breast and ovarian cancer:
- One first- or second-degree relative with ovarian cancer at any age and one first- or second-degree relative with breast cancer at any age (one should be a first-degree relative).

Note that all relatives must be on the same side of the family and be blood relatives of the patient and each other. Suspicious family histories not meeting the criteria listed, e.g. bilateral breast cancer, should be discussed with secondary care.

Breast cancer and the oral contraceptive pill

There is an increased risk of breast cancer in women who are currently or have recently used the combined oral contraceptive pill. Risk rises with age but returns to zero after 10 years' cessation of the oestrogen. Review the use of the combined pill in women over the age of 35 years with a family history of breast cancer in view of the increased risks and discuss alternatives (see National Prescribing Centre 2006; see also 2008 edition of the *BNF*).

Note HRT use: the million women study demonstrated that breast cancer is more common in users of hormone replacement therapy (HRT) than non-users and incidence was higher among oestrogen–progesterone preparations compared with oestrogen-only preparations.

Other risk factors for breast cancer

See Chapter 6.

Assessment of a breast lump

It is important when assessing a lump to consider
- Age (fibroadenoma are more common in younger women)
- The menstrual cycle: if a lump varies in size over the menstrual cycle it is most likely to be benign
- Recent trauma may cause fat necrosis
- The breastfeeding woman can develop an abscess or mastitis
- Breast buds of pubescent girls may appear at uneven rates
- Skin tethering: a poorly defined margin rather than a smooth even rubbery lump may suggest a carcinoma rather than a fibroadenoma
- A cyst may be fluctuant and a lipoma soft in consistency.

Who to refer (NICE 2005a)

Urgent referral ...
- Any patient (regardless of age) with:
  - a discrete, hard lump with fixation, with or without skin tethering
  - previous breast cancer and with a new lump or suspicious symptoms
  - unilateral eczematous skin or nipple change that does not respond to topical treatment
  - nipple distortion of recent onset
  - spontaneous unilateral bloody nipple discharge
  - a unilateral, firm subareolar mass with or without nipple distortion or associated skin changes and who are male, aged 50 years and older
- >30 s with a discrete lump that persists after their next period, or presents after menopause
- <30 s with:
  - a lump that enlarges
  - a lump that is fixed and hard
  - risk factors, e.g. family history of cancer.

Non-urgent referral ...
- <30 with a lump
- Breast pain and no palpable abnormality when initial treatment fails.

Case 1 marking schedule

This is an example of an acute presentation. The nub of the case is risk assessment and shared decision-making. Marks are awarded for the following.

Data gathering

- Takes a structured history to include the risk factors for breast cancer (see Summary), duration of the lump, changes in size, variation with menstrual cycle, history of recent trauma, nipple discharge, skin changes, pain.
- Takes a family history of breast cancer including details of the age of onset and including all first- and second-degree relatives. Documents if the affected relatives are paternal or maternal.
- Identifies the patient's ideas, concerns and expectations (ICE: I = I am at increased risk of breast cancer, C = I may need chemotherapy and lose my hair, E = I will be referred straight away for a mammogram).
- Performs a breast examination proficiently. Requests a chaperone for the breast examination. If a male the candidate offers a choice of female examiner (the examination card is revealed at this stage).

Clinical management

- Recognises the history of the lump and examination represents a low risk of breast cancer.
- Correctly identifies the patient at near population risk based on the family history (single relative affected over the age of 40) and therefore manages her in primary care in this regard.
- Addresses the patient's concerns through appropriate examination and explanation. This should include an explanation of her risk of familial breast cancer, the assessment of breast lumps and her risk of breast cancer. When discussing her expectation explain that urgent referral is not indicated and that mammography is not used in younger patients (age <35) in whom the dense breast tissue makes this technique difficult (ultrasonography or MRI is preferred).
- Discusses the management options, i.e. review after next menstrual cycle to see if nodularity resolves, or consider non-urgent referral. Agrees a shared plan based on the patient's level of concern.
- Offers advice on reducing her risk of breast cancer by addressing her risk factors (weight control, alcohol intake and use of hormonal contraception).

Interpersonal skills

- Shows empathy for the patient's concerns through active listening.
- Feeds back concerns through the assessment and management.
- Specifies conditions for follow-up.
- Offers written information (a good way of handling this in the CSA is to ask the patient to pick up a patient information leaflet on the topic from reception after the consultation).

Case 2

Candidate information

Name: Zoe Latham

Age: 5

Social and family history: two siblings aged 7 and 10

Past medical history: asthma well controlled

Drug history: Salbutamol as needed

A 5-year-old girl is brought to your surgery by her mother, complaining of a sore throat. Zoe has had two similar episodes in the last 12 months treated with antibiotics on both occasions. Mum has two older children and visits the surgery on a regular basis. The candidate's task is to find out why she has presented today and agree an appropriate management plan.

> **Role player information**
> Zoe became unwell overnight, and is pyrexial with a red throat but no other signs. Mum wants a prescription for antibiotics as 'they have worked in the past' and will press the candidate for this. She would like more information about tonsillectomy for recurrent sore throats. Mum struggles working and coping with her three children, especially when the children become unwell and are at home from school. During these episodes of minor illness she visits the surgery frequently hoping to speed the recovery of her child so she can return to work.

Topic summary: Sore throats

The majority of antibiotic prescribing in the UK occurs in general practice. However, the prescribing behaviour of GPs varies widely. Uncertainty and debate on when to prescribe antibiotics remain topical. Widespread use of antibiotics is discouraged owing to the emergence of resistant bacteria, many of which are multi-drug resistant. Antibiotic resistance is seen as a threat to public health and the central reason for limiting prescription (National Prescribing Centre 2006).

Antibiotic resistance is associated with:
- increase in the length and severity of illness
- increase in the spread of disease
- increased use of alternative drugs with lesser known, or poorer safety profiles
- increased financial cost of treatment and care.

The dilemma of whether or not to prescribe is influenced by the clinical presentation, and the knowledge and attitudes of the doctor and patient. There is also an ethical dilemma – beneficence to the patient by prescribing to relieve symptoms and prevent complications versus non-maleficence to the community by limiting prescribing and reducing the spread of drug resistance.

Preventing complications and treating symptoms

A Cochrane review (Del Mar et al. 2006) of 27 studies found that antibiotics reduced the symptoms and number of complications of acute sore throat, e.g. otitis media and quinsy. The number needed to treat (NNT) to prevent one complication ranged from 60 to 71. Antibiotics were shown to reduce symptoms of sore throat but only by an average of 16 hours, although by 1 week 90% of treated and untreated patients were symptom free. The National Prescribing Centre (2006) concludes that 'it seems reasonable to only use antibiotics where complications occur'.

Delayed prescriptions

A randomised controlled trial (RCT; Little et al. 1997) in 11 GP practices offered antibiotics, a delayed prescription for use after 3 days or no pre-scription. Of those with delayed prescriptions 60% did not use them and outcomes in terms of satisfaction and duration of symptoms were not significantly different. Those who did receive antibiotics were more likely to return for further antibiotics. Not prescribing led to the lowest number of inappropriate antibiotic prescriptions, but the strategy of offering a delayed prescription was effective at reducing the number of antibiotics prescribed. The authors found that 'explanation, reassurance and advice on symptomatic treatment are often all that is necessary'.

When are antibiotics appropriate?

A scoring system called the Centor criteria has been developed to aid the diagnosis of sore throat caused by group A β-haemolytic streptococci (GABHS), which is associated with a higher risk of complications. Presence of three or four of the clinical signs indicates a 40–60% chance of GABHS and a 1:60 risk of quinsy vs 1:400 for those without. It may therefore be reasonable to prescribe antibiotics for this group of patients. The absence of three or four signs means that there is an 80% chance that GABHS is not present and antibiotic treatment is unlikely to be necessary. The Centor scheme is not ideal, and will lead to some patients with bacterial pharyngitis not being treated and result in unnecessary antibiotic treatment for others. The Centor criteria are as follows (score 1 for each element):
• Tonsillar exudate
• Tender anterior cervical lymph nodes
• Absence of cough
• History of fever.

When is tonsillectomy indicated?

A Cochrane review 1999 concluded that there was insufficient evidence to accurately assess the effectiveness of tonsillectomy. The best available evidence indicates that children with recurrent episodes (see below for the 'Paradise' criteria) will benefit from one less episode of moderately severe or severe sore throat a year but face a postoperative complication rate of 4–7% (Paradise et al. 1984). Criticisms are that the trial was small and baseline characteristics were not controlled for. A more recent RCT by Van Staaij et al. (2004) showed no improvement in the number of recurrent episodes of fever, sore throat or quality-of-life scores (300 children aged 2–8) for those with mild symptoms (i.e. not meeting the Paradise criteria). On the current available evidence it seems reasonable to refer using the Paradise criteria after a discussion of the complication rate. Tonsillectomy is also indicated for recurrent tonsillitis with complications, e.g. quinsy or airway obstruction.

The 'Paradise' criteria are (surgery reduces the number of episodes by one a year):
• seven episodes in 1 year OR
• five a year for the last 2 years OR
• three a year for 3 years.

MEMORY BOX
• Antibiotics unnecessary for most cases
• Serious complications are rare
• 90% resolve in 1 week regardless of cause
• Centor criteria help identify those who may benefit from antibiotics
• Paradise criteria help identify those who may benefit from tonsillectomy

---

Case 2 marking schedule

This case assesses the candidate's management of acute illness in children. Communication and negotiation are important elements. Marks are awarded for the following.

Data gathering

- Establishes patients/parental ideas, concerns, expectations re cause of sore throat.
- Identifies the presence or absence of the Centor criteria through a systematic history and examination.
- Establishes the duration of the illness, and background history of previous episodes.
- Completes proficient exam of ear, nose, throat and chest (*images of oropharynx provided in exam*).

Clinical management

- Demonstrates an understanding of the causes and natural history of sore throat and the low risk of serious complications.
- Discusses the pros and cons of antibiotics for sore throat, and other management strategies including self-management of minor illness; able to discuss criteria for tonsillectomy when questioned.
- Recognises and manages significant co-morbidity, e.g. asthma exacerbation in viral illness.
- If prescribes, checks for history of adverse drug reactions.

Interpersonal skills

- Recognises the concerns of the parent and shows empathy.
- Discusses her support network.
- Comes to a shared management plan following national guidance while maintaining a good doctor–patient relationship – using a delayed prescription if necessary.
- Specifies conditions for follow-up.

An associated dilemma, the use of antibiotics for otitis media, raises similar issues. Consider the first case substituting the presenting complaint of sore throat with otitis media. A topic summary and marking schedule is provided below.

Topic summary: Acute otitis media (National Prescribing Centre 2006)

MEMORY BOX: Acute otitis media

- Antibiotics unnecessary for most cases
- Serious complications are rare
- 80% resolve in 3 days without treatment

Risk factors

Acute otitis media (AOM) is one of the most common complaints seen in children in primary care. Age and contact with other children are risk factors. Three-quarters of cases of AOM occur in those aged below 10 years. At least one in four children has an episode of AOM before they are 10 years old.

Management options

A Cochrane review (2004: 15 trials, based on 2695 children) found that there was insufficient evidence to support the use of decongestants or antihistamines in children with AOM, and both medications have undesirable side effects. There is limited evidence for the use of analgesia, but harm is unlikely and use is routinely recommended.

When are antibiotics appropriate?

A Cochrane review (Glasziou et al. 2004) compared antibiotics versus placebo in children with AOM. Antibiotics reduced pain (NNT 15) but at increased risk of side effects (vomiting, diarrhoea, rash, NNT 17). Complications were rare and antibiotics did not confer absolute protection (one child developed mastoiditis but was in the antibiotic group!). The review concluded that antibiotics are not routinely recommended for AOM. Certain subgroups had a lower NNT, e.g. children <2 years, bilateral otitis, discharging otitis, systemic illness. The benefits (pain relief and cessation of fever) are modest and antibiotic prescribing is not routinely recommended in these groups either.

Delayed prescriptions?

Use of a 48 hr delayed prescription to provide time for spontaneous resolution has proved a useful strategy for reducing antibiotic prescribing (Spiro et al. 2006) though no prescription is the most appropriate option. Where prescriptions are provided 5 days amoxicillin is recommended.

Marking schedule: acute otitis media
Data gathering
- Establishes patient's/parental ideas, concerns, expectations re ear pain.
- Identifies the signs and symptoms associated with an increase in the likelihood of AOM (ear pain, ear rubbing, cloudy eardrum, bulging eardrum, immobile eardrum, red eardrum). *Image of tympanic membrane provided.*
- Completes proficient exam of ear, nose and throat.

Clinical management
- Demonstrates an understanding of the causes and natural history of otitis media and the low risk of serious complications.
- Discusses the pros and cons of antibiotics for otitis media.
- Recognises and manages any significant co-morbidity.
- If prescribes, checks history of adverse drug reactions.

Interpersonal skills
- Recognises the concerns of the patient/parents, identifies expectations and shows empathy.
- Comes to a shared management plan following national guidance – using a delayed prescription if necessary prescribing the appropriate agent.
- Specifies conditions for follow-up.

Case 3

Candidate information

Name: Beyonce Woodbarn

Age: 19

Social and family history: Unemployed mother living in council flats with her partner Callum Woodbarn. Child, Goldie Woodbarn, 3 years of age. Callum is a patient at the practice age 20 and has a history of substance misuse.

Past medical history: Goldie had a pulled arm injury 7 months previously. Health visitor has previously documented concerns over how mum and dad are coping and so has been visiting regularly.

The health visitor asks to discuss Beyonce and her 3-year-old toddler. She has just visited this morning.

Role-player information

You have been visiting mum regularly as you have been concerned about how she is coping. Beyonce often seems disorganised and the house is a tip. She seems to get little support from her partner and has no support from her family. Neighbours have complained about shouting and loud music. Mum has poor parenting skills and you have frequently witnessed mum telling Goldie to shut up. Mum is the head of the household, she is disorganised and often runs out of money for her electric card meter. Goldie has met his developmental milestones; he often wears dirty clothes and has behavioural problems. He swears at you when he doesn't get what he wants. You visited today and found Goldie had superficial burns to his legs and bottom. No splash burns to the upper legs. Mum says he burnt himself trying to get into the bath. You have come to discuss this with the GP. You are worried that Goldie is being neglected or physically abused and want advice on how best to act.

Topic summary: Child abuse

All those who come into contact with children and families at work (e.g. GPs, nurses, health visitors, social services, teachers, etc.) have a duty to safeguard and promote the welfare of children (*Every Child Matters* 2004 and *Working Together to Safeguard Children* 2006 – see www.everychild-matters.gov.uk/publications). The appropriate action to take depends on the urgency of the need for assessment (Figure 9.1).

A golden rule for child protection

The golden principle of child protection is if in doubt to discuss the case (with a child protection lead/social services). If confidentiality is a concern withhold patient identifiable information.

What requires urgent referral?

Refer urgently where there is a risk to the life of a child or a likelihood of serious immediate harm. Neglect and abuse can fall into this category. Children can be removed for immediate protection under section 47 of the Children's Act

Information-sharing principles (*Every Child Matters* – www.everychildmatters.gov.uk/publications)

• Openly and honestly explain what, how and why information will be shared

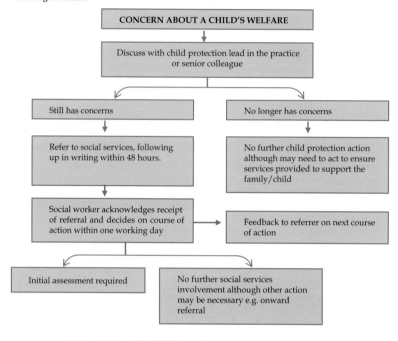

Non Urgent Action^{Working together to Safeguard children 2006 (HM Government)}

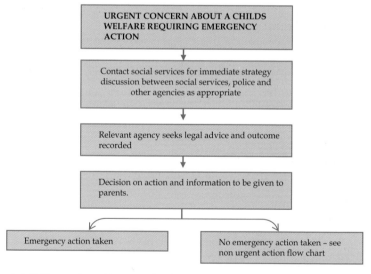

Urgent Action^{Working together to Safeguard children 2006 (HM Government)}

Figure 9.1 Child protection guidance on referral.

- Always consider a child's safety and welfare when making decisions about sharing
- Seek consent – if not secured this should be respected where possible
- Seek advice where in doubt

- Ensure that information is accurate, up to date, necessary, shared with the appropriate people and stored safely
- Record the reasons for the decision – whether it is to share or not.

Dos and don'ts
- Avoid leading questions or investigating allegations of abuse because this may undermine subsequent criminal investigation – stick to who, what, where and when
- Communicate with the child in a way appropriate to their age, understanding and preference
- Reassure the child but do not promise confidentiality as you may have to disclose information
- Record all concerns, discussions, decisions and the reasons for those decisions.

Injuries suspicious of non-accidental origin
Burns
- Patterned burns (cigarettes, irons, spoon)
- Liquid burns involving both legs and the bottom: in a non-accidental burn the child raises the legs to avoid the hot water so the feet and bottom contact first. Accidental burns usually only involve one but sometimes both legs and splash burns are usually present.

Bruises
- Inner thighs, genitals, finger mark bruising, patterned bruising, e.g. linear marks of a stick or belt.

Fractures
- Injuries not consistent with age (limb fractures in non-mobile children)
- Multiple fractures
- Rib fractures.

Other
- Trauma to lips, ear or frenulum
- Retinal haemorrhage (from shaking injury).

Forms of abuse
- Physical
- Neglect
- Emotional abuse
- Sexual abuse.

Case 3 marking schedule

This is an example of a proxy case. Proxies are commonly used for cases involving children. The nub of the case is familiarity with child protection procedures. Candidates must demonstrate that safety of the child is their paramount concern and agree an appropriate plan of action. Marks are awarded for the following.

Data gathering
- Gathers evidence from the health visitor about the current injury (who, what, where and when).
- Asks about previous injuries and discusses the information in the medical record with the health visitor.
- Asks about evidence of abuse – developmental delay, behavioural disturbances, bruising, inappropriate behaviour, previous abuse by either partner, family history of abuse, parental behaviour and parenting skills.
- Gathers information about the family's social circumstances (social support network, finances, accommodation, organisation).
- Identifies the health visitor's ideas, concerns and expectations.

Clinical management
- Recognises the burn pattern as suspicious of physical abuse.
- Identifies risk factors for abuse (poor social support network, poor parenting skills, parental substance misuse, poverty, poor parenting skills).
- Correctly identifies the need to act to protect the child and support the family.
- Agrees a management plan with the health visitor and takes responsibility for acting. The plan should involve a referral to social services and a discussion of the case to decide on whether urgent action is required. This can be achieved in several ways (referral to social services, or direct referral to paediatrician responsible for child protection). As this child has a physical injury and may need medical attention contacting, the local paediatrician may be the most appropriate.
- The candidate documents clearly and accurately, recording the discussions, concerns, decision and reasons for decision.
- The candidate agrees to contact the mum to openly and honestly explain their concerns and request consent to disclose information. Explain how and why information will be shared. (Failure to consent will not affect the need to refer but is good practice.)

Interpersonal skills
- Agrees a shared management plan respecting the health visitor's professional concerns.
- Demonstrates interest and concern in the welfare of children.
- As part of the plan states that he will send a written copy of the referral within 48 hours
- Offers to feed back any developments in the case to the health visitor.

Negative indicators
- Failure to refer or discuss the case further is a negative indicator and constitutes a clear fail.

Case 4

Candidate information

Name: Dorothy Silverman
Age: 72
Social and family history: widow. Lives alone
Past medical history: osteoarthritis, hip replacement 6 years ago
Drug history: Adcal D3, alendronate

Mrs Silverman is brought to the surgery by her neighbour following a recent bereavement. Her neighbour is concerned that Dorothy is not coping at home. The candidate's task is to establish the patient's issues and agree a management plan.

Role-player information

Dorothy's husband George died 11 weeks ago after a second stroke. George recovered good function after the first stroke and did not require additional care. Dorothy lives alone, but is close to her neighbours. She has one daughter who lives abroad and no other living relatives. Dorothy used to enjoy shopping and dancing but has stopped going out and lost her enjoyment of life. She is often tearful, low and has difficulty sleeping. She thinks that she may be 'losing her marbles' as she occasionally hears George's voice and short-term memory is poor. She is worried that she will never feel better and is frightened by her strange experiences. She does not want to burden others with her problems so has kept her feelings to herself; however, she broke into tears when her neighbour called today. Dorothy has no history of mental illness.

Topic summary: Grief (Woof and Carter 1997)
Bereavement

Bereavement is a source of considerable anguish and suffering. It can be a frightening experience, especially for those close to the dead person, who often lose an important part of their support network. Patients may need extra support to make sense of what has happened, how they feel and how to cope. Much of this is provided by family and friends. Support during the grieving process can help prevent pathological grief and psychiatric complications. Often explanation and reassurance of the normality of their experience are all that is needed. The role of the GP is to identify those requiring extra support or going through an abnormal grief process.

Normal grief (6 months)

Normal grief reactions are said to encompass the phases of:
1. Shock, numbness, blunted emotion, incomprehension (this lasts up to 2 weeks).
2. Physical distress, restlessness, withdrawal and grief. At this stage the dead person is to all intents and purposes still with her, to the point whereby the bereaved person may search for the departed, set the table for him, talk to him, hear his footsteps and even see him. There is a preoccupation with memories and idealisation and emotional reactions (depression, insomnia, anorexia, guilt) are common.
3. Gradually a more realistic memory develops, depression lifts and a process of disengagement occurs.

Normal grief reactions may last up to 6 months.

Abnormal grief (>6 months)

Abnormal grieving is said to apply when:
- grieving is *prolonged* (>6 months)
- the *intensity* of depression is extreme (patients who isolate themselves from family and friends, take a lot of time off work, attempt suicide).

Risk factors for abnormal grief
- Low socioeconomic status
- Short terminal illness with little warning of impending death
- Multiple life crises
- Severe reactions to bereavement.

(Parkes 1964; Wilkes 1983)

Post-bereavement mortality

Bereavement has a mortality:

- Morbidity and mortality are high in the first year and raised even after 2–3 years.
- Widowers aged 55 years or more have an increased mortality rate of about 40% in the first 6 months and overall 20% of widowers die in the first year compared with 4% of matched controls (Parkes 1986).
- Men are affected more than women and the risk for close relationships is greater than for distant ones.

Management of bereavement

The management of bereavement really begins with the preceding terminal illness (see Case 9):

- Help the family members prepare and recognise their new enforced roles
- Make the terminal illness as painless as possible by promoting harmony, comfort and mutual support
- Encourage family care: ideally the family should be there at the end and see the body afterwards.

Afterwards the GP must be an available and sympathetic ear. A desire to vent feelings and to search for meaning are common sequelae, as are visits with emotional problems and minor ill health. Close contact with the family also allows the pathological grief reaction to be recognised at an earlier stage. Referral to a self-help organisation (e.g. The Compassionate Friends or CRUSE) may be valuable.

A Protocol For Bereavement in Primary Care

- Offer all patients a patient leaflet about bereavement (detailing practical information, e.g. how to register the death, access support for the bereaved, i.e. CRUSE/Compassionate Friends, and a brief explanation of the bereavement process)
- Record the date of death in the bereaved notes – alerts the consulting doctor to the anniversary of the death.
- Offer a bereavement consultation:
  - ➤ the earlier the better – often appropriate when the body is certified
  - ➤ avoid contact on the day of the funeral (unless attending personally)
  - ➤ the consultation should be cathartic – GP's role is mainly listening; allow periods of silence for non-verbal communication so that the patient can express themselves and indicate empathy:
    'I will not insult you by trying to tell you that one day you will forget, I know that you will not. But at least in time you will not remember as fiercely as you do now, and I pray that time may be soon.' Rattigan (1953)
  - ➤ offer a review appointment – to assess progression of the grief and answer any questions regarding the cause of death. If ongoing support is required counselling through a bereavement organisation or locally should be offered.

(Woof and Carter 1997)

Case 4 marking schedule

This case assesses communication across psychological and social issues. Marks are awarded for the following.

Data gathering

- Establishes Mrs Silverman's symptoms (low mood, tearfulness, impaired concentration, auditory hallucinations of her husband)
- Establishes her support network (neighbour, and friends at the dancing club) and her coping strategies (stiff upper lip)
- Identifies her ICE regarding her symptoms and correctly establishes these are related to her recent bereavement (I = I am frightened by her strange symptoms and low mood, C = 'I am going mad', E = I will never get better, no one else feels like this')
- Establishes the impact of her symptoms (social isolation, loss of interest in her normal activities, difficulty coping with managing the house alone)
- Assesses for depression (two-question screen) and suicide risk ('Have you ever felt so low that you have though about harming yourself?').

Clinical management

- Discusses the grief reaction bringing her symptoms into context.
- Reassures her about the normality of her experience.
- Discusses management options:
  - ➤ personal support networks i.e. friends, family, church, dancing associates,
  - ➤ professional support networks i.e. counselling, bereavement organisations, befriending services
  - ➤ self help – bereavement support information, exercise
  - ➤ practical help – social services may provide help with financial advice, benefits, provision of carers if required
  - ➤ pharmacological – short-term hypnotic, anxiolytic.
- Offers a follow-up appointment.

Interpersonal skills

- Provides an empathic patient centred consultation.
- Listens carefully allowing periods of silence for the patient to express her grief.
- Provides written information regarding bereavement and support networks (ask the patient to pick it up from reception on the way out!).
- Confirms understanding.

The abbreviation ICE is used frequently in the chapter and stands for **i**deas, **c**oncerns and **e**xpectations. The relevant ideas, concerns and expectations from the history are then summarised after the respective initial.

Case 5

Candidate information

Name: Gemma Statham
Age: 16
Social and family history: two siblings aged 19 and 12, smokes five cigarettes a day
Past medical history: epilepsy; fit free for >12 months
Drug history: carbamazepine

A 16-year-old sixth form student presents to the surgery requesting emergency contraception – she has had unprotected intercourse 12 hours previously.

> **Role-player information**
>
> Gemma is a mature 16 year old. Her partner is 18. She has had consensual penetrative sex and has been sexually active for the last 2 years. She has had no previous partners. Her parents are unaware about the sexual relationship and she does not wish them to know because she is worried that they will be angry with her. On this occasion the condom came off during intercourse. She is worried that she might be pregnant and does not want to continue with any pregnancy.

Topic summary: Emergency contraception

In addition to emergency contraception this summary reviews the wider issues of this case; teenage pregnancy, underage sex (she has been sexually active since the age of 14), sexual abuse, child protection and consent in minors (in English Law a minor is a person less than 18 years old though the age of sexual consent is 16).

Prescribing emergency contraception

There are two main options for emergency contraception:
1. Hormonal contraception (levonorgestrel)
2. Copper IUD (intrauterine device).

Levonorgestrel 1.5 mg single dose (high-dose progesterone)

Effective up to 72 h post-intercourse
- Failure rate 1.1%
- Can be used unlicensed up to 120 h (efficacy reduces with delay)
- Available over the counter from the pharmacy (up to 72 h only)
- Patients who vomit within 2 hours of taking should take a further dose
- Enzyme-inducing drugs reduce the efficacy of levonorgestrel – a copper IUD or a 3 mg dose (unlicensed) is an alternative
- Patients should be advised that:
  - the next period may be early or late – if delayed by 1 week check status with a pregnancy test
  - barrier contraception should be used until the next period.

Copper IUD

- Effective if inserted within 5 days of:
  - unprotected sexual intercourse
  - the earliest calculated ovulation day.
- Failure rate 0.1%
- Provides ongoing contraception.

When prescribing emergency contraception, ongoing contraception and risk of sexually transmitted infection (STI) should be discussed as well.

Teenage pregnancy

The UK has the highest rate of teenage pregnancy in western Europe. Tackling this is a priority of the 2004 Children's Act (Every Child Matters). There is a multidisciplinary strategy, and for GPs this means offering an

integrated 'young person-friendly service'. Guidelines (Department of Health [DH] 2007a):
- Suitable environment: care should be delivered in a safe, suitable and young people-friendly environment. The waiting areas should be friendly, comfortable and welcoming with appropriate reading material for young people (content not stipulated!).
- Confidentiality:
  - ➤ young people should be reassured that their consultation is confidential
  - ➤ Fraser/Gillick principles should be followed when treating children under 16 without parental consent (see below).
- Sexual health services:
  - ➤ easy to understand information should be offered on sexual health issues to enable safe informed choice regarding contraception, STIs and relationships
  - ➤ check for coercion or abuse in the history and encourage confiding to parents
  - ➤ accurate information should be provided about the full range of hormonal, reversible and long-acting methods of contraception and emergency contraception
  - ➤ opportunistic chlamydia screening and treatment of young men and young women should be offered. A system for contact tracing positive results should be available (often via sexual health clinics).

Fraser guidelines (DH 2001)
In 1985, Lord Fraser said, in judgment of the Gillick case, that a doctor can give contraceptive advice or treatment to a person under 16 without parental consent provided that the doctor is satisfied that:
- The patient is competent to consent to treatment and understands the advice.
- The patient is encouraged to tell his or her parents or allow the doctor to tell them.
- It is probable that the young person is likely to begin or continue having unprotected sex with or without contraception.
- The young person's physical or mental health is likely to suffer unless he or she receives contraceptive advice or treatment.

Underage sex and sexual abuse
The Children's Act 2004 provides guidance for health professionals on underage sexual activity. Health professionals should discuss cases of concern with local child protection lead. Where confidentiality needs to be preserved, a discussion can still take place as long as it does not identify the child. The following considerations should be taken into account when assessing the extent to which a child (or other children) may be suffering or at risk of harm:
- Age of the child – young age is a very strong indicator of potential harm
- Maturity and understanding of the child
- Living circumstances or background

- Power imbalance, i.e. overt aggression or age imbalance
- Coercion or bribery
- Behaviour, i.e. withdrawn, anxious
- Family history of child sex offences
- Misuse of disinhibitors such as alcohol
- Secrecy, beyond what would be considered usual in a teenage relationship
- Response of child – denies, minimises or accepts concerns
- Methods consistent with grooming
- Whether the sexual partner is known by one of the agencies.

Penetrative sex with a child under 13 is classed as rape in law. All cases must be discussed with the local child protection lead. Thorough documentation of the history, discussions with other agencies and management plan is necessary for medicolegal purposes.

(Every Child Matters – www.everychildmatters.gov.uk/publications)

Case 5 marking schedule

This is an example of a case focused on social and prevention issues. Marks are awarded for the following.

Data gathering
- Establishes the need for emergency contraception – timing of intercourse, that it was penetrative and unprotected
- Elicits sexual history (duration of this relationship, how long sexually active, use of contraception, risk of STI, previous use of emergency contraception)
- Assesses risk of sexual abuse by establishing risk factors (see Topic summary).

Clinical management
- Reassures patient of confidentiality
- Encourages patient to tell her parents (Gemma is now 16 so Fraser competence is not in question but as a young adult it shows good practice, she may be at risk of abuse) – note that Gemma will refuse
- Raises age difference and age of onset of intercourse as factors of concern
- Correctly identifies Gemma as mature and the sex consensual, with a low risk of sexual abuse; it is acceptable to discuss the case anonymously with the child protection lead
- Demonstrates an understanding of emergency contraception and comes to an agreed management plan (levonorgestrel higher dose due to enzyme induction of carbamazepine)
- Discusses continuing contraception options
- Offers sexual health screening for *Chlamydia*
- Specifies use of emergency contraception and follow-up.

Interpersonal skills
- Provides an age-appropriate patient-centred consultation without use of technical jargon
- Recognises the concerns of the patient and addresses them in an unprejudiced consultation style
- Provides written information about contraception and sexual health
- Confirms understanding.

Example consultation model approach

This is an example of how to use the needs consultation model (see page 243) to identify the case issues.

Patient needs

- Establish a rapport
- Identify the presenting problem and consider ongoing problems
  - ➤ immediate emergency contraception
  - ➤ advice on long term contraception
- Consider ICE to achieve a shared understanding of the problems: I = wants emergency contraception, C = confidentiality, E = morning-after pill
- Consider the patient's behaviour (Adult, Child, Parent) and try to move towards an Adult–Adult consultation
- Discuss treatment options, jointly choose actions and share responsibility
  - ➤ discuss levonorgestrel vs IUD for emergency contraception
  - ➤ patient decides on levonorgestrel so increase dose to counter enzyme induction of carbamazepine
  - ➤ discuss ongoing contraception
- Safety net: specify follow-up conditions.

Practice needs

- Ensure a young person friendly practice
  - ➤ reassure regarding confidential nature of service
  - ➤ establish a suitable environment – no desk between patient and doctor, open posture, eye contact, listening without interrupting
  - ➤ explain simply without use of medical jargon and confirm understanding
  - ➤ provide appropriate patient leaflets.

Public needs

- Child protection: assess risk factors listed in topic summary – child protection
- Health promotion (sexual health – advice on STI prevention and opportunistic screening).

Practitioner needs

- Medicolegal:
  - ➤ ensure compliance with Fraser guidelines.
  - ➤ document the consultation clearly (including important positive and negative findings and plan of management/follow-up plans)
  - ➤ provide the patient with written information where appropriate
- Educational: identify any personal learning needs (review of child protection procedure)
- Organisational: contact child protection lead by telephone and if referral required confirm in writing within 48 hours
- Psychological: housekeeping (re Neighbour's model, page 17) – clear your mind to prepare for the next *case!*

Case 6

Candidate information

Name: Helena Edwards

Age: 49

Social and family history: two aged daughters 12 and 14.

Past medical history: hypertension well controlled BP 130/74

Drug history: ramipril 5 mg once daily

Helena presents today complaining of hot sweats and flushing.

Role-player information

Helena has been suffering with hot sweats for 8 months. They are affecting her quality of life but she has heard the HRT scares in the press and so has never mentioned her symptoms to a doctor. Now she has read about herbal treatment for them and wants a doctor's opinion before starting this treatment.

Examination card

BP 126/74. No abnormal findings.

Topic summary: Hormone replacement therapy

Few topics have had as much publicity and conflicting viewpoints as HRT. In the 1980s it was thought that HRT may offer a benefit to women by reducing their risk of cardiovascular disease. The Women's Health Initiative study was set up in 1991 with this as its hypothesis. It was a randomised controlled trial comparing combined HRT with placebo, set in the USA. The mean age of participants was 63 years and over 30% were obese, hypertensive or diabetic. The study was stopped early, after 5.2 years, with results showing an increase in coronary heart disease that caused adverse publicity and a swing away from prescribing. Further analysis of these data, published in 2007, showed that the increased risk was confined to older age groups and a slight reduction in cardiovascular disease in women in their 50s and those who had taken HRT in the first 10 years since the menopause. There is now renewed interest in researching further a potential cardiovascular benefit of HRT in women in the early perimenopause.

The Million Women Study recruited over a million women attending NHS breast screening over the late 1990s and was an observational study looking at incidences of cancer and death between HRT and non-HRT users. A main finding was an increased risk of breast cancer in HRT users. However, a number of criticisms have been made of this study. including the unrepresentative nature of the sample.

Your HRT questions answered!

How to diagnose the menopause?

This is usually made by the patient before attending. The average age of menopause (diagnosed in retrospect after a year of amenorrhoea) in the UK is 51 years. The diagnosis is clinical, with a typical history including irregular menstrual cycles, hot sweats, night sweats, vaginal dryness and mood/sleep disorder. Laboratory tests, including measurement of follicle-stimulating hormone (FSH), are NOT recommended due to fluctuations during the perimenopausal period and thus a lack of reliability. In women under 45 years with symptoms, it may be appropriate to measure FSH to establish a premature menopause (look for FSH >30), although this cannot be tested while on a combined contraceptive.

When to prescribe?

Eighty per cent of women in the UK experience menopausal symptoms though not all will attend their GP. Symptoms normally last 2–4 years although some can continue through to age 80. HRT is the most effective treatment for vasomotor symptoms (i.e. hot flushes). It is also beneficial for preventing osteoporosis and colorectal cancer, although these are not indications for its use. The risks should be balanced against the control of symptoms and fully discussed before prescribing.

What are the risks?

The risk of **breast cancer** increases with duration of use of HRT, and is apparent within the first 2 years. Risk returns to baseline by 5 years after stopping HRT. There is an increased risk of breast cancer in those on oestrogen and progesterone compared with those on oestrogen alone. The **cardiovascular risk** is increased in women who take HRT more than 10 years after the menopause. As cardiovascular disease is the greatest cause of death in women special consideration is required in patients with cardiovascular risk factors. In particular it is important to ensure that blood pressure is controlled before starting HRT. There is a small increased risk of **stroke** and **venous thromboembolism** (deep vein thrombosis [DVT]/ pulmonary embolism) in those taking HRT. Avoid giving HRT to those with multiple risk factors for these conditions and, before starting treatment, alert women to the signs and symptoms of DVT. There is a slight increase in **ovarian cancer** for HRT users (Table 9.2). The increase risk of **endometrial cancer** can be eliminated by treating all women who have not undergone a hysterectomy with progestogen alongside oestrogen.

What to prescribe?

All women around the perimenopause initially starting HRT are likely to have some bleeding, so they should be started on a cyclical regimen which allows a regular 'period'. If women are over 54 years or have had 6 months of amenorrhoea they can be given a continuous form of HRT. All women should receive oestrogen and progestogen unless they have had a hysterectomy. The lowest dose should be prescribed and tried for 3–6 months before swapping to an increased dose/alternative HRT, e.g. starting with Premarin 0.3 mg. A recent review of data showed that low-dose oestrogen could reduce flushes by approximately 65%, compared with 75–90% with conventional doses and 35% with placebo. Aim for the lowest dose for the shortest possible period.

Which route?

Oral treatment is usually started because it is cost-effective and well tolerated. Patches are available and the transdermal route is useful for women

Table 9.2 Risks of hormone replacement therapy (HRT) in different conditions

Risk	Age range	Oestrogen-only HRT (additional cases per 1000)		Combined HRT* (additional cases per 1000)	
		5 years	10 years	5 years	10 years
Breast cancer	50–59	10	20	2	24
	60–69	15	30	3	36
Endometrial cancer	50–59	2	4	4	–
	60–69	3	6	6	–
Ovarian cancer	50–59	2	4	<1	1
	60–69	3	6	<1	2
Venous	50–59	5	–	2	–
thromboembolism	60–69	8	–	2	–
Stroke	50–59	4	–	1	–
	60–69	9	–	3	–
Coronary heart disease	70–79	29–44	–	15	–

MHRA and CHM (2007) Risk table *Oestrogen + progestogen: http://cks.library.nhs.uk/menopause/evidence/supporting_evidence/risks_of_hrt.

with bowel disorders that may decrease absorption, or drug interactions, e.g. phenytoin or carbamazepine. If women mainly have vaginal symptoms, these can be managed with topical oestrogen without systemic treatment.

How often to review?

See women 3 months after starting HRT and then annually. Blood pressure should be measured and risks and benefits of continuing treatment discussed. Vaginal oestrogen should be reviewed annually and a break in treatment should be encouraged to assess whether it is still needed. Consideration should be given to whether to swap from cyclical to continuous combined HRT. The advantages of the latter are no need for a monthly bleed (though women should be warned to expect some bleeding in the first few months) and a single prescription charge.

What to do with breakthrough bleeding?

Refer to gynaecology to exclude endometrial cancer in women in whom:
• bleeding pattern changes
• there is breakthrough bleeding with cyclical HRT
• bleeding has not settled after 6 months of continuous combined HRT or tibolone
• bleeding restarts following a period of amenorrhoea.

How to stop HRT?

If considering stopping HRT this is normally done gradually by halving the dose for 3–6 months and then halving again for a further 3–6 months before stopping. Women should be warned that they may temporarily experience recurrence of former symptoms after stopping HRT.

How to manage side effects?

Oestrogenic symptoms include breast tenderness, nausea and headache. They may be improved by reducing the dose of oestrogen or trying a different type of oral oestrogen or different route of administration. Progestogenic symptoms include symptoms of PMS (premenstrual syndrome), back and lower abdominal ache, and low mood. Options are to change the route or preparation or try tibolone.

What about contraception?

HRT does not provide effective contraception. Women should be considered fertile until 1 year after their last period if aged over 50 years or 2 years after their last period if under 50 years. If HRT and contraception are required a Mirena coil can be used with oestrogen-only HRT to provide progestogen cover. Alternatively give a progestogen-only pill with combined sequential HRT.

What about alternatives to HRT?

The following lifestyle factors can reduce hot flushes: losing weight, taking more exercise and drinking less alcohol. A number of alternative drugs have been studied. Clonidine has been shown to have efficacy around 20–40% over placebo in reducing flushes. but has a range of potential side effects including drowsiness and dry mouth. Paroxetine and venlafaxine have been shown to help vasomotor symptoms but the effect is gradual. A 59% reduction in flushes was seen with venlafaxine at 8 weeks, but 15% of women experienced initial nausea or vomiting. Gabapentin 900 mg has been shown to decrease flushes by up to 67%. A number of complementary medicines have been used in place of HRT. Red clover seems to reduce the frequency of hot flushes, St John's wort seems to improve mild-to-moderate depression and relaxation may help hot flushes. Use of black cohosh has been shown to have evidence for use in a number of studies: it can improve sleep and improve vasomotor symptoms but there have been reports of hepatotoxicity.

MEMORY BOX: Hormone Replorement Therepy
- Control of menopausal symptoms is the indication for use of HRT
- Careful risk assessment must be made before starting HRT
- In most healthy low-risk women within the early perimenopause the benefits of symptom control will outweigh the risks
- Risks must be explained so that patients can decide if they are willing to accept them
- Use of risk charts to explain risk (e.g. the *BNF* chart) is recommended

---

Case 6 marking schedule

This case assesses the candidate's ability to discuss risks. This requires the ability to apply clinical knowledge to an individual to come to a shared understanding of risk and decision making. Marks are awarded for the following.

Data gathering

- Takes a history to diagnose the perimenopause
- Assesses risk factors regarding HRT to enable an informed discussion of risk

- Elicits adequate information to assess the risk of relevant diseases in order to safely and appropriately prescribe HRT
- Identifies the patient's beliefs, concerns and expectations of HRT.

Clinical management
- Demonstrates an understanding of the indications and contraindications to HRT
- Avoids unnecessary investigations
- Discusses risks of and alternatives to HRT in terms that a layperson can understand
- Applies the abstract concept of risk to the individual patient to demonstrate its relevance to her and aid her decision making, e.g. 'Taking HRT seems to cause one extra stroke for every 1000 patients aged 50–59. Your risk may be slightly higher than this because of your high blood pressure. If you want to take HRT we can minimise the risk to you by making sure your blood pressure is well controlled and any adverse lifestyle factors are addressed.'
- Provides written information
- Arranges appropriate follow-up.

Interpersonal skills
- Addresses the patient's reason for attending and offers to find out about efficacy of alternative treatments, if unsure
- Uses written information to demonstrate risk
- Recognises and discusses the patient's concerns
- Respects her views about the use of complementary therapies and acts to promote her health and safety in making choices about this.

Note that candidates are strongly advised to bring a current *BNF* to the exam to refer to (it includes HRT risk tables).

Case 7

Candidate information

Name: Ivor Guthrie
Age: 60
Social and family history:
Past medical history: diabetes, hypertension (well controlled)
Drug history: metformin 500 mg twice daily, Ramipril 5 mg once daily, aspirin 75 mg once daily, bendroflumethiazide 2.5 mg once daily
Results: HBA1c 6.8%, TC 5.2, HDL 1.8, LDL 1.9, TG 3

Man with type 2 diabetes and impotence over last 7 months.

Role-player information

You have noted a gradual onset of reduced turgor in your erections over the past 15 months and recently find it difficult to achieve penetrative sex. Your morning erections are now only semirigid. You are happily married and your wife is supportive regarding the problem. Although you find this topic embarrassing and difficult to talk about she has encouraged you to seek advice. Your medication is unchanged in the last 3 years. You have been reading about Viagra in a magazine article and want to try it but would like to know more about it, e.g. how much it will cost and if it's okay with your other medication. If offered a prescription you will take one today. You expect it to work but wonder if there is anything else that you can try to help.

Examination card

BP 136/80, HR regular rhythm, rate 74, normal genitalia and rectal examination.

Topic summary: Erectile dysfunction

Erectile dysfunction (ED) is a common problem in men over 40, particularly in those with cardiovascular disease (a major risk factor), which accounts for more than half of cases. There are many other causes (Ralph et al. 2000; European Association of Urology 2005).

Causes
- Physical:
  - CVD risk (hypertension, diabetes, hyperlipidaemia, smoking, coronary heart disease, atherosclerosis)
  - neurological disease (spinal injury, multiple sclerosis [MS], prostate disease, neuropathy due to diabetes, uraemia, alcohol, etc.)
  - hypogonadism and hormonal disturbance (high prolactin, thyroid disease, Cushing's disease)
- Iatrogenic:
  - cardiac drugs (antihypertensives, β blockers)
  - antidepressants
  - antiepileptics
  - antipsychotics
  - antihistamines
- Psychological: stress/depression/change in partner.

Essential ED history
- Onset and duration
- Quality of erections (morning erections, during masturbation and ability to ejaculate)
- Sexual relationship (understanding, changes in libido, changes in partner)
- Past history of ED and urogenital problems
- CVD risk factors (including lifestyle factors – smoking, exercise, weight, alcohol)
- Urinary symptoms (dysuria, frequency, urgency, hesitancy, haematuria).

Examination
- BP and pulse
- Genitalia
- PR for prostate in over 50 s.

Investigations
- Blood glucose (diabetes)
- U&Es (renal impairment)
- LFTs (liver disease)
- Urinalysis (renal impairment)
- Sickle cell screen (in African–Caribbean individuals).

Other investigations depend on the history, e.g. those with a low sex drive should have testosterone, prolactin and FSH/LH (luteinising hormone) requested and those with flow symptoms PSA.

Management
Physical causes
- Address lifestyle factors:
  - ➤ increase exercise
  - ➤ weight reduction
  - ➤ stop smoking
  - ➤ reduce alcohol intake.
- Control CVD risk: hypertension, diabetes, hyperlipidaemia, smoking, coronary heart disease, atherosclerosis.
- Prescribing for symptom relief:
  - ➤ first-line treatment = phosphodiesterase inhibitor, e.g. sildenafil (50 mg about 1 hour before sexual activity, subsequent doses adjusted according to response to 25–100 mg as a single dose as needed; maximum one dose in 24 hours – *BNF* 2009)
  - ➤ vacuum pumps.

Iatrogenic causes
- Review medication; consider alternatives: dose reduction or stopping medication.

Psychological causes
- Treatment of underlying causes (depression, anxiety)
- Psychosexual counselling referral.

Prescribing in ED
Many patients with ED come expecting a prescription for symptom relief. Before issuing a prescription, check if a private script is required and the patient's CVD risk profile. Patients can have an NHS script if they meet the SLS (Selected List Scheme) criteria, otherwise they should be issued with a private script. Patients with mild-to-moderate stable angina, an old MI, controlled hypertension and well-controlled heart failure are considered safe. Patients with other categories of cardiovascular risk should be referred for specialist assessment.

SLS criteria (*Drug Tariff* – DH 2009)
NHS prescriptions are available to patients with impotence in the following conditions: diabetes, MS, Parkinson's disease, poliomyelitis, prostate cancer, severe pelvic injury, single gene neurological disease, spina bifida, spinal cord injury, prostatectomy, radical pelvic surgery, or renal failure treated by transplantation or dialysis.

MEMORY BOX: Erectile Dysfunction

Indicators of a physical cause:
- Gradual onset
- CVD risk factors
- Failure of morning erections

Indicators of a psychological cause:
- Sudden onset
- Morning erections unaffected
- Change in partner
- Stress/Psychiatric history

Case 7 marking schedule

Good communication skills are necessary to handle this sensitive issue. A good candidate will put the role-player at ease enabling them to elicit a full sexual history. A frank structured discussion of the issues and treatment options in an empathic and positive attitude will achieve high marks. Marks are awarded for the following.

Data gathering

- Establishes an ED history as outlined in the topic summary.
- Examines the BP, pulse and rectal examination (examination card given at this point)
- Investigates Ivor's ICE (I – Viagra is the cure; C – I've heard it is expensive; E – the doctor probably won't let me have any).

Clinical management

- Discusses the nature of ED and the likely cause for him (i.e. history indicates a physical cause most likely due to cardiovascular and neurological damage secondary to his diabetes and possibly exacerbated by other factors– his current medication, lifestyle factors)
- Assesses safety of prescribing for Ivor based on his CVD risk and agrees that a trial of medication would be safe.
- Shares the treatment options and agrees a management plan with Ivor, e.g.:
  - ➤ offers routine investigations (see Topic summary) to identify other causes
  - ➤ discusses lifestyle modification
  - ➤ discusses pros and cons of changing his antihypertensive medication (pros – may be a cause of his impotence and lead to an improvement; cons – well-controlled on current medication; no ED on same medication for first 15 months makes this a less likely cause)
  - ➤ offers a choice of prescription of a phosphodiesterase inhibitor or a trial of lifestyle factors, with review following investigation results
  - ➤ agrees follow-up.
- Ivor will want a prescription today:
  - ➤ explain that the prescription is free of charge to Ivor (he is entitled to an NHS prescription under the SLS rules and as he is over 60 there is no charge)
  - ➤ explain how to take the medication and confirm understanding
  - ➤ correctly issue a prescription, marking SLS on it.

Interpersonal skills

- Empathises with the patient's concerns and establishes rapport
- Agrees a follow-up appointment
- Offers and shares management decisions by presenting information in an accessible manner appropriate to the patient's level of understanding
- Offers written information.

Case 8

Candidate information

Name: Sharon Whittington
Age: 20
Social and family history: university student
Past medical history:
Drug history: Depo-Provera (next injection due in 4 weeks)

Sharon last attended your practice 8 weeks ago and was seen by the nurse for her Depo injection. At that time she reported no medical problems. She attends today saying she thinks that she may have thrush.

Role-player information

You are very embarrassed about seeing the doctor today. Over the last 6 weeks you have developed a vaginal discharge. The discharge is a yellow-stained mucus. You have also noticed some bleeding after sex in the last few weeks. You have tried over-the-counter thrush medication (7 days ago) but it has not resolved. You have a long-standing partner but 4 months ago you had unprotected sexual intercourse with a different partner while on holiday. Your boyfriend is unaware and you do not regularly use condoms. You have no abdominal pain. You don't want to go to the genitourinary medicine clinic – you would be too embarrassed and cannot be convinced to go. You are reluctant to have a pelvic examination but will agree if the risk of infertility and STI is explained. You will become upset and withdrawn if not handled sensitively. You are worried that your partner will find out about your one-night stand.

Examination card

Mucopurulent vaginal discharge, abdomen non-tender

Topic summary: Vaginal discharge

Infection is the most common cause of a pathological discharge in a sexually active woman. Of the infective causes, bacterial vaginosis (BV) and candida infection are the most common. It is important to make an adequate assessment to assess risk of STIs, which are on the rise. Untreated STIs are a risk factor for PID (pelvic inflammatory disease) and infertility.

(Mitchell 2004)

Causes
Physiological

Clear or white in appearance and varies in appearance and quantity throughout menstrual life. Asymptomatic and non-offensive.

Infective

- Non-sexually transmitted:
  - *Candida* sp. (itchy creamy discharge associated with recent antibiotics, dyspareunia and diabetes)
  - BV (offensive fishy, grey, thin discharge)
- Sexually transmitted
  - *Chlamydia* sp. (asymptomatic in 80%; those with symptoms may complain of discharge, intermenstrual or postcoital bleeding, and lower abdominal discomfort)
  - *Trichomonas* sp. (offensive yellow discharge, dysuria, itch and abdominal pain)
  - *Neisseria gonorrhoeae* (purulent discharge, half of cases asymptomatic).

Other non-infective causes account for a minority of cases (e.g. ectropion, polyps, malignancy and pre-malignancy).

Focused history

- Discharge (onset, duration, consistency, smell, colour, bleeding, past episodes)

- Pelvic symptoms (itching, dyspareunia, dysuria, abdominal pain, fever)
- Sexual history (change in partners, use of barrier contraception, symptoms in partner).

When to examine and swab
- Risk factors in the history for an STI
- Change in normal discharge not typical of thrush or BV
- Failure to respond to a treatment course for thrush or BV.

Focused examination
- Abdominal exam
- Smell
- External genitalia and PV for adnexal pain and cervical excitation
- Speculum exam (to inspect cervix, vagina and take swabs)

Investigations
Triple swabs:
- High vaginal for BV, candida infection and *Trichomonas vaginalis* (TV)
- Endocervical for gonorrhoea
- Endocervical DNA swab for *Chlamydia* sp.

Management
Offers to test and treat or referral to a sexual health clinic for further investigation. Avoid sexual intercourse during investigation and treatment period.

Advantages of investigating in the surgery
- Avoid stigma of attending a sexual health clinic
- Convenience and choice
- Same-day testing.

Disadvantages
- Lack of contact tracing
- Less effective at picking up some STIs – gonorrhoea
- Less time available for counselling
- Unable to offer extended full sexual screening.

The chlamydia screening programme
(www.chlamydiascreening.nhs.uk)
This was established in 2003 with the aim of controlling chlamydia infection through early detection of asymptomatic infection, therefore preventing further complications and onward transmission:
- Opportunistic screening of 15- to 24-year-old males and females
- Both health- and non-health-care settings, e.g. universities, youth clubs or outreach events
- Men: urine sample
- Women: urine sample or vaginal swab
- Results can be texted, posted, emailed or sent to GP
- Positive in around 10%.

Case 8 marking schedule

This is an acute presentation assessing risk management, and communication skills as well as core knowledge of the management of women's health. Marks are awarded for the following.

Data gathering

- Takes a focused history of the discharge as outlined in Topic summary
- Identifies Sharon's ICE.

Clinical management

- Recognises the risk factors for STIs, discusses the possible causes, consequences if left untreated and the methods of investigation
- Reassures that many STIs are readily treatable
- Explains the management options and their advantages and disadvantages (test and treat, or refer to sexual health clinics for screening)
- Respects Sharon's decision to have investigation at the surgery
- Examines and investigates appropriately (the candidate will have to state her plan and then will receive the examination card details)
- Reassures Sharon that her consultation is confidential but there may be a need for contact tracing if the results are positive to protect others from infection; Sharon would refuse contact tracing (her confidentiality should be respected)
- Agrees follow-up.

Interpersonal skills

- Offers a non-judgemental approach
- Respects patient's decisions and agrees a shared plan
- Listens carefully to concerns and offers empathy
- Confirms understanding and offers to answer any queries
- Offers a female doctor to perform the examination (if male) and requests a chaperone.

Case 9

Candidate information

Name: Dennis Hull

Age: 43

Social and family history: lives with his wife Lorna 41, has two adult children who have left home, smoker 40 a day

Past medical history: COPD

Discharge note: metastatic small cell lung cancer diagnosed on CT scan and bronchoscopy; oncology follow-up appointment 1 week

Dennis has recently been discharged from hospital with a diagnosis of lung cancer. He has come to talk to you about his prognosis. The candidate's task is to gather information about Mr Hull's concerns and agree a plan of action.

Role-player information

Dennis has been told that he has extensive disease and that his prognosis is poor – 3–4 months. Although his diagnosis is recent he has been losing weight for some time and suspected that he had a serious illness. Dennis is pain free but breathless on exertion. He has been offered chemotherapy and has an appointment in 4 days' time to start treatment. Mr Hull has decided, however, that he does not want to go ahead with it. His reason for refusal is that he saw his uncle go through a terrible time 4 years ago with chemotherapy for cancer (oesophageal). The oncologist has estimated his survival to be improved by 1–2 months with treatment. Mr Hull is adamant about his decision, has discussed it with his wife and will not change his mind whatever the candidate says. Mr Hull had a bad experience in the hospital and does not want to go back. He would like to be looked after at home and die there, but is worried that his wife won't be able to cope. He wants to make sure that if he stops breathing or if his heart stops no one tries to resuscitate him.

Topic summary: Death and dying
Attitudes to death
In the Middle Ages, when life expectancy was only 30 years or so, death was readily accepted as an everyday event. But with increasing life expectancy a taboo has grown up around the subject.

Doctors' attitudes
Doctors' attitudes are complicated by uncertainty (of true diagnosis, of accurate prognosis, of whether the patient really wants to know). Questionnaires of the early 1960s and late 1970s suggest a complete reversal of doctors' attitudes from compounding the taboo to fighting it. In practice, however, and in part because of the uncertainty element, there is reluctance to tell.

Patients' attitudes
Patients' attitudes are complex. Most patients harbour suspicions about dying. Thus, Hinton (1980) interviewed patients in the 10 weeks before death and found that:
- 66% recognised death as a possibility
- 8% were non-committal
- 26% talked only of recovery.

Most patients wish to be enabled to die in the place of their choice (Gott et al 2004; NICE 2004a), often their own home. They want to be assured that their families and carers will receive support during their illness and after their death. Most patients want detailed information about their condition, possible treatments and services. They wish to be treated as individuals with dignity and respect and to be involved in decisions about treatment and care. Good face-to-face communication is highly valued. Should they need it, patients expect to be offered optimal symptom control and psychological, social and spiritual support.

These are of course generalities in the very individual experience of dying. Other interesting generalisations have been made about the so-called *awareness patterns* and *stages of dying.*

The four awareness patterns
1. Closed awareness: the patient does not recognise death, although everyone else does.
2. Suspected awareness: the patient suspects that others know and tries to confirm it.
3. Mutual pretence: all sides know but pretend that the others do not.
4. Open awareness: everyone knows and openly admits it.

Stages of dying
1. Denial and isolation: shocked and numbed: 'It can't be me'; It's a mistake'; intense isolation.
2. Anger: 'Why me?' Anger may be displaced or projected on to staff.

3. Bargaining: a phase of good behaviour to try to postpone death.
4. Reactive depression: due to physical suffering or impending loss (of health, life, family, etc.).
5. Acceptance.

(Kubler Ross 1969)

Palliative care in the community

The Gold Standards framework (developed by the Gold Standard Framework Centre – an NHS organisation responsible for developing systematic evidence-based palliation) outlines the key tasks (the seven Cs) that need to be addressed for effective palliation:
1. Communication
2. Coordination
3. Control of symptoms
4. Continuity of care (out of hours)
5. Continued learning (keeping up to date)
6. Carer support
7. Care in the dying phase.

(www.goldstandardsframework.nhs.uk)

The place of death

Home care is still considered natural and preferable to most patients, relatives and families, once they share the problem. There must be adequate support for the carer, often a close family member readily available. Night sitting services are available to provide respite. The concerns of the family and carer should be assessed and addressed:
1. The patient often prefers the home but worries that he will be a burden.
2. The relatives often prefer the home but worry that they will be unable to cope.
3. The GP prefers the home but worries about both these things!
   It is a balanced judgement because good-quality terminal care depends on:
1. Available resources (GP time, nursing time, aids and appliances, the ability to provide 24-h care)
2. The nature of the problem
3. The attitudes of patient and carers.

Communication and coordination

Palliative care often requires a multidisciplinary approach including teamwork between the GP, district nurses, palliative care nurses, secondary services, social services, patient and patient's relatives. NICE recommend the nomination of a key worker who is the main point of contact for the patient, family and team. Their role is to coordinate the care, ensure that the seven Cs are being addressed and prevent duplication. This role may fall to the GP, palliative nurses or a case manager.

During terminal illness patients, families and doctors tend to endure unpleasant feelings that they fail to share and that hinder effective communication.

The patient's feelings

Common reactions are:

1. *Anxiety*:
   (a) for himself ('What is it like? Will there be pain and suffering? Will I lose control?')
   (b) for his family ('Will they cope? Will they suffer and feel abandoned?')
   (c) about his disease (ignorance and fear of the unknown).
   This anxiety is totally understandable, but it may also become maladaptive and hence pathological.
2. *Depression*: a mourning reaction for loss of health, life, family, station, etc.
3. *Anger*:
   (a) 'Why me? Can't the doctors do more?'
   (b) frustration born of impotence
   (c) anger displaced on to the family or medical staff.
4. *Guilt*: at letting dependants down or being a burden.
5. *Denial*: 'There's been a mistake; I need a second opinion.'
6. *Dependence and regression.*
7. *Bewilderment* and the search for meaning.
8. *Withdrawal.*
9. *Paranoia*: patients who cannot cope with 'I'm dying' sometimes substitute 'They're killing me'.
10. *Isolation*, loneliness and loss of worth.

Family problems

1. All of the reactions felt by the patient may be experienced by the relatives in their own right or observed in their loved one. Inevitably they cause distress, particularly the upsetting tendency of some patients to withdraw from their family.
2. Attempts from both sides to protect their loved ones from stress actually exacerbate the situation: deceit and tension disrupt family bonds.
3. Relatives particularly feel the sense of impotence and frustration.
4. A long terminal illness is exhausting.
5. Bereavement forces new roles on to the survivors.
6. Guilt feelings are very common:
   (a) guilt if illness occurs at a juncture when relationships were strained
   (b) guilt in wanting a terminal illness to end
   (c) guilt because of the human but selfish tendency to dwell most on one's own problems, etc.
7. Practical problems:
   (a) financial hardship
   (b) time off work
   (c) loss of the family driver, etc.

The doctor's problems

1. Should I tell?
   (a) Does the patient really want to know?
   (b) Do the relatives agree?
   (c) Will they cope with the information?

Evidence suggests that the majority do want to know; however, the patient should be given the chance to refuse knowledge. This can be achieved through a stepped approach to breaking bad news by the use of a warning shot, e.g. reveal that you have the results of tests and ask if the patient would like to know them. If the patient gives permission then reveal that the news is not good (this gives the patient time to prepare for the results and allows a second opportunity to refuse); finally reveal the information.

2. Do I really know?
   (a) uncertainty about diagnosis
   (b) uncertainty about prognosis.
3. Can *I* cope? Terminal illness highlights to doctors:
   (a) their own failure and impotence
   (b) their own mortality; it also brings out their own defence mechanisms, e.g. *avoidance* by:
      − the detached scientific approach
      − limiting contact to ritualistic conversational gambits
      − false cheeriness.
   On top of these psychological problems there are the physical ones such as:
      − control of symptoms
      − continuity of care (ensure handover to out-of-hours care of palliative patients − a proforma should exist for this)
      − continued learning

Control of symptoms
Useful resources include the knowledge base of the palliative care nurse, local hospice and the *BNF's* palliative care chapter. See also the Gold Standard Framework for Community Palliation (www.goldstandardsframework. nhs.uk).

General principles
• Try to use the oral route as long as possible
• Regularly ask about the need for pain relief
• Reassure that pain control is achieved in the majority
• Aim to prolong life not prolong the dying phase.

Carer support
• Assess how the carer is coping and offer support/respite care
• Encourage discussion of practical issues (funeral arrangements, financial affairs) with the patient
• Explain what to do when death occurs (call the surgery, if out of hours contact the undertaker to collect the body or wait for the surgery to open)
• Offer an appointment in the surgery to discuss concerns.

Management of death and the dying
The *objectives* of care are to:
• promote the patient's self-esteem (emphasise value and role)
• promote the patient's emotional comfort (relieve anxiety, depression and guilt)

- promote mutually supporting family relationships.

Needless to say these objectives are easier said than done and require a deft touch, but certain management pointers are probably valid:

1. Listen to the patient:
   (a) this shows the patient that he is valid (understood and not abandoned)
   (b) it allows him to ventilate unpleasant feelings (anger, frustration, guilt, shame, fear)
   (c) it enables the GP to gain a sense of what the patient knows and what he wants to know.
2. Encourage him to retain his role and responsibilities and to participate in decision-making. This emphasises that he still has worth and importance, undiminished by illness. Try to preserve his dignity above all.
3. Work with the family:
   (a) encourage openness
   (b) promote insight into the family's own feelings and those of their loved one
   (c) allow the family to vent their feelings
   (d) encourage family care where this is possible
   (e) prepare the family members for their new roles and responsibilities.
4. Control physical symptoms.
5. Remember practical problems, e.g. if the patient is the family bread-winner, financial hardship may require the social worker's attention.

Liverpool Care Pathway (www.mcpcil.org.uk/frontpage)

Candidates should be aware of the Liverpool Care Pathway (LCP). The pathway is an evidence-based framework for providing palliative care. It is aimed at terminally ill patients without reversible causes for improvement who have entered the dying phase. To enter the pathway the team should agree that the patient is dying and meets two of the criteria:

- bed-bound
- semi-comatose
- only able to take sips of fluids
- unable to take tablets.

The LCP provides a tick list of the tasks that need to be completed and the order and timing in which they should be addressed. The tasks encompass physical, psychological and spiritual care of the dying patient. Ideally the pathway documentation will replace all existing notes and guide health professionals to deliver best care. Patient progress and any variance from the pathway guidance (with an explanation of the rationale) should be recorded in the pathway.

Advance directives (Mental Capacity Act 2005; Age Concern 2008)

Advance directives (also called living wills) allow the patient to record their wish to refuse certain types of medical treatment, and are binding on the people providing care if the patient loses the capacity to make the decision at the relevant time. They were set out in the Mental Capacity Act 2005 and came into force in 2007. People commonly use them to specify treatment decisions for end-of-life care, and mental incapacity due to episodes of mental illness.

Guidance
- An adult with mental capacity can refuse treatment for any reason, even if the consequences are fatal.
- Although good practice, advance directives do not have to be in writing unless concerning refusal of life-sustaining treatment.
- A record should be kept in the notes.
- A refusal of life-sustaining treatment must be signed, witnessed and include a statement that the decision is to apply to the specific treatment even if death may result from refusal.
- It is advisable to keep a copy at home, and give a copy to a close family member and the GP.

The person providing treatment must decide whether the advance directive is valid and applicable, i.e.
- not been withdrawn (including subsequent actions by the patient suggesting that it no longer represents his wishes)
- made at a time in which the patient had mental capacity
- not overruled by someone given Lasting Power of Attorney who can make decisions of consent on the patients behalf
- the current situation meets the conditions specified in the directive
- changes have not occurred that could not have been anticipated at the time of the decision and that could have affected the decision (e.g. new treatments or changes in personal circumstances).

Patients cannot refuse:
- an offer of food and drink in advance
- basic nursing care (including pain relief)

A downloadable directive proforma is available at the Age Concern website.

Case 9 marking schedule

This case assesses management of the dying patient and ethical issues. Marks are awarded for the following.

Data gathering
- Establishes Mr Hull's understanding of his diagnosis, prognosis and treatment options
- Identifies the nature of his uncle's illness and treatment
- Identifies Mr Hull's ICE (I = I want to spend what time that I have left with my family without losing the quality of life I have to chemotherapy and I want to die at home; C = my family won't be able to cope, I will be sent to hospital, someone might try and resuscitate me, I will suffer a painful death; E = the doctor will try to make me go back to hospital, nothing can be done to help me)
- Establishes current symptoms and treatment
- Identifies Mr Hull's support network (professional and personal) and what information he has disclosed.

Clinical management

- Confirms that any treatment offered would be palliative and not curative. Tempers this bad news by offering hope in the form of high-quality palliative care enabling symptom control and a 'good death' for most.
- Discusses the pros and cons of chemotherapy as a treatment option. Highlights that his uncle's cancer was of a different type and probably a different chemotherapy regimen.
- Respects Mr Hull's right as an adult with capacity to refuse treatment.
- Reassures that dying at home is acceptable and that support for him and his wife is available.
- Offers further appointment with his wife to discuss their needs and concerns.
- Suggests use of advance directive or Lasting Power of Attorney to help ensure that his wishes for care are met if he loses capacity.

Interpersonal skills

- Provides an empathic patient-centred consultation.
- Shows good listening skills and practical problem-solving addressing the patient's health beliefs.
- Respects Mr Hull's autonomy to refuse treatment and assists him in achieving his goals.

Case 10

Candidate information

Name: Lisa Pearson
Age: 42
Social and family history: married with two children.
Drug history: Micronor
Results: TSH, FBC, U&Es, fasting glucose, LFTs all in normal range
Examination findings: BP 124/72, normal cardiovascular and abdominal exam

A 49 year old complaining of tiredness comes for a second appointment with you. She mentioned her tiredness at a consultation for contraception the previous week and your colleague examined her and requested some investigations (above). She has returned for the results. The candidate's task is to review the results, identify and discuss possible causes for her symptoms, and agree a management plan.

Role-player information

Lisa's father has Alzheimer's disease and has been increasingly demanding. Her mother is finding it difficult to cope with him at home and Lisa is the main support. She is struggling to split her time between caring for her teenage children and caring for her elderly parents. She works in a bank, and has supportive colleagues. Her husband is also supportive but very busy and they have little time together. Lisa feels exhausted throughout the day. She has no difficulty sleeping, is not tearful and enjoys her work and home life. She does not feel depressed. She has no other symptoms or signs. Lisa wants a diagnosis and treatment.

Topic summary: Tired all the time

Generalised tiredness is a non-specific symptom which may be psychological, physical or physiological in origin. Only a minority of cases have a physical cause (approx 20–30%) with 75% attributable to psychological distress. A systematic approach will help to identify the underlying cause and enable appropriate management.

(Moncrieff and Fletcer 2007; Willacy 2008)

Aetiology
Physical
- Anaemia
- Endocrine (hypothyroid, diabetes, Addison's disease, hypopituitiary)
- Organ failure (heart, liver, renal)
- Malignancy
- Medication related (antidepressants, β blocker).

Psychological
- Depression
- Psychoses (e.g. schizophrenia)
- Adjustment reaction.

Physiological
- Sleep deprivation
- Acute stress reaction (following a stressor, i.e. pressure at work, home)
- Increase in physical activity.

Focused history
- Listen without interrupting to the history offered
- Define the onset, duration and nature of the tiredness (generalised, specific muscle groups, mental or physical)
- Review changes in medication
- Ask patient what she thinks is the cause and if she has noted other symptoms
- Ask specifically about:
  - weight loss/appetite loss (thyroid disease, diabetes, malignancy, depression)
  - urinary symptoms (renal disease, diabetes)
  - menstrual changes, i.e. menorrhagia (secondary to hypothyroidism, anaemia secondary to menorrhagia), absence of menstruation (pregnancy, anorexia)
  - bowel habit change (thyroid disease, malignancy)
  - sleep disturbance – physiological (young children, carer for sick); psychological – depression related
  - stressors (home/work).

Focused examination
- General inspection (affect for anxiety and tearfulness, pallor for anaemia and systemic features, i.e. oedema, ascites)
- Further examination will be guided by the history, e.g. depression screening, examination for evidence of thyroid disease (heart rate, tremor, sweaty palms, eye disease) or malignancy.

Baseline investigations
- FBC – ? anaemia
- Glucose – ? diabetes
- LFT – ? hepatitis, alcohol abuse

- U&Es – ? renal impairment
- ESR (erythrocyte sedimentation rate) – ? underlying inflammatory disease
- TFTs – for those with features of thyroid disease
- Two-question depression screen/PHQ9/HADs depression screening tools.

Treatment options

This will depend on the cause. Whatever the cause there is often a psychological component (NICE 2007a):

- Sleep hygiene (avoid stimulants, e.g. caffeine, nicotine, use bedroom only for sleeping, quiet period 30 min before bed, avoid sleeping in daytime, write worries down on to-do list before bed time)
- Counselling (six to eight sessions over 10–12 weeks)
- Exercise (three sessions per week of moderate exercise of 45 minutes to 1 hour)
- Social support (support groups, family support, GP and counselling interaction)
- Self-help leaflets (depression, anxiety).

Case 10 marking schedule

This case is an example of an undifferentiated presentation. The candidate needs to work through systematically to exclude physical causes and identify that the underlying cause is likely to be due to social factors. An empathic and person-centred consultation is necessary to score highly. A management plan should be tailored to the patient's health beliefs, preferences and social circumstances. Marks are awarded for the following.

Data gathering

- Establishes the duration, nature and character of the tiredness through a focused history. If elicited adequately the history will indicate that no further examination is required.
- Identifies ideas, concerns, expectations re cause of her tiredness. Addresses whether the patient recognises social factors as a possible cause and what actions she has taken if any to improve her situation.
- Enquires about the social impact on the patient's work and family.
- Establishes the social support network for the patient and her parents.

Clinical management

- Correctly identifies social factors as the most likely cause of her tiredness.
- Demonstrates an understanding of the causes and natural history of tiredness presentations in general practice.
- Correctly interprets the investigations in the context of the history and does not order unnecessary tests.
- Explores practical solutions to her problems (increasing support for father by using day centres, carers, meals on wheels, Alzheimer's disease support groups), as well as general management strategies (sleep hygiene, counselling, exercise, social support, self-help plans).
- Offers a follow-up consultation for herself and her parents to discuss the issues further (assuming parents are registered at the same surgery).

Interpersonal skills
- Recognises the concerns of the patient and shows empathy.
- Discusses likely cause in a patient-centred manner. Takes a holistic approach to management incorporating the patient's ideas.
- Provides written information regarding support groups (tells the patient to pick this up from reception).

Case 11

Candidate information

Name: Donna Longford

Age: 52

Social and family history: lives in Mencap-supported living accommodation, unemployed and receives Disability Living Allowance. Independent in many of her activities of daily living. Attends the local day centre and is supported by her family who live nearby, including her sister and elderly parents. Non-smoker.

Drug history: omeprazole 20 mg once daily

Past medical history: Down's syndrome, learning disability, gastro-oesophageal reflux, early stage cataracts. No cardiovascular history

Donna attends morning surgery with her sister who is waiting outside. Your colleague who normally sees her is away. She is complaining of her chest feeling funny and sometimes hurting.

Role-player information

You have mild-to-moderate learning difficulties and find it difficult to explain what is wrong with you. You can, however, understand explanations provided that they are given clearly in simple terms with no technical language. You are keen to please the doctor and if asked leading questions you will agree with him or her. Your sister brought you to the surgery today and is waiting outside. You have attended the appointment alone as you value your independence. You can only describe your chest as feeling funny and sometimes hurting. It started this week and can happen at any time. You have not blacked out though you have felt faint at times. You are otherwise well and have no history of heart problems. You spend your time at the local day centre, with family or out around the local town. You are not sure what is causing the symptoms and wondered if it was an infection. You have come to find out, and expect the doctor to tell you what is wrong.

Examination card

Regular heart rate. Auscultation reveals a midsystolic click followed by a systolic murmur heard loudest over the apex. Lung bases clear. Respiratory exam normal. No other abnormal findings.

Topic summary: Learning difficulties and mitral valve prolapse

Down's syndrome (trisomy 21) is a common cause of learning difficulties, which can range from severe to low normal cognitive impairment. Principles of management for patients with learning difficulties are outlined in the RCGP curriculum and should be applied to this case:

Learning disability – principles of management
(RCGP curriculum map 2008 – www.rcgp-curriculum.org.uk)

- Realise that physical and mental illness may present differently in those with communication difficulties.
- Understand the need for additional enquiry, appropriate investigation and careful examination (in this case, although the patient is unable to clearly verbalise her symptoms, careful examination provides the information required to make the diagnosis and arrange appropriate investigation)
- Be aware of associated conditions (note that Down's syndrome is specifically mentioned in the syllabus, as are fragile X syndrome, cerebral palsy and autistic spectrum disorder)
- Understand how health problems can be overlooked in people with learning difficulties
- Know where to obtain specialist help and advice: community learning disability teams, specialist learning disability nurses and support workers, speech and language therapy, consultants specialising in learning disability
- Appreciate that such patients may have reading, writing and comprehension difficulties
- Respect autonomy
- Be aware of the roles of those involved with learning disability including the voluntary sector (e.g. Mencap, Down's syndrome associations)
- Consider the need for more time in order to deal effectively with people with learning disability
- Demonstrate equality, i.e. all citizens should have equal rights to health and access to health care according to need.

Common associated conditions
Down's syndrome (Saenz 1999; Draper 2007)

Cardiological
- Mitral valve prolapse 46%
- Atrioventricular canal defect 45%
- Ventral septal defect 35%
- Aortic regurgitation 17%.
  (Mitral valve prolapse and aortic regurgitation present in adults without known congenital heart disease; the others are congenital and usually identified on childhood screening.)

Gastrointestinal
- Reflux
- Pyloric stenosis
- Duodenal atresia.

Endocrine
- Hypothyroidism.

Fragile X
- Strabismus
- Hypermobile joints

- Autistic features
- Mitral valve prolapse.

Cystic fibrosis
- Respiratory tract infection
- Bronchiectasis
- Pneumothorax
- Pulmonary fibrosis
- Pancreatic insufficiency
- Gynaecomastia
- Cirrhosis
- Gallstones
- Subfertility
- Diabetes.

Autistic spectrum disorder
- Social abnormalities
- Language and communication abnormalities (limited development and communication)
- Behavioural abnormalities (rigid stereotyped behaviour and repetitive patterns).

Mitral valve prolapse
Mitral valve prolapse presents with non-specific symptoms including palpitations, tiredness, chest pain, breathlessness and syncope. On examination a mid systolic click and murmur loudest in expiration over the apex is typical of the condition. The diagnosis is confirmed by echocardiography. ECG is useful to exclude arrhythmia or ischaemic causes of chest pain. The majority of patients do not require any treatment. Prophylaxis against infective endocarditis is recommended during exposure prone procedures and β blockers are used for those with distressing palpitations. There is a small increased risk of thromboembolic events and in some cases antiplatelets are used (e.g. a history of TIA).

Case 11 marking schedule

This nub of the case is communication and the application of the principles of management for individuals with learning disability. Marks are awarded for the following.

Data gathering
- Establishes the onset, duration, nature and severity of each of the symptoms as far as possible with the patient.
- Asks the patient to explain further when she uses ambiguous terms (i.e. a funny feeling) but is understanding if unable.
- Avoids leading questions or putting words into the patient's mouth.
- Understands that the history may represent an atypical presentation of illness due to her learning disability and demonstrates this through careful enquiry.
- Records the patients symptoms in her own words avoiding assumptions (i.e. funny feelings should not be documented as palpitations but 'funny feelings'? palpitations).

- Establishes risk factors for cardiac disease (smoking, family history, sedentary lifestyle).
- Asks Donna about any ideas, concerns and expectations.
- Asks to perform a cardiological and respiratory examination including auscultation of the heart and lungs, and assessment of the cardiac rhythm. May also request to examine the abdomen in view of the non-specific history.

Clinical management
- Identifies mitral valve prolapse as the most likely cause in view of the typical examination findings and its strong association with Down's syndrome.
- Explains in simple terms the cause of the problem and agrees a management plan with Donna, which should include:
  - ➤ an ECG to look for evidence of arrhythmia and exclude ischaemia
  - ➤ an echocardiogram to confirm mitral valve prolapse as the cause.
- Arranges follow-up.
- Offers written information – this can be quite brief and should include the name of the problem and any key features/investigation (e.g. 'I think this is a heart condition common in people with Down's syndrome called mitral valve prolapse. It usually doesn't cause any serious problems and can be checked for using a test called an echo. This involves putting jelly on your chest and using a machine to look at your heart').

Interpersonal skills
- Establishes the severity of her learning difficulty by listening carefully during the opening of the consultation to judge an appropriate level of communication.
- Asks if she would like her relative to be present during the explanation but respects her autonomy if she says no.
- When taking a history or explaining the possible cause uses simple terms and seeks to confirm understanding.
- When explaining the need to examine her requests a chaperone and asks if she would like her sister to be present to reassure her.
- Understands the need for careful examination due to her inability to verbalise her symptoms.
- Checks her ability to read before providing written information and explains its use even if she can't read (i.e. to help explain to others).
- Respects equality and provides her with equal access to health care irrespective of her learning difficulty.
- Avoids a paternalistic or patronising approach.
- Provides a positive outlook.

Case 12

Candidate information

Name: David Lyons
Age: 58
Social and family history: divorced, two children, advertising executive, drinks 44 units/day, smokes 15/day, BMI 31
Past medical history: intermittent low back pain

A 58-year-old executive comes to see you. He rarely attends and was last seen 1 year ago for his back. His ex-wife is concerned that he is not eating properly or looking after himself.

Role-player information

Over the last 6 months you have developed a lot of upper abdominal pain particularly after meals and at night. The pain is heavy and often burning. There is no radiation and it can leave you feeling sick. Recently you have bought a belt because your trousers are falling down despite no change in diet. You eat restaurant meals or takeaways three to four times a week. You work long hours, eat late at night and do little exercise. Your back has also been hurting a lot more and you have started to take some ibuprofen in addition to paracetamol. Your bowels are regular and you don't suffer from constipation, although you have noticed that your stools have become darker of late. The only thing that seems to ease the pain has been Gaviscon. You are concerned that you might have an ulcer caused by stress at work and expect a prescription for a PPI (as your friend has had this for a similar problem).

Examination card

Abdominal examination – epigastric tenderness (mild). Otherwise no abnormal findings.

Topic summary: Dyspepsia (NICE 2004b)

Dyspepsia is a general term covering gastro-oesophageal reflux disease, peptic ulcer disease and non-ulcer dyspepsia. It is common and estimated to affect between 23 and 41% of the population. Around a quarter of those will consult with a GP. It is important to distinguish dyspepsia from cardiac and biliary disease.

Presentation

Dyspepsia is typically a pain in the upper abdomen and described as being heavy, achy or burning in sensation. Associated symptoms include nausea, belching or feeling full. Depending on the site symptoms can improve or worsen with food and are usually improved by antacids. In addition there are a number of alarm features that should prompt urgent referral.

Alarm symptoms
- Age >55 years with unexplained and persistent recent-onset dyspepsia
- Chronic gastrointestinal bleeding
- Unintentional weight loss
- Progressive difficulty swallowing
- Persistent vomiting
- Epigastric mass
- Suspicion of a gastric cancer after a barium meal.

Investigation and management of dyspepsia
With alarm symptoms (NICE 2005b)
- Urgent endoscopy within 14 days
- FBC (iron deficiency anaemia is a risk factor for gastric cancer)
- Stop all NSAIDs
- Prescribe an alginate or antacid while waiting for the appointment (not a PPI or H_2-receptor antagonist – patients being referred urgently for endoscopy should ideally be free from acid suppression medication, including PPIs or H_2-receptor agonists, for a minimum of 2 weeks)
- Explain how to avoid lifestyle factors that exacerbate dyspepsia.

Without alarm symptoms (NICE 2004a)

Two important management points:

1. 'Routine endoscopic investigation of patients of any age presenting with dyspepsia and without alarm symptoms is not necessary.'
2. *Helicobacter pylori* testing? There is no evidence that testing and treating for *H. pylori* is superior to a trial of a PPI. It is therefore reasonable to routinely use a PPI trial without testing.

Lifestyle advice for dyspepsia (as set out by NICE)

- Weight loss
- Smoking cessation
- Alcohol intake reduction
- Avoidance of precipitants, e.g. spicy and fatty foods
- Avoid having meals 3–4 h before going to bed (for reflux symptoms)
- Try to raise the height of the bed by a few inches (for reflux symptoms).

Review medication

- Nitrates, SSRIs, corticosteroids, calcium channel blockers, iron, NSAIDs, anti-platelets, and bisphosphonates are potential causes of dyspepsia.
- Offer alternatives (e.g. paracetamol or codeine for NSAIDs) or if unable to stop add a PPI to reduce the risk of GI bleeds (e.g. add PPI to aspirin for those with established CHD).

Prescribing plan

- One-month course of a PPI at full dose (OR test and treat for *H. pylori*)
- If no response to a PPI then test and treat for *H. pylori* (OR if no response to *H. pylori* treatment then prescribe a PPI for 1 month)
- If no response, trial a prokinetic (metoclopramide or domperidone) OR a H_2-receptor antagonist for 1 month
- If still no response consider referral to secondary care.

Follow-up

Following successful treatment with a prokinetic or acid-suppressing drug, the lowest dose possible to control symptoms should be prescribed. A limited number of repeat prescriptions should be issued and a medication review should take place on at least an annual basis.

H. pylori

There are three tests available to diagnose *H. pylori*:

- Urea breath test
- Stool antigen test
- Laboratory serology testing (where performance has been locally validated).

Before the test the patient should be PPI free for 2 weeks and have had no antibiotics in the last 28 days. Retesting should be with a urea breath test (as the other tests may remain positive).

Eradication treatment

First-line treatment is a 7-day course of PPI, clarithromycin and either amoxicillin or metronidazole, e.g. a 7-day course of twice daily omeprazole 20 mg, amoxicillin 1 g and metronidazole 400 mg/clarithromycin 500 mg.

Case 12 marking schedule

The nub of this case is the recognition of alarm criteria and action using urgent referral guidance. Marks are awarded for the following.

Data gathering

- Establishes the nature of the abdominal pain (site, severity, radiation, previous episodes, precipitating factors)
- Assesses alarm symptoms (see topic summary)
- Identifies risk factors for dyspepsia in his lifestyle
- Reviews medication
- Identifies David's ICE regarding dyspepsia and treatment
- Performs proficient abdominal examination.

Clinical management

- Identifies the need for urgent referral (unintentional weight loss in a patient over 55) and agrees a management plan.
- Discusses David's ICE in a positive manner, i.e. could be an ulcer but need to investigate to ensure that it is not upper GI cancer. Reassure that most referrals do not find cancer but urgent investigation is needed to provide prompt treatment for the unfortunate minority. Explain that a PPI is not appropriate for those having endoscopy so prescribe an antacid or alginate.
- Stops NSAID use.
- Requests a FBC.
- Explains lifestyle changes to reduce exacerbations.

Interpersonal skills

- Empathises with the patient's concerns
- Follow-up appointment offered for support
- Shares management decisions by presenting information in an accessible manner appropriate to the patient's level of understanding (seeks to confirm understanding of the plan)
- Offers written information.

Case 13

Candidate information

Name: Peter Cuniculus
Age: 22
Social and family history: single man, shop fitter
Drug history: Nil
Hospital discharge note: fracture of wrist. Immobilised. Alcohol-related injury. Fracture clinic appointment in 6 weeks (signed Dr Johnson SHO)

Peter Cuniculus is a recently registered patient. He presents for the first time today requesting a sick note. He has broken his wrist.

Role-player information

Peter broke his wrist after drinking heavily. He drinks mostly at weekends and on average 6 pints a night on Fridays, Saturdays and Sundays. He thinks that his drinking level is okay as his mates drink similar levels. He has had 1 day off work in the past 6 months as a result of drinking. Peter has no features of dependency. When raised as an issue Peter is interested in the guidelines on safe alcohol intake. He recognises the impact that alcohol has had on his present situation (unable to work for 6–8 weeks). Peter will agree to reduce his alcohol intake but not stop. If a confrontational interview style is adopted Peter will respond negatively 'my mates all drink the same and they're okay – my dad drinks more than me'.

Alcohol abuse (*National Alcohol Strategy* – DH 2007b)
Size of the problem
Ninety per cent of adults in England drink alcohol, a quarter drink above recommended limits and 4% are dependent. Excessive drinking costs the UK £20bn annually in health, crime and disorder. There were 180000 hospital admissions in 2007 due to alcohol-related injuries or illness costing the NHS £1.7bn. Alcohol-related death rates have doubled since 1979, affecting more and more people at a young age. Over 4000 people died of alcoholic liver disease in 2005 in England and Wales. Alcohol dependency affects more than one generation: children grow up in an environment affected by social, family and marital strife, and are more likely to become or marry an alcoholic themselves. Only the tip of the iceberg has been recognised: in some studies one-fifth of 'healthy' men attending screening programmes have abnormal LFTs, and probably 1 in 10 heavy drinkers is known in general practice.

Identifying the problem drinker
In June 2007 the DOH initiated an updated alcohol strategy. This identifies three target populations:
1. Under 18s
2. 18- to 24-year-old binge drinkers
3. Harmful drinkers (those who unconsciously drink over their safe limits).

The strategy focuses on early identification and intervention in these groups. GPs are well placed to spot problem drinkers because two-thirds of their patients see them in a year, almost 90% in 5 years, and the alcoholic person probably sees his GP twice as often as other patients. Other advantages that the GP has in this respect (Acres 1979) are:
1. A long-standing and detailed knowledge of many of his patients and their families.
2. An opportunity to observe changes in behaviour, attitudes and attendance patterns.
3. A chance to visit and see the patient's home environment.

Despite this less than a quarter of alcohol referrals come from primary care. The DH has suggested that primary care is not fulfilling its responsibility in this area, and this is a matter of topical interest.

Why are GPs poor at identifying the problem drinker?
1. *Definitions.* There is inconsistency of advice on 'safe' drinking levels:
    (a) The BMA, and Royal Colleges recommend 21 units per week for men and 14 units per week for women. Controversially a DH

working party advised that a 'benchmark' 50% higher in women and a third higher in men would not incur significant health risk. (Several studies had suggested that moderate alcohol intake had a beneficial effect on risk of heart disease in older men and women.)

(b) During pregnancy, NICE (2008) recommends no more than 1–2 units once or twice a week, the government recommends 0 units, and The Royal College of Obstetricians says <2 units twice a week.If expert advice is contradictory, is it so surprising that GPs find difficulty in recommending limits to their patients?

2. *GPs' attitudes*. There are many problems:

(a) On average GPs themselves consume more than they should (standardised mortality ratio from cirrhosis 311), so they may not be best placed to advise.

(b) GPs often lack the experience of handling problem drinkers, and the sensitive counselling skills needed have been neglected in traditional medical school training.

(c) it is easier to avoid potential conflict and embarrassment in a consultation which is, in any case, too short.

(d) alcoholism will be exacting to deal with, problems will be difficult and time-consuming, GPs are generally pessimistic about outcome, and people with alcohol problems are help-rejecting complainers, leaving most GPs feeling helpless and frustrated.

(e) Doctors are taught at medical school to distrust the drinking history that they obtain – given a sensitive line of questioning and dubious returns it is simpler not to ask.

(f) The diagnosis is not straightforward – vague and protean patterns confuse the unwary, and making a connection between apparently unrelated events requires a methodical record system (when often there is none).

3. *Patients' attitudes*: patients face many problems in common with their doctor:

(a) ignorance about safe drinking levels

(b) a variety of vague effects that may not be linked to alcohol

(c) psychological barriers (anxiety, guilt, shame, embarrassment) that result in denial

(d) the perception of a negative, censorious or uninterested attitude in the family doctor

(e) underestimation of true consumption: due to tolerance or cognitive impairment (if volunteers drink in simulated restaurant surroundings, the heaviest drinkers tend subsequently to underestimate their drinking by up to 12%).

4. *The unknown drinker*: not all problem drinkers present to their doctors:

(a) Teenagers may be better known to the police.

(b) Professional people in competitive jobs may drink away from home.

(c) Older people may drink in complete isolation.

The tools of detection

Unfortunately there is another barrier to detection: the absence of a cast-iron diagnostic test. The DH recommend rapid screening using an abbreviated version of the WHO 'AUDIT' questionnaire called FAST (sensitivity 93%, specificity 88%, mean time to screen using the FAST test = 12 seconds; on the face of it a sensitivity of 93% and a specificity of 88% looks pretty good, but, if the prevalence of problem drinking is say 1/4, then the positive predictive value will be under a third).

FAST alcohol screening test (Table 9.3)
A score of three or more indicates hazardous drinking.
    Other tools of detection are:
1. *The honest question*: useful only if you get an honest answer in return.
2. *Blood tests* (raised MCV, GGT): these are markers, but they are not particularly sensitive and have a high false-positive rate. (MCV is mean corpuscular volume; GGT, γ-glutamyl transaminase.)
3. Alternative screening questionnaires include the full AUDIT questionnaire, CAGE and MAST:
   – AUDIT is 92% sensitive and 93% specific
   – the brief MAST questionnaire (scores >6) has a sensitivity of 85% and a specificity of 86%
   – the CAGE test (scores >2) has a sensitivity of 93% and a specificity of 76% (Bernadt et al. 1982).

Table 9.3 FAST alcohol screening test

Questions	Scoring system					Your score
	0	1	2	3	4	
How often do you have eight (men)/six (women) or more drinks on one occasion?	Never	Less than monthly	Monthly	Weekly	Daily or almost daily	
Only answer the following questions if your answer above is monthly or less						
How often in the last year have you not been able to remember what happenned when drinking the night before?	Never	Less than monthly	Monthly	Weekly	Daily or almost daily	
How often in the last year have you failed to do what was expected of you because of drinking?	Never	Less than monthly	Monthly	Weekly	Daily or almost daily	
Has a relative/friend/doctor/health worker been concerned about your drinking or advised you to cut down?	No		Yes, but not in the last year		Yes, during the last year	

Hodgson et al. (2002).

What can GPs do about harmful drinking?

Brief alcohol interventions as short as 5 minutes have been shown to be effective in reducing alcohol consumption to guideline levels (NNT 8) within primary care settings (Kaner et al. 2007). This compares favourably with behavioural change after interventions for smoking cessation (NNT 20 advice alone and NNT 10 with nicotine replacement therapy). It is estimated that this simple intervention, if applied nationally, could reduce harmful drinking in 310000 adults annually. Unfortunately dependent drinkers respond very poorly to interventions to change drinking behaviour – hence the importance of early intervention in the pre-dependent problem drinker. The DH (Health Development Agency 2002) suggests brief intervention using the mnemonic BRIEF to prompt patients along the cycle of change (page 151):

Benefits: advise the patient of the benefits of sensible drinking

Risk factor: link alcohol as a risk factor for the patient's present symptoms/ situation

Intentions: discuss the patient's future intentions and options for cutting down, i.e. target setting

Empathise: motivational interviewing (empathise and retain a non-judgemental attitude)

Feedback: feedback on their levels of consumption.

SIGN recommendations (SIGN 2003)

1. Elicit patient's concerns
2. Regular review to offer encouragement
3. Monitor (see or telephone patient, information from family/GGT)
4. Reassess with patient the costs and benefits of change
5. Enlist support of family and friends
6. Consider use of local alcohol services, although there is little evidence to demonstrate the effectiveness of any of the following (group therapy, Alcoholics Anonymous, counselling) in patients with harmful drinking (Ferri et al. 2006)
7. Offer encouragement for any successes.

What can GPs do about dependent drinkers?

In addition to the guidance for harmful drinkers:

- Plan medically assisted withdrawal if indicated, at home or in hospital
- Consider specific pharmacotherapy: acamprosate (reduces intensity of and response to cues and triggers to drinking) and/or disulfiram (deterrent)
- Initiate active intervention if other psychiatric problems (depression/ anxiety) persist >2 weeks, i.e. SSRI
- Refer to alcohol support programmes, e.g. Aquarius, Alcoholics Anonymous and GPs with a specialist interest.

Managing patients in crisis (SIGN 2003)
Suicidal behaviour

Suicidal threats or demands for immediate but undefined 'help' require assessment, preferably within the surgery or by the out-of-hours service.

Listening to the patient's concerns may help to alleviate the pressure on the health-care professional to take additional action. Immediate admission is rarely indicated or possible but, if suicidal ideation persists, it may be needed, in which case referral to psychiatric services is appropriate.

Threatening behaviour

Physically threatening behaviour should be dealt with by calling the police. Drunken patients should be listened to politely and with courtesy, because showing frustration may inflame the situation. The patient may respond to being listened to politely and may be gently encouraged to go home. Drunken patients on the telephone can be disruptive to surgery function and also out-of-hours services because they may block the line. Having given due consideration and advice on who to contact when the patient is sober, it may be appropriate to terminate the call. At times, it may be quicker to see these patients.

Domestic abuse

The domestic violence/abuse liaison officers at police stations provide advice to victims of domestic abuse and can put them in touch with support systems, whether or not they wish to prosecute their partner. Sometimes the police arrest and charge the aggressor, even if the victim will not give evidence. The victim may need to be removed to a place of safety such as a refuge.

Motivational interviewing

A systematic review has shown a motivational interviewing technique to have a significant effect on reducing alcohol consumption in primary care (Dunn et al. 2001; SIGN 2003). The principal points are:
- Portraying empathy:
  - use of open-ended questions expressing interest/concern
  - reflective listening so that patients sense that you are trying to 'get on their wavelength'.
- Highlighting discrepancy:
  - patients are helped to see the gap between the drinking and its consequences and their own goals/values - the gap between 'where I see myself' and 'where I want to be'
  - weighing up the pros and cons of change and of not changing.
- Avoiding argument ('rolling with resistance'): resistance, if it occurs (such as arguing, denial, interrupting, ignoring), is not dealt with head-on, but accepted as understandable, or sidestepped by shifting focus
- Sharing decision making (from a menu of options).
- Facilitating and reinforcing 'self motivating statements':
  - being optimistic about change.
  - 'People believe what they hear themselves say'.

Case 13 marking schedule

The nub of this case is prevention and lifestyle intervention. Candidates using motivational interviewing techniques, a recommended alcohol screening tool and the principles of the 'BRIEF' intervention tool are likely to score best. Marks are awarded for the following.

Data gathering

- Clarifies the primary reason for attendance – sick note request.
- Identifies alcohol intake as an important issue, takes a focused history and relates this to an alcohol screening tool (ideally FAST test).
- Once raised as an issue, identifies ICE relating to alcohol intake: I = I didn't think I had a problem; C = have I caused any harm, will I have to stop drinking? E = the doctor will stop me drinking altogether.
- Excludes physical features of dependence (sweats, tremors within 12 hours of last alcohol intake).

Clinical management

- Issues Med 5 sick note for a maximum forward period of 4 weeks.
- Advises on the guideline levels for safe alcohol intake and safe patterns of drinking (ensuring understanding of the concept of units of alcohol).
- Feeds back on patient's level of consumption and health risk.
- Links alcohol to his current injury and past days off work.
- Discusses the patient's future intentions and the costs/benefits of change. May offer options for cutting down – not buying rounds, drinking every other round, alcohol intake diary, setting targets.
- Enlists support of family and friends (if appropriate).
- Agrees a review appointment.

Interpersonal skills

- Agrees a shared management plan modified to patients preferences.
- Adopts a motivational technique avoiding confrontation (a confrontational approach is a negative indicator).
- Respects individual differences, and shows interest/concern.
- Provides encouragement and is optimistic about change.
- Facilitates the recognition that alcohol has caused adverse consequences.

Case 14

Candidate information

Name: Martin Mathews
Age: 29
Social and family history: lives with his mother. Currently unemployed, single
Past medical history: DVT (deep vein thrombosis) 4 years ago
Drug history: nil

Martin is relatively new to the practice and is seeing you today for the first time. At the last appointment it was written in the notes 'appears dishevelled and when asked about drug misuse was evasive'. The candidate's role is to identify the reasons for Martin Mathew's attendance today.

Role-player information

You are attending today because you are worried that you may have hepatitis C. You are an intravenous opiate drug user and have been for the past 8 years. You spend £175–250 weekly on heroin and can't afford it. You inject into the groin so you don't get track marks. You have shared needles in the past and one of your friends recently found out that he had hepatitis C. Your concerns are that you have hepatitis C and that this will cause you cancer. As a result of this scare you want to stop using heroin but are not sure how to go about it. You have never tried to stop before. You smoke 10–15 cigarettes a day. Occasionally you smoke cannabis. Your main questions are: How can I stop? Can you tell me if I've got hepatitis C and what that means?

Topic summary: Drug abuse

GP practices are required to provide as a minimum:

- Drug treatment screening and assessment
- Referral to specialised drug treatment
- Drug advice and information
- Partnership/'shared care' working with specialised drug treatment centres to provide specific drug interventions.

  Practices may also provide more specialised services including:

- Triage assessments
- Drug interventions to minimise harm
- Psychological interventions
- Drug-related support.

(National Treatment Agency for Substance Misuse (NTA) 2006 Models of Care framework)

Drug abuse in the UK

Heroin is the most common problem drug in the UK cited by two-thirds of clients receiving drug treatment as their main drug of abuse. The mortality in this group is 12 times that of the general population (Oppenheimer et al. 1994). Most of these enter treatment through self-referral to drug centres. It is unclear why GPs are failing to identify and refer more cases, making this a potential hot topic (see also Alcohol abuse for a similar background). Drug abuse is associated with a wide range of health and social problems. There are higher rates of social deprivation, smoking and lifestyle behaviours associated with negative health outcomes. Risk behaviour has been increasing in recent years with 25% of injecting drug addicts reporting sharing needles in 2005. Younger drug users (<18 years) are most likely to use cannabis.

Drug abuse and blood-borne viral infection

Drug abusers (particularly injecting users) are at high risk of contracting and spreading blood-borne viruses. Almost half of injecting drug users (IDUs) in the UK have been infected by hepatitis C and 1 in 75 injecting drug users is said to be HIV infected (Health Protection Agency 2006). Treatment plans should assess and reduce risk through needle exchange programmes, controlled opiate substitution programmes, education strategies and advice on avoiding exposure to viruses.

Hepatitis C

- Most cases are asymptomatic
- Eighty per cent will develop chronic infection and are at increased risk of developing cirrhosis or liver cancer
- No vaccine available
- Treatment options include retroviral medication, most commonly interferon and ribavirin
- Transmission is blood borne and sexual.

Hepatitis B
- One in five injecting users is hepatitis B positive
- Ninety-five per cent will clear the infection without treatment
- Five per cent develop chronic infection and 20% of those develop cirrhosis
- A vaccine is available and should be offered to all drug abusers (the accelerated schedule is recommended, i.e. 0, 7 and 21 days)
- Partners and children should also be immunised against hepatitis B
- Transmission is blood borne and sexual.

Hepatitis A
Immunisation against hepatitis A should be encouraged. Combined vaccines with hepatitis B may improve uptake but single component vaccines are more effective. If immunisation against tetanus is in doubt it may be worth offering a booster.

Initial assessment
Where drug misuse is identified a first consultation should aim to recognise the issues, identify risks and agree a shared plan of follow up, ideally engaging the patient with specialist services.

Assessment points:
- **Habit**: what drugs, how much, mode of use, cost, duration of abuse, impact psychosocially, previous treatment
- **Motivation to change**: what stage of the cycle of change (see Chapter 6) is the patient in? If not ready to change offer brief intervention along the lines of alcohol abuse to promote change
- **Risk behaviour**: sharing habits, safe supply and disposal of equipment, awareness of blood borne viruses and advice on prevention, i.e. immunisation and reducing risk behaviour, safe sex
- **General health**: screening questions, e.g. 'Do you feel well in yourself?' 'Do you or have you recently had any symptoms that concern you?'
- **Mental health**: past history and two-question depression screen (see page 219)
- **Examination**: brief exam to include injection sites for infection, oral hygiene, chest exam (increased risk of chest infection/TB).

If there is time, or in further consultations, assess social support network, accommodation, income and legal issues.

Driving
The DVLA must be informed if an individual is drug dependent. The minimum ban is 6 months.

Travelling abroad
In general all controlled drugs should be carried with their original packaging. They must be accompanied by a letter stating the patient's name, destination, amount and details of medication. Special licences may be required if abroad for more than 28 days.

Register of drug abusers (see Chapter 3)

Drug abuse is notifiable and must be registered with the regional drug misuse database.

Case 14 marking schedule

The case focus is the initial assessment of drug misuse. This is a time pressured consultation with a lot of data gathering required. Success depends on a systematic approach. Marks are awarded for the following.

Data gathering
- Brief assessment of habit, motivation, risk behaviour, general health and mental health as discussed in the topic summary.
- Examination to include a brief oral, injection site and chest exam.
- Identifies the patient's ideas, concerns and expectations regarding hepatitis C.

Clinical management
- Discusses risks of drug abuse and risk reduction options (immunisation, testing for viral infection, safe sex, substitution treatment with methadone/buprenorphine, avoidance of injecting drugs if possible, and if not the use of clean equipment through drug centre schemes).
- Agrees a plan of action, e.g. viral testing, and referral to local drug centre to access specialist support services (detoxification, substitution treatment, psychological support).
- Addresses patient's concerns about hepatitis C by explaining the risks of transmission. Gives a realistic but positive outlook that should the result be positive treatment is possible.
- Notifies drug abuse to local register.
- Arranges a follow-up appointment to discuss his results, offer continued support, arrange immunisation and monitor progress.

Interpersonal skills
- Empathises with the patient's concerns.
- Provides an unbiased and non-judgmental consultation.
- Encourages his plan to change his behaviour and offers continued support.
- Shares management decisions by presenting information in an accessible manner appropriate to the patient's level of understanding (seeks to confirm understanding of the plan).

Case 15

Candidate information

Name: Declan Hartford
Age: 32
Social and family history: single
Past medical history: nil
Drug history: nil

A 32-year-old man complains of headache and nasal congestion.

Role-player information

You have had a previous episode to this 2 years ago and a course of antibiotics led to a speedy resolution. You would like a further course today. You have had symptoms for 5 days and a fever in the last 2 days. You are otherwise well. The symptoms are affecting your ability to concentrate at work. You are a police officer.

Topic summary: Acute sinusitis (NPC 2006)

> **MEMORY BOX:** Acute Sinusitis
> - Antibiotics unnecessary for most cases
> - 80% resolve in 2 weeks without antibiotics
> - Antibiotics indicated in patients with systemic illness or severe persistent symptoms >7–10 days
> - Delayed prescriptions appropriate
> - Complications are rare

Diagnosis

Acute sinusitis is usually diagnosed after symptoms (nasal discharge, congestion, headache, earache, facial pain, fever and maxillary tooth pain) are present for >5 days (because coryzal symptoms usually resolve within this period). Sinusitis is chronic if symptoms persist >90 days. More than a third of patients with clinically suspected infection have no evidence of infection on radiography or needle aspiration. The best predictors of sinusitis are maxillary toothache, poor response to nasal decongestants, history of coloured discharge, purulent nasal secretion and abnormal transillumination (Williams and Simel 1993). Acute sinusitis resolves in 80% of cases within 2 weeks without antibiotics and the complication rate of acute sinusitis is low (<1/10 000).

Management options

Antihistamines, decongestants and topical intranasal steroids have all traditionally been used for symptomatic relief of acute sinusitis. However, there is no robust evidence to support their use (NPC 2006). Simple analgesia is recommended for symptom relief. A review (Williams and Simel 1993) concluded that: 'antibiotics have a small treatment effect in patients with uncomplicated acute sinusitis in a primary care setting with symptoms for more than seven days. However, 80% of participants treated without antibiotics improve within two weeks. Clinicians need to weigh the small benefits of antibiotic treatment against the potential for adverse effects at both the individual and general population level.'

Red flags for referral

- Suspected periorbital infection
- Suspected sinonasal tumour (persistent unilateral symptoms including bloodstained discharge, crusting or facial swelling).

The MeReC bulletin review of prescribing 2006 recommends the following:

- Antibiotics are reserved for patients with systemic illness, or several severe signs and symptoms which have lasted longer than 7–10 days, or worsened after 5–7 days.
- A period of watchful waiting or delayed prescription may be appropriate.
- First-line antibiotic choice: amoxicillin or phenoxymethylpenicillin, three times daily for 7 days.

(CKS 2006 – www.cks.nhs.uk/sinusitis/drugs_in_this_topic/scenario_acute_sinusitis#-367874)

CSA marking schedule: acute sinusitis
Data gathering
- Establishes patient's/parental ideas, concerns, expectations re acute sinusitis.
- Establishes the duration and background history, and excludes red flag features (persistent unilateral symptoms, such as bloodstained discharge, crusting, or facial swelling).
- Identifies the signs and symptoms associated with an increase in the likelihood of acute sinusitis (maxillary toothache, poor response to nasal decongestants, history of coloured discharge, purulent nasal secretion and abnormal transillumination).
- Completes proficient exam of ear, nose and throat.

Clinical management
- Demonstrates an understanding of the causes and natural history of acute sinusitis and the low risk of serious complications.
- Discusses the pros and cons of antibiotics for acute sinusitis.
- Recognises and manages any significant co-morbidity.
- If prescribes checks history of adverse drug reactions.
- Recognises that further investigations are not warranted in an acute presentation.

Interpersonal skills
- Recognises the concerns of the patient/parents, identifies expectations and shows empathy.
- Comes to a shared management plan following national guidance – using a delayed prescription if necessary, prescribing the appropriate agent.
- Specifies conditions for follow-up.

Case 16
Candidate information
Name: Lucy Overton
Age: 62
Social and family history: lives with partner 64. Delivers milk for a living
Past medical history: hypertension

Mrs Overton comes in complaining of headache and a painful red eye on the left side. The candidate's task is to assess the cause and agree an appropriate management plan.

Role-player information
Mrs Overton complains of pain in her left eye and intermittent blurring of vision, which started in the morning and has worsened throughout the day. She now has persistently blurred vision in the affected eye, it is very painful and she sees haloes around lights. She feels nausea but has not vomited. She has had no previous episodes. Mrs Overton is hypermetropic (long-sighted). She is worried that she might be having a stroke and could lose her vision.

Examination card
Eye appearance
Clouded cornea, dilated oval pupil, corneal and scleral injection.
If acuity is tested = left eye decreased visual acuity to hand movements, right eye normal.

Topic summary: The red eye (Figure 9.2)

The red eye is a common presentation (in clinical practice and the exam). Although most red eyes are due to minor causes it is important to recognise red eyes that require urgent treatment. Document findings clearly, including important negative findings (visual acuity, photophobia, erythema). It

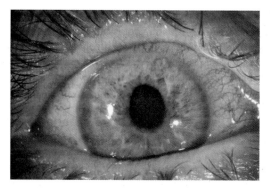

Figure 9.2 Examination card showing the patient's red eye.

can be helpful to categorise causes into painful and painless and their typical features.

Acutely painful red eye (Table 9.4)
Refer for same day specialist assessment.

Painless red eye (Table 9.5)
Painless red eye conditions should usually be managed in primary care. Episcleritis should be referred on if not resolving within a week. Direct irritants may also cause a red eye, e.g. entropion, or reaction to ocular medication.

Case 16 marking schedule
This is an example of a common acute presentation. The case describes acute glaucoma. A systematic approach to identifying the cause of a red eye will gain most marks. Marks are awarded for:

Data gathering
- Identifies the time of onset and progression of symptoms.
- Specifically asks for key symptoms (pain, haloes, photophobia, headache, nausea, blurring of vision, epiphoria, trauma, foreign bodies, discharge).
- Asks about exposure to irritants, allergens and the use of contact lenses and hygiene.
- Establishes past eye history (e.g. hypermetropia increases risk of glaucoma as does a family history of glaucoma).
- Establishes patient's ICE (I – worried about loss of vision; C – am I having a stroke? E – I am going to be disabled and out of work as my job involves driving).
- Investigates social situation – transport to hospital, ability to take treatments if provided.
- Examines the eye systematically, starting anteriorly and working through. Identify site and type of any erythema, visual acuity, red reflex and papillary response. If a foreign body or keratitis history, stain with fluorescein.

Clinical management
- Explain the likely cause (acute glaucoma) and treatment (urgent referral to hospital for eye pressure-lowering medication – intravenous acetazolamide and topical β blocker). Avoid covering the eye because this promotes dilatation of the pupil which can prolong the attack.
- Address the patient's ideas, concerns and expectations and answer any queries.
- Offer pain relief and an antiemetic if required.
- Arrange hospital transport and consider any social support if required (is she a carer for someone?). Are there other considerations that she is concerned about – impact on work/life –she is an occupational driver.

Interpersonal skills
- There are no real treatment options in this case but discussion about treatment should be shared and a paternalistic approach avoided. Good communication is needed to ensure that the explanation addresses the concerns and expectations of the patient and takes into account the social factors (work).
- A realistic but positive outlook should be offered.

Table 9.4 Acutely painful red eye

Pathology	Symptoms	Signs
Foreign body	Pain around the site of Trauma Usually the history indicates a foreign body as the cause	Dependent on the site and severity of the trauma
Acute angle glaucoma	Haloes around objects Headache and nausea Blurred vision (moderate to severe) Pain ++	Reduced visual acuity Sluggish dilated oval pupil Cloudy cornea Conjunctival injection (erythema)
Keratitis (corneal inflammation)	Photophobia Foreign body sensation Blurred vision (mild) History of contacts use	Circumcorneal injection Staining with fluorescein reveals lesion (trauma/ulcer) Hypopyon may be present (white cells in the anterior chamber)
Acute iritis (anterior uveitis)	Lacrimation Photophobia Headache	Irregular pupil Circumcorneal injection (engorgement of the deep vessels around the limbus) Reduced visual acuity
Scleritis	Pain ++ ± blurred vision	Red scleral patch ± reduced visual acuity
Irritant conjunctivitis due to acid/alkali/cement	Pain	Conjunctival injection

Table 9.5 Painless red eye

Pathology	Symptoms	Signs
Conjunctivitis	Mild-to-moderate irritation	Conjunctival erythema
	One or often both eyes	Discharge on lashes ± papillae on eyelids
Episcleritis	Asymptomatic	Red scleral patch (pain free)
Subconjunctival haemorrhage	Asymptomatic	Film of blood under conjunctival surface

From Farina and Mazarin 2006; NHS Clinical Knowledge Summary 2008, Scott 2008.

Case 17

Candidate information

Name: Vicky Taylor
Age: 34
Social and family history: mother – obesity, father – hypertension
Drug history: Cerazette
BMI: 32

Vicky mentioned in a previous consultation that she would like to lose weight. She has come back today to discuss this. The candidate's task is to discuss her weight and agree a weight loss strategy.

Role-player information

Vicky has had her first child 15 months ago and feels that she never lost the weight that she gained afterwards. She is a part-time receptionist. Her job is sedentary and she takes no regular exercise. She has take-out meals three times a week because she is busy caring for her child. She has heard about a pill for weight loss on the radio and would like to try it.

Topic summary: Obesity (NICE 2006b)
The problem

In 2005 23% of men and 25% of women were obese, a rise of approximately 10% over the previous decade. Levels of obesity are predicted to hit 33% by 2020. Obesity is also rising in young people. Prevalence in children under 16 has increased from 11% to 18% over a similar time period. Frighteningly, obesity is becoming the norm. A study in the *British Medical Journal* in 2005 (Jeffery et al. 2005) found that only 25% of parents correctly identified their child as overweight and a third of mothers failed to recognise their children as obese.

Morbidity

Jack Sprat eats lots of fat
His wife eats lots of sweeties
Jack has had his coronary
And his wife has diabetes!
Jung (2005)

Obesity is a risk factor for common diseases including diabetes, ischaemic heart disease, stroke, hypertension, DVT, cancers, sleep apnoea and osteoarthritis. Obese women are 13 times more likely to develop type 2 diabetes and men 5 times more. *Psychological sequelae* are also common in this stigmatising condition. The financial cost to the NHS directly and indirectly is considerable.

Obesity can be assessed by a variety of means including measures of:
- weight
- corrected weight (weight as a percentage of ideal weight for similar height, age, sex and build: 'ideal' according to insurance data)
- skinfold thickness
- waist:hip ratio.

The (currently) preferred method for classifying body weight is the Quetelet index, also known as the *body mass index* (BMI). This is calculated by dividing weight (in kilograms) by the square of height (in metres). However, BMI is not as accurate at predicting cardiovascular risk as waist:hip ratio (see Table 8.7, page 206).

Management of obesity

The pros and cons of whether a disorder such as obesity should occupy medical time need to be considered. Obesity is not a disease but a social/behavioural problem with medical complications, and hence the solution is not necessarily a medical one. The condition is so common that an undertaking to treat all obesity will be a great drain on medical resources. However, currently obesity has reached epidemic proportions with an upward trend. If not tackled the health burden and cost may be even greater. In this context NICE have issued guidance on the prevention and treatment of obesity (NICE 2006b).

Management of obesity in primary care

General principles
- Tackling obesity is a NICE priority
- Multicomponent interventions are the approach of choice
- Offer regular follow-up and tailor treatment to the patients preferences (fitness, lifestyle, co-morbidity)
- Target a loss of 5–10% of original weight every 3 months
- Document the plan and give the patient a copy
- Praise successes.

Adults obesity guidance
Assessment:
- Calculate and inform patients of their BMI and associated risk.
- Assess:
  - lifestyle (environmental, social and family factors, eating behaviour, diet and physical activity)

- co-morbidity (type 2 diabetes, hypertension, cardiovascular disease, dsylipidaemia, osteoarthritis, sleep apnoea; check lipid profile, BP and blood glucose).
- willingness to change (see cycle of change, page 151 – potential health gain).

Treatment options:
- Multicomponent interventions (increased physical activity, improved eating behaviour, improved diet) for all patients.
- Drug treatments (only to be used in addition to multi-component interventions after failure to lose weight).
- Bariatric surgery (reserved for patients with a BMI >40. In those with co-morbidity, e.g. diabetes, hypertension, a BMI >35 is adequate to recommend surgery. Non-surgical measures must have been tried for 6 months without adequate weight loss. Bariatric surgery is the first-line treatment for adults with a BMI >50).
- Referral to obesity clinic (if conventional treatment has failed, BMI >50, surgery required or complex co-morbidity requiring secondary care).

Multicomponent interventions
- Behavioural intervention (goal setting, self-monitoring of behaviour, slowing rate of eating, increasing physical activity, reinforcement of changes, relapse prevention)
- Physical activity (30 min, 5 days a week); supervised activities and activities that can be incorporated into everyday life, e.g. gardening, cycling, are encouraged.
- Dietary intake – aim for a balanced diet consistent with normal healthy eating advice.
- Encourage the partner to lose weight if they are also overweight.
- Offer weight management programmes, e.g. Weight Watchers, exercise programmes.

Drug treatments
For those who are overweight and have not achieved target weight loss on dietary, activity and behavioural changes alone.

Orlistat
Orlistat is an intestinal lipase inhibitor that reduces absorption of lipids from the gut. It is licensed for prescription only as part of an overall plan for managing obesity in adults who have a BMI >30 (or >28 with co-morbidity). Only continue after 3 months if the patient has achieved at least 5% weight loss. Continuation is dependent on maintenance of weight reduction. Potential side effects include rectal leakage of oily fats.

Sibutramine
Sibutramine is a serotonin and noradrenaline reuptake inhibitor (SNRI). It is licensed for use only up to 1 year for patients with a BMI >30 (or >27 with co-morbidity). Only continue after 3 months if the patient has achieved at least 5% weight loss.

Rimonobant

Rimonobant acts on cannabinoid receptors. It was withdrawn from weight loss guidelines in October 2008 because of reports of increased incidence of psychiatric disorders and suicide.

Childhood obesity
- Tackle lifestyle within the context of the family and social setting
- Use BMI adjusted for age
- Refer to obesity specialists for overweight children with co-morbidity or learning difficulties
- Drug treatment not recommended in under-18s in primary care.

Case 17 marking schedule
This case assesses management of the obesity and primary prevention. Marks are awarded for the following.

Data gathering
- Identifies lifestyle factors (diet, exercise, eating behaviour) and co-morbidity/risk factors (family history of diabetes, obesity, IHD, hypertension, smoking).
- Informs the patient of her BMI and discusses the associated risk.
- Discusses previous weight loss interventions and successes/failures.
- Assesses patients ICE (I = I've heard I can take a pill to lose weight; C = I might have to pay for it, I don't want to look fat; E = I can lose weight without having to exercise).

Clinical management
- Discusses the treatment options and tailors a weight loss plan to the patient's lifestyle (e.g. decreased use of the car, increased walks with the pram, regular meals, food diary, reduced take outs/processed food, Weight Watchers programme, exercise programme).
- Sets an agreed realistic weight loss goal (5% of body weight loss in 3/12 months).
- Offers drug treatments if reduction in weight not achieved by measures after 6 months. Explains side effects.
- Emphasises the potential health benefits of weight loss.
- Agrees follow-up.

Interpersonal skills
- Agrees a shared management plan with regular planned follow-up.
- Respects the patient's negative self-image and offers a positive plan of action.
- Provides written information of the agreed plan and dietary leaflets.
- Offers encouragement and motivation for any successes past or present.

Case 18

Candidate information

Name: John Blowdon
Age: 17
Social and family history: lives with parents. Two younger siblings. A-level student at local sixth form college

> **Past medical history**: nocturnal fit 2 months ago – investigated at local hospital, FBC, electrolytes, MRI of brain normal
> **Drug history**: nil
> **Discharge letter details**: nocturnal seizure. Second episode. No structural abnormality. EEG shows epileptiform activity. Outpatient follow-up in 3 days. Sodium valproate 600 mg twice daily commenced.
>
> John's dad has come in and explains that John has had a second admission with a night-time fit and the investigations confirm epilepsy. He says that he has started treatment and has a follow-up appointment with the specialist later in the week. John's dad has come in wanting practical advice about epilepsy.
>
> ### Role-player information
> John had his first nocturnal seizure 2 months ago and now has had a further fit. Dad is sensible and well educated. He has had advice about the medication and possible side effects at the hospital but feels overwhelmed by the whole episode. He knows that epilepsy is to do with fitting but no more, and wants to know what has caused it. Could it have been caused by his appendix operation 2 years ago? He has come to discuss the diagnosis with you because, as his GP, he knows you and trusts your judgement. He is particularly interested in what this means for the family, i.e. 'What can he do, what can't he do? Will he be able to start his driving lessons for his birthday in 2 months time? What does this mean for his younger brothers?'. Mum is worried that she may have to give up work as a teaching assistant to help look after John with his medications and hospital appointments. Dad is worried about the stigma of epilepsy and how he will cope at school.

Topic summary: Advising the person with epilepsy

Epilepsy is a very common problem. It is estimated that 1 in 20 people has a non-febrile seizure at some stage and 1 in 200 will have chronic epilepsy. In a practice list of 2000 this means that 100 patients will have a non-febrile seizure and 10 will have epilepsy.

The psychological and social impact of the diagnosis may pose more problems than simple stabilisation to a fit-free state. Advice will be required on drugs and concordance, the likely restrictions on activity and employment, the genetic implications and to the carers in the first-aid situation. People with epilepsy will need intensive education and emotional support. Some of these points are now considered.

Driving

People with epilepsy cannot legally drive until entirely fit free for 1 year (or experiencing fits only while asleep for 3 years). People who have a 'liability to seizure' are ineligible to hold a vocational (group 2) licence (to qualify they would need to be fit free and off medication for 10 years, and have no underlying pathology). After a single fit it is recommended not to drive for a year, and not to resume until medically reviewed. People with epilepsy should not drive while treatment is being altered and this should ideally be managed by a specialist in view of the implications (social, medical, legal) should fits resume.

Work

Certain occupations exclude people with epilepsy, e.g. air traffic controllers, the armed forces and police, and those debarred by driving restrictions.

Activities

Most young people with epilepsy risk being cocooned in a restrictive environment by overprotective relatives. Activities should be as free as possible with the exception of a few commonsense guidelines:

- Do not swim alone
- Do not climb trees/ropes or take up mountaineering
- Do not bathe babies while alone, etc.
- Avoid using heavy machinery
- If alone showers are safer than having a bath.

Bicycle riding (wear a helmet) is generally felt to be an acceptable risk, and little restriction is advised on games and school activities.

Genetic advice

If one parent has epilepsy the chance of producing an affected child is about 3%, although there are some variations. The risk is higher if the epilepsy is idiopathic or generalised, and lower if focal or structural. However, it is still less than 5%, and therefore no reason to advise against child-bearing. The incidence of congenital malformation is increased from about 2.7% to 7.5% (although abnormalities are often mild).

Women with epilepsy should be managed by a specialist when planning pregnancy. Most continue taking their drugs in pregnancy. Although there is a small teratogenic potential, the risk to pregnancy is greater from uncontrolled epilepsy.

Some of the drugs used in treatment (e.g. carbamazepine, phenytoin, phenobarbital) are potent inducers of liver microsomal enzymes and may interact with oral contraceptives, reducing their effectiveness (a high-dose pill or barrier method may be required to avoid pregnancy).

Precipitants

Patients should be aware that triggers can increase the likelihood of a seizure, i.e.

- Tiredness
- Drugs (antidepressants, illegal drugs, alcohol)
- Flashing lights
- Menstruation
- Infection.

First-aid advice (British Epilepsy Association 2008)

Simple guidelines are required to help carers cope with a frightening situation, e.g.:

- Move any dangerous objects
- Place a cushion under the head
- So not try to restrain them during the fit unless in a dangerous location

- If the fit continues for >5 min, or the person is injured, call an ambulance
- After the fit place them in the recovery position and check their breathing, pulse
- Reassure them while waiting for them to regain their orientation

Emotional support and education

The patient should be treated as normally as possible. Remember that he (and especially his family) may be experiencing a variety of emotions, e.g.:

- anger and rejection
- anxiety
- a sort of bereavement reaction (following loss of health, job, etc.)
- shame or embarrassment.

Offer easy access and a sympathetic ear. Educate at every opportunity. Referral to the British Epilepsy Association (www.epilepsy.org.uk) and books such as *Epilepsy – the Facts* may help.

Follow-up

- Drugs and concordance
- Side effects
- Control
- Social and psychological problems.

Case 18 marking schedule

This proxy case encompasses the continuing education and management of epilepsy (including general advice and support). An effective consultation will elicit and address the family's concerns as part of a general education and management plan. Marks are awarded for the following.

Data gathering

- Establishes what is understood currently by dad with regard to epilepsy, its causes and management.
- Identifies his ICE about epilepsy and its treatment.
- Investigates the psychosocial impact that this has had on the family (e.g. mum's concerns about having to give up work, dad's worry about the stigma of epilepsy)/
- Uses this information to gain rapport using a combination of verbal and non-verbal communication skills.
- Gathers sufficient information to address the concerns/

Clinical management

- Has a sufficient understanding of management of epilepsy and practical issues to provide an explanation of epilepsy (explains in this case that the cause is unknown despite investigations).
- Discusses the core areas, tailoring the discussion to the family's concerns (driving, work, activities, genetic advice, precipitants, first aid, emotional support and education, follow-up):
  - dad should be reassured that the appendix operation is unrelated, that in most cases people with epilepsy lead a full and active life and that mum should not have to give up work.

- Confirms understanding and offers follow-up appointment with John to discuss the issue further.
- Offers written materials and details of support groups.

Interpersonal skills
- Provides a level of information appropriate for the patient while avoiding, or explaining, jargon.
- Uses appropriate empathy and offers a positive outlook.
- Allows time for questions and input from the family on their thoughts and ideas.
- Respects dad's ideas and concerns.

Case 19
Candidate information
Name: Violet Blunt
Age: 38
Social and family history: retail assistant with two children aged 1 and 3, living with her partner
Past medical history: depression – paracetamol overdose 2 years ago, 10 months SSRI following episode
Drug history: nil current

Violet comes to see you today to ask for advice on smoking cessation.

Role-player information
Violet tried to stop smoking 3 years ago during her first pregnancy. A lot of her friends have recently stopped after the introduction of the smoking ban in work and public places in England. She has heard about a new treatment called Champix and wants to give it a try. She also wonders about trying hypnotherapy.

Topic summary: Smoking cessation
NICE guidance (NICE 2002, 2006c, 2007b)
- Only offer smoking cessation therapy to patients who commit to a stop date.
- Offer brief interventions to promote progression along a cycle of change:
  - opportunistic advice to stop
  - assessment of patient's commitment to quit
  - offer of medication and/or behavioural support
  - self-help material.
- Patients should be reviewed 2 week after the agreed stop date.
- Prescriptions should only last until the time of first review (2 weeks of nicotine replacement therapy [NRT], 4 weeks of bupropion and varenicline)
- Failed treatment should not be restarted for 6 months (although this is flexible)
- Treatment choice should be based on patient's preference and contraindications; combination therapy is not recommended
- Cessation is most effective when behavioural support forms part of a smoking cessation plan (e.g. at a practice stop smoking clinic).

Treatment options
Nicotine replacement therapy
- **Action**: direct nicotine replacement.
- **Prescription**: continue for 8 weeks after the stop date and stop. Dose dependent on method of replacement and number of cigarettes smoked (refer to *BNF*). Available over the counter.
- **Modes of replacement**: patch, gum, spray, inhaler, lozenge, sublingual tablet.
- **Contraindications**: unstable cardiovascular disease. *Note that it is used in pregnancy as an adjunct to smoking cessation.*

Bupropion (Zyban)
- **Action**: atypical antidepressant.
- **Prescription**: start 1–2 weeks before target stop date, initially 150 mg daily for 6 days then 150 mg twice daily. Continue for 7–9 weeks. Prescription only.
- **Contraindications**: pregnancy, breastfeeding, seizures, bipolar disorder.

Varenicline (Champix)
- **Action**: nicotine receptor partial agonist and partial antagonist.
- **Prescription**: start 1–2 weeks before target stop date, initially 500 mcg once daily for 3 days, increased to 500 mcg twice daily for 4 days, then 1 mg twice daily for 11 weeks.
- **Contraindications**: pregnancy, suicidal behaviour.

Other interventions (White et al. 2006)
- **Hypnotherapy**: no evidence of superiority to other interventions or no treatment.
- **Exercise programme**: weak evidence that exercise programmes help reduce cravings and promote cessation.
- **Acupuncture and acupressure**: no consistent evidence of efficacy greater than placebo.
- **Self help material**: superior to no intervention but efficacy small. More effective if tailored to the individual (e.g. their stage in the cycle of change).
- **Group-based cessation programmes**: double the chance of quitting compared with self-help materials alone.

Case 19 marking schedule

Preventive care and lifestyle intervention are the focus here. The treatment plan should be tailored to the patient's preferences and risk factors. Marks are awarded for the following.

Data gathering
- Smoking history (how many, how long, previous attempts to quit, motivation, smokers around her, i.e. home/work, general health issues relating to prescribing, i.e. CVD, pregnancy, breastfeeding, depression and suicidal ideation).
- Identifies ICE (I – I want to give up, will varenicline help me, perhaps I could try hypnotherapy on the NHS? C – cost; E – I will leave with a script today).

- Examination: nil required but a chance for opportunistic screening, e.g. BP, weight and pulse.

Clinical management
- Discusses the different pharmacological and non-pharmacological treatment options and their efficacy. Her ideas regarding hypnotherapy, varenicline and cost should be specifically addressed (i.e. hypnotherapy not available on NHS and evidence of efficacy poor).
- Identifies that varenicline is contraindicated in view of her history of suicidal ideation and depression; explains this and offers a choice of NRT or bupropion.
- Agrees a stop date.
- Emphasises that success rates are higher if combined with behavioural counselling and encourages her to attend the surgery smoking cessation clinic.
- Addresses her concerns regarding cost (free) and her expectation of treatment (provide a script today if stop date agreed)
- Agrees follow-up 2 weeks after the stop date
- Issues a correct prescription for the treatment of choice.

Interpersonal skills
- Encourages patient's effort to stop smoking by emphasising the advantages – savings from cost of cigarettes, health benefits for her and her children.
- Offers ongoing support.
- Shares decisions and respects ideas regarding treatment options.

Case 20

Candidate information

Name: John Dunn
Age: 32
Social and family history: married with two children
Past medical history: previous episode of low back pain 15 months ago. Infrequent attendee
Drug history: nil

A 32 year old presents with back pain at your surgery. He has had several episodes of back pain over the last 12 months but on this occasion he has been unable work. John says that he needs a sick note to claim benefits. He would like some pain relief and wants to know if a chiropractor might help. The candidate's task is to assess his back pain, discuss the treatment options and agree a management plan.

Role-player information

John is a self-employed plumber; he hurt his back lifting a radiator 2 days ago. His episodes of low back pain in the last year have been mild and self-limiting. He did not present to the surgery on these occasions. His pain is felt over his back and buttocks with no paraesthesia or weakness. Pain is aggravated by movement. John's main concern is the impact on his work and income.

Topic summary: Low back pain
The scale of the problem

Back pain is very common; 40% of adults will have experienced an episode of back pain over the previous 12 months. The cost to the NHS is more than £1bn a year. The cost to the economy through lost work is estimated at £3.5bn a year.

The natural history
- Some 50–80% recover completely in 4 weeks without treatment and 90% in 6 weeks
- In 80% of cases no specific diagnosis is made
- However, almost 70% of patients who ever experience an episode will suffer three or more recurrences.

Should cases be referred?
Of the 3–7 million people who consult with backache annually:
- 1.5 million (about one-third) are referred for an opinion
- a similar number have a radiograph
- 1 million attend NHS physiotherapy departments
- 100 000 people are admitted and 24 000 undergo surgery (<1 in 200 of the original sufferers, and 1 in 60 of the referrals).

Many patients are referred for primarily social reasons: patient insistence on a second opinion; to reassure the patient that all possible avenues have been explored; to demonstrate continuing concern; or to reassure the doctor that no serious pathology has been missed. However, as relatively few cases are amenable to specialist help this represents a questionable use of orthopaedic resources.

The element of referral due to medical ignorance could be reduced by the NICE (2009) guidelines.

When to refer
Immediate
Evidence of cauda equina syndrome or widespread neurological disorder (disturbed micturition/anal tone, saddle anaesthesia, widespread progressive motor weakness, gait problems).

Urgent
'Red flag' signs suggestive of serious pathology.

No referral
Simple backache and non-progressive nerve root entrapment should *normally be managed within general practice*, but referred if prolonged (not returned to normal activities in 3 months) and unresolved.

Red flags of low back pain
- Backache in <20 years or >55 years
- History of cancer
- Non-mechanical back pain (i.e. not related to movement)
- Thoracic pain
- Systemic features (weight loss, night sweats)
- Widespread neurological signs (not limited to one nerve root)
- Progressive neurological signs
- Structural deformity associated with backache
- Steroid use or drug abuse
- Severe nocturnal pain.

Investigations?

The yield from lumbosacral radiographs is low. Thus:

- In one district general hospital where there were 3000 such radiographs per year; 30–40% were reported normal and about 40% showed degenerative changes only.
- Many large studies have found a very poor correlation between degenerative changes and symptoms.

Despite these drawbacks, surveys indicate that a high percentage of backache sufferers eventually present to the radiology department, e.g. in the UK there are half a million lumbar spine radiographs taken annually.

Why then are so many patients referred for radiographs at great cost in terms of personnel, money and convenience? In general many of the social reasons for referral are mirrored in the use of radiographs and other investigative procedures. Important factors include:

1. The insistence of poorly counselled or impatient patients
2. Impatience or ignorance on the part of the doctor
3. The fear that something important may be missed
4. The psychological benefit that patients (and doctors) gain from a normal radiograph report.

What treatment should be given?

Initial management strategies for patients with simple acute low back pain include reassurance as to the benign nature of the pain, avoidance of bed rest, encouragement to maintain their normal activity, education on posture and lifting, manipulation therapy, physical therapy and exercise programmes to help restore function. Drug treatment typically includes effective analgesia. In a patient with simple low back pain radiographs are best avoided (NICE 2009).

Mobilisation

Active exercise and rehabilitation often promote recovery: the particular type of exercise may be less important (Chou and Huffman 2007a).

Manipulation

1. A Cochrane review (Assendelft et al. 2004) of 39 trials found that spinal manipulation was more effective in reducing pain and improving the ability to perform everyday activities than sham (fake) therapy and therapies already known to be unhelpful. However, it was no more or less effective than medication for pain, physical therapy, exercises, back education or the care given by a GP.
2. Manipulation requires some expertise and is potentially harmful in the presence of neurological complications and certain pathological conditions (fractures, metastases, osteoporosis).
3. Some patients derive comfort from manipulation and believe in it.

Pharmacological treatment options

There is evidence for the use of NSAIDs, paracetamol and muscle relaxants for acute low back pain. Chronic back pain sufferers may benefit from use of a tricyclic antidepressant (Chou and Huffman 2007b).

Primary prevention

A number of studies in industry have shown initial benefits from lifting training programmes, but the benefit generally diminishes with time (HSE 2008).

MEMORY BOX: Low back pain
- Triage cases into – mechanical, nerve root or serious spinal pathology
- Exclude serious pathology (cauda equina, inflammatory arthritis)
- Avoid investigation in acute simple low back pain
- Reassure – 90% resolve in 6 weeks
- Analgesia, exercise, physiotherapy, education and spinal manipulation are equally effective

---

Case 20 marking schedule

This case assesses the candidate's management of a common recurrent illness. The candidate must safely assess the patient with a targeted history and examination. The request for a sickness certificate encourages the candidate to demonstrate their ability to investigate the social aspects. It also assesses the correct use of medical statements. Marks are awarded for the following.

Data gathering

- Establishes the character of the back pain (type, radiation, aggravating factors) and excludes cauda equina or red flag features indicative of serious pathology.
- Establishes the duration of the illness, and background history of previous episodes including current or previous treatment.
- Enquires about the patient's job and the impact of his symptoms on his work and home life.
- Identifies his ideas, concerns, expectations re cause of his low back pain and sickness certification.
- Completes proficient examination (inspects back for deformity, palpates for tenderness, tests range of movement, performs straight-leg raise and femoral stretch tests).

Clinical management

- Correctly identifies pain as simple low back pain, and reassures re prognosis.
- Demonstrates an understanding of the causes and natural history of low back pain through explanation to the patient.
- Avoids investigation.
- Explains treatment options and comes to a shared management plan in line with guidance.
- Explains sickness certification and advises patient to self-certify for the first 7 days.
- Specifies conditions for follow-up and alerts patients to red flag signs requiring urgent review.

Interpersonal skills

- Recognises the concerns of the patient and shows empathy. Emphasises the good prognosis for return to work.

- Takes a holistic approach to management incorporating the patient's ideas regarding back manipulation and complementary therapy into the management plan.
- Confirms understanding and provides written information.

Case 21

Candidate information

Name: Jenny Whitson
Age: 15 years
Social and family history: lives with younger brother, mum and dad
Past medical history: no recent attendances and nil of significance in the past history

A 15 year old attends the surgery with her mother. She has not been seen at the surgery since the computer records began. She is upset about her skin although her mother believes that she is making a fuss about something all teenagers go through. The candidate's task is to take a history and agree a management plan.

Role-player information

Jenny is extremely upset about her mild-to-moderate acne. She has been teased at school and is convinced that the spots are being caused by something that she is doing. She feels that she has tried every over-the-counter treatment available, as well as dietary and lifestyle changes, and is very keen for 'the strongest treatment possible'.

Topic summary: Acne vulgaris

Acne is a common problem affecting 80% of 11–30 year olds at some point and, although many self-medicate, up to 60% will consult a GP. Psychological distress caused by acne can be considerable and should be weighed up when deciding on appropriate management. Given this patient's demographics consideration should be taken of whether there is a hidden agenda of wanting a contraceptive. Antibiotics are commonly used in acne treatment and with increasing resistance this poses a prescribing dilemma for GPs.

Diagnosis of acne vulgaris

Diagnosis is by clinical examination which may reveal closed comedones (whiteheads), open comedones (blackheads) or inflammatory lesions, including pustules, inflamed papules or nodules. There may also be scarring or post-inflammatory hyperpigmentation (especially seen in dark skin). These occur most commonly on the face but can also be on the shoulders and back.

Underlying causes of acne should be considered, e.g. medication and androgen excess. Relevant medication includes steroids and antidepressants. Signs of androgen excess (irregular periods, hirsutism, infertility, obesity) should precipitate investigation for underlying hormonal abnormalities.

Any doubt about the diagnosis is an indication for referral.

Management of acne vulgaris

The patient should be graded according to the severity of her acne and the psychological impact that it is having on her. Severe social problems or failure to respond to treatment is an indication for referral. A patient's acne should be categorised as mild, moderate or severe according to the type of lesions, risk of scarring (e.g. increased with FH) and amount of skin affected. For most patients the prognosis is good with treatment improving symptoms and for most teenagers acne will clear.

Address acne myths:

- There is no evidence that any foods worsen acne.
- Acne is not due to poor skin hygiene (in fact excessive washing of the skin or use of abrasive washes can stimulate oil production and worsen acne, instead patients should be encouraged to wash the skin twice a day without these products)
- Acne is not contagious.

Mild acne

The mainstay of treatment is topical. Topical treatments should be applied to the whole area in order to treat quiescent lesions. Topical preparations in an alcohol base should be avoided with sensitive skin but may help greasier skin. A gel can be better for oily skin or cream for dryer skin. Most topical treatments initially cause skin irritation and warning patients will improve concordance. Patients should be warned that benzoyl peroxide and topical tetracycline can bleach clothes.

Benzoyl peroxide is the first-line treatment and many over-the-counter (OTC) remedies contain this. Skin irritation can be decreased by titrating up from a lower strength and using the treatment at night. If benzoyl peroxide has already been used in an OTC treatment without success an alternative should be offered rather than increasing the strength.

Alternatives include topical retinoids (vitamin A derivatives, e.g. tretinoin). Retinoids are considered most effective against comedomal lesions. However, they do have some anti-inflammatory effect (Gollnick et al. 2003). They also have a role in long-term maintenance where use can reduce the need for chronic antibiotics. Patients should be warned about skin irritation associated with topical retinoid use, especially likely at the start of treatment. Retinoid strength should be chosen as a balance between achieving efficacy and avoiding inflammatory response. Retinoids are teratogenic (even topical preparations) and women using them should be on contraceptives where appropriate and not pregnant or breastfeeding.

Topical antibiotics (erythromycin or clindamycin preferred) are good for treating inflammatory lesions. Of the topical antibiotics erthromycin and clindamycin have most evidence for their use (Sarah and DeBerker 2008). Resistance can develop where topical antibiotics are used alone.

Combination therapy is helpful to manage resistant acne. For increased efficacy where both comedones and inflammatory lesions are present treatments can be combined, e.g. using a topical retinoid before bed and a topical antibiotic on waking. Benzoyl peroxide plus an antibiotic is more effective than either alone, and less skin irritation is seen than with using benzoyl peroxide alone. Combination products exist (benzamycin R is erythromycin and benzoyl peroxide). However, these are often more expensive and come in an alcoholic base which can irritate the skin.

Review should be after 8 weeks although it can take up to 4 months to see a maximal benefit. If a treatment is effective it should be continued for 6 months. Subsequent courses maybe needed to control flares.

Moderate acne

First-line treatment is a topical antibiotic in combination with benzoyl peroxide. Where this fails or the back or shoulders are affected or there is a risk of scarring, oral antibiotics should be used. Oral erythromycin is the most effective agent (Sarah and DeBerker 2008). However, it is not recommended as a first-line choice because of concerns over resistance. Tetracyclines are the first-line choice. Doxycyline has the most evidence of efficacy, although it can cause photosensitivity and as other tetracyclines should not be used in pregnancy, breastfeeding or under 12 s (stains growing teeth). Minocycline, while as effective as other tetracyclines, is associated with safety concerns (Garner et al. 2003). If other antibiotics cannot be used trimethoprim is an option. An improvement with oral antibiotics is normally seen over 3–6 months. The Global Alliance to Improve Outcomes in Acne (Gollnick et al. 2003) has recommended that if antibiotics are used for longer than 2 months benzoyl peroxide should be used for a minimum of 5–7 days between antibiotic courses to help reduce resistance. Attempts to stop antibiotics should be made after 12 weeks, with further courses given as needed, and a topical retinoid used in between. Some patients may need to continue oral antibiotics for longer to prevent acne returning.

Severe acne

Consider oral antibiotics as the first line. Refer if considering an oral retinoid (Roaccutane). This treatment is highly effective, but given its teratogenic nature it should be prescribed only by a specialist. NICE advises referral if there is no improvement over a 6-month period after treatment with several topical and oral antibiotics. Failure of treatment in this definition is by subjective assessment by the patient.

Oral contraceptive pill

There is some evidence from a Cochrane review that the combined oral contraceptive pill can help improve acne, but there is no evidence for use of a particular pill. The progesterone-only pill may worsen acne. Dianette (an anti-androgen) can be used for acne treatment if oral antibiotics do not work, and will also provide effective contraception. There is an increased risk of venous thromboembolism with this treatment and an assessment of risk factors for venous thromboembolism should be made first.

MEMORY BOX: Acne
- Consider psychosocial factors (i.e. impact on the patient's life and well being)
- Grade acne and treat accordingly
- A topical retinoid is often a good starting point for mild or moderate acne or in combination for severe acne
- Combination treatment is key (e.g. topical retinoid before bed and topical benzoyl peroxide in the morning)
- Using benzoyl peroxide alongside antibiotics helps to reduce resistance
- Only refer after using a variety of topical and oral treatments over a minimum of 6 months

Case 21 marking schedule

This is an example of a common problem. The impact on the patient may be disproportionate to the severity of the acne. Good communication is necessary to achieve a shared understanding and plan. Concordance with long-term treatment relies upon this. Marks are awarded for the following.

Data gathering

- Establishes symptoms, duration and treatments used to date.
- Explores the patients ICE (I = why is the acne continuing even though I've stopped eating chocolate: C = I'll have this my whole life and it'll keep getting worse; E = if I could get a treatment maybe it'll resolve before next week's school disco).
- Elicits psychological effects of acne, e.g. embarrassment, social isolation, bullying.
- Confirms expectations in terms of contraceptive pills (e.g. 'Some people find the pill can help with skin and also cover for contraception. Is that something you had wondered about?' – in this instance she does not want this)
- Excludes other relevant symptoms, e.g. of androgen excess, other medication including over-the-counter/complementary (Chinese medicines often contain steroids) ones.
- Examines to confirm the diagnosis.

Clinical management

- Addresses the patient's ICE through discussion and explanation of the natural history of acne.
- Gives a realistic timescale for improvement.
- Empathises and offer hopeful prognosis.
- Agrees a joint management plan appropriate to disease severity and psychological impact with realistic expectation of treatment duration.
- Discuss antibiotic use and balances treatment decision.
- Agrees follow-up for review at an appropriate time, e.g. 8 weeks.

Interpersonal skills

- Listens and empathises with patient giving appropriate weighting to the problem for the effect it is having on the patient's life.
- Is patient centred in approaching treatment options.
- Offers realistic but positive prognosis.

Case 22

Candidate information

Name: Mary Hawberry
Age: 48
Social and family history: solicitor, lives with husband
Past medical history: high BP reading 8 months ago, DNA's follow-up.
Drug history: nil current
Test results: TSH 3.6, T_4 14, ESR 7, Hb 12.8, MCV 86, WCC 6, Na^+ 140, U 6, K^+ 3.9, creatinine 86, eGFR 45
Repeat test: Na^+ 141, U 6, K^+ 3.9, creatinine 87, eGFR 47

This woman saw a colleague the previous week complaining of feeling 'tired all the time'. Some routine blood tests were requested. Following her test results she was contacted by the surgery and told that she needed a repeat blood test and then an appointment for the results. She attends today for her repeat appointment.

Role-player information

Since her first appointment Mary has been feeling a bit better and wonders if she was recovering from a viral episode. She sees herself as being in good health and attends the doctor's as little as possible. Mary is well educated and busy at work. She is not happy at having to attend the surgery for no apparent reason now that she is feeling better, especially as the receptionists have told her that most of her blood tests were normal. Mary wants clear and detailed information about any problem. She is not keen on medication, especially if the only reason seems to be 'because the doctor says'.

Chronic kidney disease (CKD) – the facts (NICE 2008b)

Since estimated glomerular filtration rate (eGFR) became widely reported and easily available to GPs and, with its inclusion in the QOF in 2006, there has been a change in the primary care management of CKD. Many practices are still finding their way around this area and a clear understanding and interest in this may pay off in job interviews as well as for the exam.

The rationale behind use of eGFR is to detect kidney disease in its earlier stages where urea and creatinine may be normal and patients are asymptomatic. Intervention at this early stage may slow or prevent the progression to more serious kidney disease or reduce the risk of cardiovascular disease. The eGFR is an estimate, as the name suggests, of how well the kidneys are filtering (Table 9.6).

CKD 1&2 (eGFR >60)

In stages 1 and 2 the estimation of GFR is much less accurate in assessing how well the kidneys are functioning. Renal disease may be present despite a normal eGFR (CKD1) and is identified by the presence of one of the following: persistent microalbuminuria/haematuria/proteinuria, structural kidney abnormalities on ultrasonography/other radiology or chronic

Table 9.6 The estimated glomerular filtration rate (eGFR) and action to take

Stage	eGFR (mL/min per 1.73 m^2)	Monitoring/Action[a]
1	>90[b]	Annual eGFR
2	60–90	Annual eGFR
3	30–60	*Stable* annual eGFR
3a	*45–59*	*Unstable* 6-monthly eGFR
3b	*30–44*	
4	15–30	*Stable* 6 monthly eGFR
		Unstable 3 monthly eGFR
		Refer to renal team[c]
5	<15	3-monthly eGFR (specialist monitoring)

[a]At all stages address CVD risk and lifestyle factors.
[b]Normal renal function plus another indicator of renal disease e.g. proteinuria.
[c]For planning for end stage renal failure.
Note that stable eGFR = change <2 over 6 months. If proteinuria is present the suffix p is added to the stage, e.g. eGFR 68 with proteinuria is categorised as stage 2p.

glomerulonephritis on biopsy. If CKD is suspected at this stage dipstick urine, assess CVD risk factors, review medication for nephrotoxic drugs and monitor eGFR annually.

CKD 4&5 (eGFR <30)
Refer for specialist care and investigate as for CKD stage 3.
  Refer immediately if:
- GFR <15
- acute renal failure
- accelerated hypertension
- potassium >7.

CKD 3 (eGFR 30–60)
This leaves CKD 3, the main area for GP management.

Initial assessment (newly diagnosed eGFR <60)
Exclude acute renal failure (though majority will be chronic):
- Consider sepsis, hypovolaemia, heart failure, urinary retention (the abdomen should be examined to exclude bladder enlargement). Medication should be reviewed for iatrogenic causes of acute renal failure such as NSAIDs. The urine should be dipped, because the presence of blood or protein may indicate glomerulonephritis which may be rapidly progressive. A further eGFR reading should be taken within 5 days.
- Any of the following are diagnostic of acute renal failure (or acute-on-chronic renal failure) and should be referred immediately: a drop of 25% or more in eGFR, a rise of 1.5 times the previous creatinine (if unknown baseline creatinine should be assumed to be 75) or oliguria (<0.5 ml/kg per h) in the context of acute illness.

Further management of CKD 3
The main risk for those with early CKD is from cardiovascular disease rather than specific kidney problems.

Management checklist
- Assess CVD risk
  - lifestyle factors (smoking, alcohol, exercise, weight reduction)
  - BP control
  - CVD risk >20% over 10 years add statin (SHARP study [Baigent and Landry 2003] on lipids in CKD without other risk factors reports in 2010; note that myositis on statin more likely in renal failure)
- Medication review (stop nephrotoxic drugs)
- Immunize (influenza and pneumococci)
- Check PTH (renal failure-induced hyperparathyroidism – if PTH >70 then check 25-hydroxyvitamin D; if vitamin D normal then refer, if low then start treatment and repeat PTH after 3 months)
- Monitor annually:
  - FBC for anaemia (if Hb <11 exclude other causes; if none found treat with iron and erythropoietin to maintain Hb 11–12)

> renal function
> calcium, phosphate (renal failure-induced hyperparathyroidism)
> urinalysis.

Proteinuria should be confirmed by requesting an MSU to exclude infection and an early morning sample for protein:creatinine (or albumin:creatinine ratio). The sample should be early morning to exclude postural proteinuria. Testing for protein (or albumin):creatinine ratio is a recent QOF indicator for patients with CKD. Refer if ratio >100 or >45 with haematuria.

Note that, if there are lower tract symptoms, progressive fall in eGFR or refractory hypertension, request renal ultrasonography.

Blood pressure

Blood pressure should be measured at least annually. Treatment should be started if BP is >140/90 or >130/80 if proteinuria is present. The targets to aim for, although in practice they may be difficult to achieve, are <130/80 or <125/75 with proteinuria.

ACE inhibitors (or angiotensin receptor blockers – ARBs) are first-line treatments for hypertension in patients with renal disease because they have proven efficacy in minimising deterioration in kidney function (unless you have renal artery stenosis, when they may make things worse!). A conventional approach is to start all patients on an ACEI/ARB and monitor their renal function (before starting and 2 weeks after). If there is a fall in eGFR by 15% or more, or an increase in creatinine by 20% or more, which is sustained, then referral to a specialist is advised, without stopping the ACEI. ACEIs should not be given in pregnancy, so use caution when prescribing to women of child-bearing age. If a patient still has a BP >150/90 on three antihypertensive agents they should be referred.

Case 22 marking schedule

The focus here is a candidate's ability to carry out the initial assessment of a chronic disease and lay the groundwork for a long-term therapeutic relationship. Marks are awarded for the following.

Data gathering
- Establishes what is understood currently by patient with regard to kidney and CVD.
- Uses this information to gain rapport using a combination of verbal and non-verbal communication skills.
- Gathers sufficient information to complete a CVD risk assessment.

Clinical management
- Has a sufficient understanding of management of CKD, and in particular CKD 3, to explain to the patient the risks and relationship to cardiovascular risk.
- Discusses all core areas including monitoring of BP, urine, lifestyle changes, role of medication with explanation for the reason for the relevance of these factors on the kidneys.
- Agrees which of these are acceptable to start treating initially, considering the impact for a patient of a new chronic diagnosis and need for life-long medication.
- Advises on follow-up as appropriate for the agreed strategy.

> **Interpersonal skills**
> * Provides a level of information appropriate for the patient while avoiding, or explaining, jargon.
> * Uses appropriate empathy and breaking bad news skills as this may be for this patient.
> * Allows time for questions and input from the patient on their thoughts and ideas about such a 'silent' condition to allow them to feel ownership of their health
> * Provides written information on CKD.

Acknowledgements

To Dr S. Westmore for Cases 1, 8, 12 and 14, and to Dr S. Ball for Cases 6, 21 and 22.

References

Age Concern. *Arranging for Others to make Decisions about your Finances or Welfare.* Factsheet FS22. London: Age Concern, 2008.

Assendelft WJJ, Morton SC, Yu EI, Suttorp MJ, Shekelle PG. Spinal manipulative therapy for low-back pain. *Cochrane Database Syst Rev* 2004;**1**:CD000447.

Baigent C, Landry M. Study of Heart and Renal Protection (SHARP). *Kidney Int* 2003;**63**:S207–10.

Bernadt MW, Mumford J, Taylor C, Smith B, Murray RM. Comparison of questionnaire and laboratory tests in detection of excessive drinking and alcoholism. *Lancet* 1982;**i**:325–8.

British Epilepsy Association. First Aid for Seizures. Available at: www.epilepsy.org. uk/info/firstaid.html (accessed 2008). Cochrane review. *Cochrane Database Syst Rev* 2004;**3**:CD001727.

Chou R, Huffman LH. Nonpharmacologic therapies for acute and chronic low back pain: a review of the evidence for an American Pain Society/American College of Physicians clinical practice guideline. *Ann Intern Med* 2007a;**147**:492–504.

Chou R, Huffman LH. Medications for acute and chronic low back pain: a review of the evidence for an American Pain Society/American College of Physicians clinical practice guideline. *Ann Intern Med* 2007b;**147**:505–14.

Del Mar C, Glasziou PP, Spinks A. Antibiotics for sore throat. *Cochrane Database Syst Rev* 2006;**4**:CD000023.

Department of Health. *Reference Guide to Consent for Examination or Treatment.* London: DH: 2001.

Department of Health. *You're Welcome Quality Criteria, Making health services young people friendly.* London: DH, 2007a.

Department of Health. *National Alcohol Strategy.* London: DH, 2007b.

Department of Health. *The National Health Service Drug Tariff 2009 for England and Wales.* London: DH, 2009.

Draper R. Patientplus article: Down's. Patient.co.uk, 2007.

Dunn C, Deroo L, Rivara FP. The use of brief interventions adapted from motivational interviewing across behavioural domains: a systematic review. *Addiction* 2001;**96**:1725–42.

Edwards G, Grant M (eds), *Alcoholism: New knowledge and new responses*, 3rd edn. London: Croom Helm, 1979: 324–5.

European Association of Urology. *Guidelines on Erectile Dysfunction.* The Netherlands: European Association of Urology, 2005.

Farina GA, Mazarin GI. Red eye evaluation. 2006; online. Available at: http://emedicine.medscape.com/article/1216540-overview.

Ferri MMF, Amato L, Davoli M. Alcoholics anonymous and other 12-step programmes for alcohol dependence. *Cochrane Database Syst Rev* 2006;**3**:CD005032.

Garner SE, Eady EA, Popescu C, Newton J, Li Wan Po A. Minocycline for acne vulgaris: efficacy and safety. *Cochrane Database Syst Rev* 2003;**1**:CD002086.

General Medical Council. *Good Medical Practice*. London: GMC, 2006.

Glasziou PP, Del Mar CB, Sanders SL et al. Antibiotics for acute otitis media in children. *CochraneDatabase Syst Rev* 2004;**1**:CD000219.

Gollnick H, Cunliffe W, Berson D et al., Global Alliance to Improve Outcomes in Acne. Management of acne: a report. *J Am Acad Dermatol* 2003;**49**(1 suppl):S1–37.

Gott M, Seymour J, Bellamy G et al. Older people's views about home as a place of care at the end of life. *Palliat Med* 2004;**18**:460–7.

Health Development Agency. *Alcohol Consumption and Alcohol Related Behaviour*. London: HAD, 2002.

Health Protection Agency. *Shooting Up. Infections in injecting drug users in the United Kingdom*. London: HPA, 2006.

Health and Safety Executive. *Better Backs Campaign*. London: HSE, 2008.

Hinton J. Whom do dying patients tell? *BMJ* 1980;**281**:1328–30.

Hodgson R, Alwyn T, Bev J, Thom B, Smith A. The FAST alcohol screening test. *Alcohol and Alcoholism*. 2002;**37**(1):61–6.

Jeffery AN, Voss LD, Metcalf BS, Alba S, Wilkin TJ. Parents' awareness of overweight in themselves and their children: cross sectional study within a cohort (EarlyBird 21). *BMJ* 2005;**330**:23–4.

Jung R. Obesity, the most important nutritional problem in Scotland. Presentation at The Royal Society of Edinburgh, 2005. Available at: www.rse.org.uk/events/reports/2004-2005/jung.pdf.

Kaner EF, Dickinson Ho, Beyer FR et al. Effectiveness of brief alcohol interventions in primary care populations. *Cochrane Database Syst Rev* 2007;**2**:CD004148.

Kubler Ross E. *On Death and Dying*. New York: Macmillan, 1969.

Langewitz W, Denz M, Keller A, Kiss A, Rüttimann S, Wössmer B. Spontaneous talking time at start of consultation in outpatient clinic: cohort study. *BMJ* 2002;**325**:682–3.

Little P, Gould C, Williamson I, Warner G, Gantley M, Kinmouth AL. Reattendance and complications in a randomised trial of prescribing strategies for sore throat: the medicalising effect of prescribing antibiotics. *BMJ* 1997;**315**:350–2.

Medicines and Healthcare products Regulatory Agency and the Commission on Human Medicines. *Drugs Safety Update*, vol 1, Issue 2. London: MHRA, CHM, 2007. Available at: http://cks.library.nhs.uk/menopause/evidence/supporting_evidence/risks_of_hrt.

Mitchell H. Vaginal discharge – causes, diagnosis and treatment. *BMJ* 2004;**328**: 1306–8.

Moncrieff G, Fletcer F. Tiredness. *BMJ* 2007;**334**:1221.

National Institute for Clinical Excellence. *The Clinical Effectiveness and Cost Effectiveness of Bupropion (Zyban) and Nicotine Replacement Therapy for Smoking Cessation*. London: NICE. 2002.

National Institute for Health and Clinical Excellence. *Supportive and Palliative Care*. London: NICE, 2004a.

National Institute for Health and Clinical Excellence. *Dyspepsia – Management of dyspepsia in adults in primary care*. London: NICE, 2004b (updated 2005).

National Institute for Health and Clinical Excellence. *Referral Guidelines for Suspected Cancer*. London: NICE, 2005.

National Institute for Health and Clinical Excellence. *Familial Breast Cancer: The classification and care of women at risk of familial breast cancer in primary, secondary and tertiary care.* London: NICE, 2006a.

National Institute for Health and Clinical Excellence. *Obesity: The prevention, identification, assessment and management of overweight and obesity in adults and children.* London: NICE, 2006b.

National Institute for Health and Clinical Excellence. *Brief Interventions and Referral for Smoking Cessation in Primary Care and Other Settings.* London: NICE, 2006c.

National Institute for Health and Clinical Excellence. *General Management Strategies for Mild–Moderate Psychological Distress.* London: NICE, 2007a.

National Institute for Health and Clinical Excellence. *Varenicline for Smoking Cessation.* London: NICE, 2007b.

National Institute for Health and Clinical Excellence. *Antenatal Care, Routine Care for the Healthy Pregnant Woman.* London: NICE, 2008a.

National Institute for Health and Clinical Excellence. *Chronic Kidney Disease: Early identification and management of chronic kidney disease in adults in primary and secondary care.* London: NICE, 2008b.

National Institute for Health and Clinical Excellence. *Low Back Pain: Early management of persistent non-specific low back pain.* London: NICE, 2009.

National Prescribing Centre. Contraception – current issues: summary. *MeReC Bulletin* 2006;**17**(2):1–9.

National Prescribing Centre. The management of common infections in primary care – Sore Throat. *MeReC Bulletin* 2006;**17**(3):12–14.

NHS Clinical Knowledge Summary. Red eye, revised Sept 2008. Available at: www.cks.nhs.uk/red_eye#332545001.

Office for National Statistics. *Cancer Statistics Registrations: Registrations of cancer diagnosed in 2004.* London: National Statistics, 2007.

Oppenheimer E, Tobutt C, Taylor C, Andrew T. Death and survival in a cohort of heroin addicts from London clinics: a 22-year follow-up study. *Addiction* 1994;**89**:1299–308.

Paradise J, Bluestone C, Bachman R et al. Efficacy of tonsillectomy for recurrent throat infection in severely affected children: results of parallel randomised and nonrandomized clinical trials. *N Engl J Med* 1984;**310**:674–83.

Parkes CM. Recent bereavement as a cause of mental illness. *Br J Psychiatry* 1964;**110**:198–204.

Parkes CM. *Bereavement: Studies of grief in adult life*, 2nd edn. Basingstoke: Taylor & Francis, 1986.

Ralph D, McNicholas T. UK management guidelines for erectile dysfunction. *BMJ* 2000;**321**:499–503.

Rattigan T. *Collected Works*. London: Hamilton, 1953.

Royal College of General Practitioners. *nMRCGP: the CCT and new Membership Assessment.* London: RCGP, 2007. Available at: www.rcgp-curriculum.org.uk/examinations_and_assessment.aspx (accessed 2007).

Royal College of General Practitioners. CSA Information For Candidates v.5 MSSRJAC 271108. London: RCGP, 2008. Available at: www.rcgp-curriculum.org.uk/docs/CSA%20Info%20For%20Candidates%20v%205%20MSSRJAC%20271108.doc.

Saenz RB. Primary care of infants and young children with downs syndrome. *Am Family Physn* 1999;**59**:381–90, 392, 395–6.

Sarah P, DeBerker D. Acne vulgaris – skin disorders. *BMJ Clinical Evidence*, online May 2008.

Scott O. The red eye. Patientplus article for Patient UK, 2008. Available at: www. patient.co.uk/showdoc/40000850.

Scottish Intercollegiate Guidelines Network. The Management of Harmful Drinking and Alcohol Dependence in Primary Care. Edinburgh: SIGN, 2003 (updated 2004).

Spiro DM, Tay K-Y, Arnold DH et al. Wait-and-see prescription for treatment of acute otitis media. A randomised controlled trial. *JAMA* 2006;**296**:1235–41.

van Staaij BK, van den Akker EH, Rovers MM et al. Effectiveness of adenotonsil-lectomy in children with mild symptoms of throat infections or adenotonsillar hypertrophy: open, randomised controlled trial. *BMJ* 2004;**329**:651.

White AR, Rampes H, Campbell J. Acupuncture and related interventions for smoking cessation. *Cochrane Database Syst Rev* 2006;**1**:CD000009.

Wilkes E. *The Dying Patient: The medical management of incurable and terminal illness.* Ridgewood, NJ: GA Bogden, 1982.

Willacy H. Fatigue and tired all the time. Patient UK, 2008, online publication.

Williams JW, Simel DL. Does this patient have sinusitis? Diagnosing acute sinusitis by history and physical examination. *JAMA* 1993;**270**:1242–6.

Woof WR, Carter YH. The grieving adult and the general practitioner. *Br J Gen Pract* 1997;**47**:509–14.

Appendices

The appendices provide relevant background information on General Practice. This information, though less likely to feature in the examination, may nevertheless be of interest to candidates.

Notes for the MRCGP: A curriculum based guide to the AKT, CSA and WBPA, 4th edition.
By K. Palmer and N. Boeckx. Published 2010 by Blackwell Publishing,
ISBN: 978-1-4051-5724-7.

Appendix I – The structure of the health service

This appendix relates to curriculum statement 4 (Management in primary care)

The primary health-care team is only one cog (albeit a central one) in the complex machinery of the country's medical services. Many other bodies provide support for primary care and for patients, directly or indirectly, through administration, fiscal planning, resource provision and other activities. Although confusing it is important to understand where general practice lies in the bigger picture and this is our attempt to explain it, with considerable help from the information sheet of The Royal College of General Practitioners (RCGP 2004) on the structure of the NHS.

Tiers of management

The NHS organisation can be divided into national organisations (focusing on strategy and planning) and local organisations (focusing on local implementation of clinical care) (Figure AI.1).

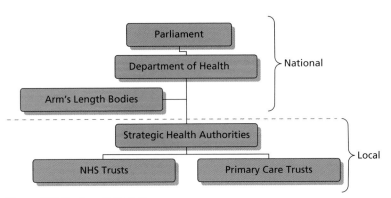

Figure AI.1 Structure of the NHS.

Notes for the MRCGP: A curriculum based guide to the AKT, CSA and WBPA, 4th edition.
By K. Palmer and N. Boeckx. Published 2010 by Blackwell Publishing,
ISBN: 978-1-4051-5724-7.

Parliament

The government allocates funding to the Department of Health (DH) and indicates priorities for health-care spending.

Department of Health

The DH is run by the Secretary of State for Health and is accountable to parliament for the performance of the NHS. It sets national standards and strategies, and allocates resources to the different parts of the NHS aided by the arms' length bodies.

Arms' length bodies

These are independent bodies such as NICE (National Institute for Health and Clinical Excellence) that are funded by the DH. Their role is to help the DH develop and manage its strategies and national standards. There are four branches.

The Modernisation Agency

- The National Primary Care Trust Development Team (organisational support for primary care trusts [PCTs])
- The National Primary Care Development Team (NPDT – developing primary care – new Quality Outcome Framework [QOF] targets, etc.)
- And others … .

Executive agencies

- NHS Pensions Agency
- Medicines and Healthcare products Regulatory Agency (MHRA)
- And others … .

Executive non-departmental public bodies

- Commissions, e.g. CHAI – Commission for Healthcare Audit and Inspection – responsible for clinical governance in the NHS.

Special health authorities

- NICE
- NHS Direct
- National Blood Service.

Strategic health authorities (SHAs)

There are 28 SHAs which oversee the PCTs. They monitor their perform- ance and help them develop local health plans (in line with national priorities).

Primary care trusts

PCTs run the local health services, i.e. they commission GP, community and hospital services, and monitor their performance. PCTs are responsible for developing the local health services to meet local health needs, e.g. drug misuse services in areas of high drug dependency. Seventy-five per cent of the NHS budget is allocated to PCTs.

Other organisations

Local medical committees
These are professional groups representing local doctors. The local medical committee (LMC) advises the PCT on medical matters. They also have links with the British Medical Association (BMA), and provide support for GP practices and individual GPs.

Practice commissioning groups
These are groups of practices that have clubbed together to share the burden of practice-based commissioning (see Chapter 5).

NHS trusts
The NHS Act allowed hospitals and community care units to assume managerial independence from PCTs. There are six types:
1. Acute trusts (general medical and surgical services)
2. Care trusts (specialist mental health and care of older people services)
3. Mental health trusts (mental health service provision)
4. Ambulance trusts (emergency and transport services)
5. Children's trusts (integrated children's services, i.e. health, education and social services)
6. Foundation trusts (similar to acute trusts but with more local control over the running and development of services).

Local authorities
Local authority responsibilities include the promotion of social care and a healthy environment for daily living. Provision includes:
- social services (meals on wheels, social workers, home helps, childminding and fostering services, etc.)
- special educational facilities for learning disabled individuals
- environmental health services
- rented housing for general needs, sheltered housing for older people and residential homes for children in care.

Voluntary associations
Numerous voluntary associations (Samaritans, Alcoholics Anonymous, Diabetes UK, etc.) have been formed to provide support and advice for families and individuals with a wide range of problems. Referral to a voluntary association is a valid, often valuable, adjunct to other treatment. They may be of particular use when the GP has limited knowledge of a condition (i.e. rare genetic disease) because the voluntary body can often offer the patient specialist advice, contacts and support. Consider referral on as an adjunct to management in CSA (Clinical Skills Assessment) and CBD (case-based discussion) cases. You can search for recognised UK-based patient support groups using the patient UK website (www.patient. co.uk and click on the link support groups).

Prescription Pricing Authority (PPA)

Within the NHS the PPA has the status of a special health authority. Its functions include:

1. Feedback to prescribers – comes in several forms the most useful of which is PACT data: Prescribing Analysis and CosT (PACT) data – a report that summarises what GPs have prescribed and the cost of their prescribing. Data from individual GPs and practices are compared against other GPs in the PCT and also against national prescribing data. PACT data are provided quarterly.
2. Information for the DH on high prescribers and prescribing patterns and costs.
3. Pricing arrangements that enable pharmacists and dispensing doctors to be paid.
4. Assistance in research, post-marketing surveillance and even police investigations!

The Royal College of General Practitioners
Function

The main function of The RCGP since inception has been to serve as a think-tank for the setting of standards and the improvement of general practice. The RCGP seeks to achieve this broad aim through its main activities, important among which are:

- the setting of a postgraduate examination as a benchmark of expected standards
- the organisation and conduct of general practice research
- the publication of an academic journal based on original research and frequent special reports
- the provision of reference and advisory material to aid good practice
- the stimulation of debate through policy statements and its national and local educational meetings
- the promotion of continuing professional development (CPD)
- direct influence on the structure of vocational training.

The RCGP represents the academic voice of general practice. It has contributed significantly to the state of improved esteem and morale that exists within general practice. It has proved a successful breeding ground for fresh and innovative thinking, and is likely to remain at the forefront when it comes to future developments within the profession. All GPs training in the UK from 2007 will have to achieve membership status to practice.

Reference

Royal College of General practitioners. *The Structure of the NHS*. RCGP Information Sheet No. 8. London: RCGP, 2004.

Appendix II – Social medicine

This chapter relates to Curriculum statement 5 (Healthy people, subsection Inequalities in health)

Social class

The Registrar General's classification of social class is based on *occupation*:

- for men and single women on their own occupation
- for married women on their husband's occupation
- for children on their father's occupation
- for the retired and unemployed on their last significant period of employment.

Classification has five divisions ranging from professionals (Class 1) at the top of the scale to unskilled manual workers (Class 5). This system is widely accepted and is comprehensive for the whole population, although it is clearly not precise to label people on the basis of their job alone, and even less precise to label women on the basis of their partner's job.

Social inequalities related to class

Various studies (e.g. those by the Office of Population Censuses and Surveys [OPCS] and by the Department of Employment and the Royal Commission on the Distribution of Income and Wealth) have highlighted class inequalities in areas such as wealth, income, living and working conditions. Typical findings were illustrated in Table 5.2.

In wealth terms the gap between rich and poor has been widening over the 10 years to 2007 with the disposable income of class 1 being six times greater than class 5 (Office of National Statistics).

Health inequalities related to class

Unfortunately there is no perfect measure of health: self-reported symptoms are often unreliable and, although death is an unequivocal event, it does not help in the measurement of minor and chronic illness. Field

Notes for the MRCGP: A curriculum based guide to the AKT, CSA and WBPA, 4th edition. By K. Palmer and N. Boeckx. Published 2010 by Blackwell Publishing, ISBN: 978-1-4051-5724-7.

workers have attempted to circumvent this problem by examining a variety
of parameters. In fact, the relationship of health to social class is so clear
that it is borne out for *all* the parameters considered. Similar gradients have
been shown for nearly all leading causes of death, and for common chronic
musculoskeletal, circulatory and respiratory complaints, and there is a clear
gradation through the classes that applies to all ages and both sexes: class
5 has the worst health, class 1 the best, and the other classes are in between,
in the exact order that they appear in our class structure. This is equally
true in international and prospective studies, when the comparison is
between geographical units of comparative affluence and deprivation, and
even after smoking is taken into account of (see Delamonthe 1991; Eachus
et al. 1996; Watt 1996).

On the tenth anniversary of the Black Report commentators pointed out
that socioeconomic differences in health, such as those in wealth, were
widening (Davey et al. 1990). Similar patterns can be seen in all industrialised countries collecting relevant data (Lynge 1981).

Two contradictory theories have been proposed to explain these
findings:

1. *Health determines social class*, e.g. sickly individuals fail to hold down
   good jobs, or ill health over several generations produces a similar social
   drift – there is no great evidence to support this theory.
2. *Social class determines health*, e.g. exposure to disease-producing agents
   and access to medical resources is class related. There is some evidence
   in favour of this model:
   (a) lower social classes use the preventive services less than classes 1 and
       2
   (b) lower social classes are more likely to indulge in unhealthy habits
       such as smoking
   (c) the lower classes live in less healthy environments and suffer more
       deprivation.

The distinction between these two theories is of more than academic
importance: if social class *does* determine health it suggests that health
inequalities are best combated by tackling social inequalities, and this
approach would be sociopolitical rather than medical. (Many commentators and epidemiologists indeed believe this to be true.)

Inequalities of access to health care

Tudor Hart (1971) argued that the 'inverse care law' applies in the UK, i.e.
the *provision* of health care is inversely related to the need for it. He
attributes this to market forces in a free economy: prosperous areas attract
more resources and more highly skilled personnel.

There is some evidence in favour of this 'law':

- Some depressed areas with high morbidity receive poorer facilities than
  the so-called affluent areas.
- The higher social classes, who appear to be the least in need of preventive
  services such as cervical screening, are the highest users of the service
  (so-called worried well).

- According to OPCS surveys, the upper social classes are more likely to be referred to hospital than their working-class counterparts in the event of chronic handicapping illness.
- According to Cartwright and Anderson's (1981) survey, practices in middle-class areas are more likely to employ doctors with higher qualifications, and less likely to use deputising arrangements than practices from working-class areas; they are also more likely to have extra equipment such as an ECG machine.
- On average, middle-class patients have longer consultations with their GP than working-class patients; they ask more questions and cover more problems; doctors in working-class areas have heavier surgery loads.

Deprived areas

Nowhere is the inequality of access to health care more clearly illustrated than in inner cities, where there are problems in the recruitment of health-care personnel because of high overheads, vandalism, vagrant or highly mobile populations, and social problems such as alcohol and drug addiction. This has also led to GPs living outside their practice areas, the heavy use of deputising services and the use of hospital accident and emergency departments by patients for basic primary care problems. The need for a deprivation payment has generally been acknowledged and is included in the General Medical Service (GMS) contract. See also APMS contracts (Chapter 5).

Illness behaviour

The clinical iceberg

Many minor conditions are extremely common and it is normal for people to feel ill a lot of the time, e.g.:
- In one survey more than 90% declared themselves to have been ill in the last 2-week period (only 20% consulted their GP);
- A review (Zollman and Vickers 1999) estimates that about a third of the population had used some form of complementary medicine and 10% had consulted a complementary practitioner in the last year. Levels of use in patients with chronic disease are twice as high.
- White found, in an audit of 588 primary care patients with chronic back pain, that 46% used complementary therapies to control symptoms (White 2008).

The level of self-care is high.

It is clear from these data that a clinical iceberg exists and that most symptom episodes do not reach medical attention.

Social definitions of illness

It is a basic tenet of medical sociology that definitions of illness and health *vary*, depending on socially determined perceptions, e.g. whether you regard tension headaches, hypertension, alcoholism or premenstrual tension as illnesses depends on your viewpoint: doctor and patient may disagree, and one generation may disagree with another.

Illness behaviour

Given the foregoing comments it is interesting to consider what prompts a person to consider him- or herself in need of medical advice – a complex decision that sociologists call illness behaviour. Factors shown to be important include:

1. *Culture*, e.g. some people of Italian, Jewish or Mediterranean origin have been shown to have lower thresholds for reporting pain.
2. *Symptom presentation*: symptoms presenting in a striking way are more readily perceived as illness, as are those deemed to be 'severe'.
3. *Lay beliefs*.
4. *Sex and social class*: women and social classes 4 and 5 consult more often.
5. *Stress levels*, e.g. mothers who have high scores on anxiety–depression rating scales consult more often, for themselves and for their children (Leach et al. 1993).
6. *Accessibility of medical care*, e.g. as the distance between home and the surgery increases, the likelihood of consultation decreases.
7. *Learned behaviour*: much anecdotal experience suggests that high usage of medical services runs in families, perhaps because members learn their illness behaviour from each other and pass it on to future generations.
8. *Trigger factors*: Zola (1973) identified five triggers that influenced the timing of decisions to consult:
   (a) another interpersonal crisis
   (b) perceived interference with personal and social relations
   (c) perceived interference with job or leisure activities
   (d) the pressure of other family or friends (approximately 75% conduct lay consultations before the professional one)
   (e) the setting of an arbitrary deadline ('If I feel the same next week').

The Health Belief model, developed by a group of social psychologists in the 1950s, proposes that people vary individually, and for different conditions, in:

- health motivation
- perceived vulnerability
- the perceived seriousness of the condition
- the perceived costs and benefits of obtaining medical care
- cues for action (new symptoms, TV article, friend's advice, etc.).

The decision to consult does not correlate with:

- the true seriousness of the illness
- the doctor's perception of a need to consult.

In other words, a patient's judgement of illness and decision-making is often at variance with what doctors believe to be an appropriate use of the service. It is, fortunate therefore that only 1 in 37 symptom episodes receives medical attention, because the health service would otherwise surely be overwhelmed!

Stress

Stress rating scales

Several attempts have been made to quantify the amount of stress attached to important life events. Holmes and Rahe's Social Readjustment Rating Scale (SRRS) was obtained by asking a large sample of people to score 42 life events, pleasant and unpleasant, according to the amount of readjustment needed (Holmes and Rahe 1967). Taking marriage as the midpoint (50) on a scale of 1–100, typical ratings were:

- death of a spouse: 100
- divorce: 73
- marriage: 50
- major change at work: 29
- change of house: 20
- holiday: 13.

Stress and physical illness

The SRRS shows a crude correlation with physical illness, e.g.:

- One study classified doctors into high-, medium- and low-risk groups, based on their stress scores: the ratio of self-reported illness over the next 9 months was approximately five times greater (49%) in the high-risk than in the low-risk group (9%).
- Another study found a linear relationship between stress scores and illness in naval personnel (Holmes and Masuda).

Other studies suggest that major life events can affect physical problems such as peptic ulceration, urticaria and diabetes control.

Stress and psychiatric illness

There is a relatively poor correlation with the SRRS here, but much empirical experience in general and psychiatric practice indicates that stress is a vital precipitant of psychiatric ill health. The failure of the SRRS has been blamed on the relative crudity of a scale that ascribes the same rating to an event without examining the individual and the context of the event, e.g. stressors are likely to be more significant if they were believed to have long-term threatening implications (major loss or potential loss of health, marriage, job, etc.). Painful but self-limiting stresses were less important (Brown and Harris 1978).

Stress and human givens

The 'human givens' approach was published in 1997 based on the work of Joe Griffin and a group of psychologists and psychotherapists (www.hgi.org.uk). The human givens model works on the principle that there are basic needs and resources that, if not met, may lead to psychological distress, antisocial behaviour and mental health problems.

The human givens
Emotional needs
- Security (a stable home life and safe territory to live in):
  - ➤ financial
  - ➤ employment
- Intimacy and friendship
- Attention (received and given)
- A sense of autonomy and control
- Social interaction (as part of a wider community)
- The need to feel competent (which comes from successful learning and effectively applying skills); privacy (to reflect on and consolidate our experiences); housing
- Achievement (through facing and overcoming challenges).

Resources
- The ability to learn and add new knowledge to innate knowledge
- Memory and the ability to forget
- Curiosity, imagination and the ability to problem solve
- The ability to focus attention
- The ability to understand through metaphor (pattern matching)
- Self-awareness (an observing self)
- Resilience
- The ability to empathise and connect with others
- A dreaming brain that dearouses the autonomic nervous system.

The aim is to identify where needs are lacking and to help patients to meet them by developing their resources. This biopsychosocial model has been used by as an alternative to cognitive–behavioural therapy to tackle a range of mental health problems, including stress and depression. Many of the emotional needs listed in the model are recognised in the literature as important stress factors.

Bereavement (loss of security, intimacy, friendship and social interaction)
A review in *The Lancet* (Stroebe et al. 2007) confirmed a much higher morbidity and mortality in the recently bereaved, e.g.:
- Widowers had a 21% increased risk for all-cause mortality and widows a 17% increased risk.
- Risks were further increased in the first 30 days after bereavement.
  The absolute numbers of deaths were, however, low.

Work (loss of security, sense of competence and achievement)
Retirement does not appear to be a major stress factor, assuming that it is planned; redundancy by contrast is a great source of stress, so:
- Self-reported illness, including chronic ill health, is more common.
- In the short term, blood pressure and serum cholesterol can be raised.

- Loss of work, or threat of it, is associated with markedly higher consultation rates, for both the individual and the partner (and GPs in areas of high unemployment can therefore expect to have higher caseloads).
- Longitudinal mortality studies from 1971 to 1981 showed, after adjustment for social class, an excess of mortality rate of 20–30% among unemployed individuals (Moser et al. 1984).
- Important effects on mortality have also been described in Italy, Denmark and Finland. In Finland the effect was still evident after adjustment for background variables, and it showed a dose–response relation – mortality increased with duration of unemployment (Martikainen 1990).
- Deaths from suicide, lung cancer and ischaemic heart disease are more common, and so too are depression and parasuicide.

Unemployment is concentrated in the lower social classes and this may partly account for the observed class inequalities in health.

Marriage (provision of security, attention, intimacy and friendship)

Clearly this can be a positive or a negative force, e.g.:
- Married people have a lower mortality rate than unmarried, widowed or divorced people (this effect is greater for men than for women).
- However, marital problems are a well-recognised precipitant of alcoholism, suicide, accidents and psychiatric illness, and the constrained role of mother and wife, in particular, may cause depression in housewives.

Family problems (loss of security, intimacy and friendship)

Problems within the family are a potent source of stress that can affect more than one generation, e.g. child abuse and alcoholism are often passed from parents to children.

Social upheaval (loss of security, and most of the emotional needs may occur)

Migrant and other studies suggest that major upheaval can predispose to physical and mental ill health.

As a relatively new concept the body of evidence (other than positive anecdotal reports) to support its efficacy in clinical practice is lacking but this model is gaining popularity. It neatly draws together known stress factors.

The value of social support (social integration)

Integration into a social community or family is generally protective, e.g.:
- lower mortality rates in married men
- lower death rates in Mormons and Seventh Day Adventists.

Support of a family can:
- reduce the impact of stress (e.g. following enforced redundancies men supported by family and friends experience fewer stress-related symptoms)

- influence the course and outcome of physical illness (e.g. orthopaedic patients rehabilitate more quickly if they are married and have children at home)
- influence the course and outcome of mental illness (e.g. the studies of Brown and Harris [1978] suggest relapse in schizophrenia is higher when patients come from families with high expressed emotion)
- provide vital care for those with chronic illness and handicap.

Families can also constitute a *pathological* influence (as described earlier).

The structure of family life is changing (more divorces, more single-parent families, working women and mobile populations). This threatens to undermine the supporting role of the family, especially with respect to their ageing relatives.

Stress and the role of personality

Friedman and Rosenman (1974) proposed two types of personality related to cardiovascular risk:

1. *Type A* people show:
   (a) impatience
   (b) competitiveness
   (c) a sense of the pressure of time and responsibility.
2. *Type B* people do not exhibit any of these traits.

Some studies suggest that type A men have twice the risk of heart disease when compared with type B men.

Attempts have been made to link physical illness to personality type for other conditions such as peptic ulceration, but the results have not been corroborated. Vulnerable personalities are certainly a well-established concept in psychiatric illness (e.g. the schizoid personality is linked to schizophrenia, and the cyclothymic to bipolar depression).

Ethnic minorities

There are two main patterns of migrant-community relationship:

1. 'Integrated' or 'assimilated' (e.g. many African–Caribbean communities).
2. Culturally separate and isolated (e.g. some Asian communities).

Historically there is strong evidence that racial prejudice places immigrant groups in a position of social inequality. The inequality in health in ethnic minority groups is in part explained by behavioural traits (e.g. less use of antenatal and postnatal services; restrictive diets), in part by genetic vulnerability, and in part by social disadvantages such as unemployment, poor housing and discrimination.

As in the case of social class, social inequalities are mirrored by inequalities in physical and mental health:

1. *Physical health*: migrants have:
   (a) lower-birthweight babies
   (b) a higher perinatal mortality rate
   (c) more anaemia (sometimes dietary, sometimes due to diseases with an ethnic element such as sickle cell and thalassaemia)

(d) more rickets

(e) more imported and tropical diseases.

2. *Mental health*: it is sometimes difficult to distinguish between cultural beliefs that seem bizarre to the western mind and true mental illness. However, some studies on African–Caribbean migrants suggest that the stress of social upheaval, alien culture and racial discrimination cause more mental breakdowns.

Cultural differences also pose problems in the *doctor–patient relationship*, e.g.:

• language barriers
• completely different values and beliefs
• different (culturally determined) patterns of illness behaviour
• taboos concerning the physical examination of women.

It is therefore difficult to ensure that these patients are not also disadvantaged in the medical care they receive.

Elderly people

The size of the problem (ONS 2007)

1. The percentage of the population aged over 65 years is now approximately 16%, with 2% of those being over 85 years old.
2. This represents a considerable growth in the elderly population (the percentage of over-65s was only 6% in 1901 and the over-85 group has risen by 84% in the last 25 years).
3. There are three reasons for this growth:
    (a) a slight increase in life expectancy
    (b) a fall in birth rates (which means that young people are a relatively smaller percentage of the whole)
    (c) a present glut of older people produced by the dramatic decline in perinatal mortality at the turn of the century.

Characteristics of older people

1. More often women than men: mean life expectancy of women is approximately 3 years greater than men
2. Multiple physical problems
3. Drug problems:
    (a) polypharmacy and drug interactions
    (b) impaired drug handling and clearance
    (c) sensitivity to drug effects.
4. Financial status. On the *plus* side older people gain:
    (a) a statutory retirement pension
    (b) certain exemptions and concessions, e.g. on prescription charges and travel fares.

On the *debit* side of course they lose their earning power. On balance the latter is not compensated for and National Audit Figures (2004–5) suggest that about 17% of the over-65s live below, or occasionally far below, the official poverty level. This is an improvement from 27% in 1995, largely due to changes in the benefit system.

State benefits may help in part, but they are under-claimed because:

(c) the benefits system is complicated and confusing
(d) older people fear the humiliation of means testing and the stigma of 'scrounging'.

5. Other problems:

(a) inadequate housing
(b) subnutrition
(c) social isolation and apathy
(d) physical handicap.

A combination of these factors renders the elderly population prone to an increased risk of hypothermia.

Support for older people

Family trends (fewer children, a more mobile population, more working women) mean fewer carers nowadays. Also society's current values place older people in relatively low esteem when compared with the right of other family members to exercise their independence. Consequently the proportion of older people living with family or friends has dropped over the last two decades (over 50% of over-85s live alone – ONS 2006). Help the Aged raises valid concerns about an increase in social isolation, although relatively better health at older ages means that many more in this generation of older people remain independent through personal choice.

Where family support is provided, there is a cost, e.g.

• loss of paid work, social life and holiday opportunities
• family discord
• impaired health of the carers.

Alternative support systems are provided through the social services departments:

• *Home help*: for more than 700 000 older people, who pay according to their means, home helps perform many important services – cleaning, washing, shopping, and collecting prescriptions and pensions. They also provide companionship and are an early warning system for the primary health-care team.
• *Meals on wheels*: hot meals provided from central kitchens to the home on a subsidised basis. Voluntary organisations also contribute to this service.
• *Social services day centres*: these provide a more stimulating environment and a social outlet for isolated older people and day relief for their carers.

These support systems are considerably under-used in relation to the need, e.g. in one study 6% of the 65–75-years age group and 19% of the over-75s used these services, but this supplied only one-quarter of the perceived need for home helps and one-sixteenth of the need for meals on wheels. Similarly there is evidence that aids and adaptations for the home are under-provided, under-used and under-maintained.

Under-use of aids and support services arises because of:

- ignorance regarding their availability
- the reluctance of a largely stoical elderly population to ask for help
- the limited provision of resources
- the high level of commitment of many carers, despite personal difficulties and stress.

Institutional care

Options *include*:

- private nursing homes
- private residential care
- social services Part 3 accommodation
- voluntary association non-residential homes
- local authority sheltered housing (including warden-controlled and other flats for older people).

Primary care services and social services aim to maintain independence at home through the use of home carers, adaptations, aids and day services. Where the patient's needs exceed the level of care available at home or the patient is unsafe in their own home despite maximum home care/adaptation, institutional care may be required. The provision made by local authorities is determined by Part 3 of the National Assistance Act 1948, which imposes a duty to 'provide for those who by reason of age or infirmity need care and attention not otherwise available'. Many homes include a short-stay bed quota for trial periods and respite care.

Disability and handicap

Problems of disabled individuals

Disabled individuals encounter various problems that include:

- poor mobility (and hence reduced leisure opportunities)
- difficulties with basic self-care
- disadvantage in employment and difficulties in education
- the need for a modified environment at home, at work and in public places
- poverty
- the stigma label and other psychological problems.

Mobility and disabled people

Resources that are available include:

- physiotherapy
- the provision of walking aids
- home adaptations (handrails, stairlifts, etc.) through the advice of a domiciliary occupational therapist
- the provision of a wheelchair
- Disability Working and Living Allowances
- sometimes a grant towards a specially adapted car
- advice, e.g. from the Directory for the Disabled, on the help that travel agencies, car-hire firms, British Rail and the airlines can provide
- voluntary or paid visitors, home helps and day centre attendance to combat the problem of isolation.

Employment and disabled people

Unemployment levels are higher among disabled people. The 1995 Disability Discrimination Act made it illegal to discriminate against disabled job applicants and those who become disabled in the course of employment, provided that reasonable accommodation can be made for their condition.

Employment benefits for disabled people

- Sheltered workshops are provided by local authorities and voluntary bodies.
- Under the Sheltered Placement Scheme a host company provides an opportunity for disabled workers to integrate with able-bodied ones: the host company provides tools and training and pays according to output, with the balance of salary provided by an employing sponsor.
- The government provides PACTs (Placement Assessment Counselling Teams) and residential retraining courses to help disabled people find work.
- Grants are available for adaptation of premises and equipment to meet the needs of disabled people, assistance with fares to work (when inability to use public transport incurs extra expense) and a 'job introduction' grant to promote trials of employment.
- A government-sponsored company, Remploy, provides 3000 jobs for disabled people, and in 2007–8 found 6500 jobs for disabled people and those facing complex barriers to work. It is committed to supporting 20 000 people per year into mainstream employment by 2012–13.
- Certain groups of visually handicapped people can be helped at the cost of engaging a sighted reader at work for their assistance.

Poverty and disabled people

Surveys indicate that disabled people often suffer financial hardship, e.g. a 2004 report by the New Policy Institute found that almost a third of disabled adults are living in poverty (Palmer et al. 2004).

The *reasons* for greater financial hardship among the disabled include:
- restricted employment
- extra expenses (living costs are quoted as 25% higher than for able-bodied individuals), e.g. special diets, higher fuel bills, transport costs, home adaptations.

Although welfare benefits are available they do not adequately compensate because:
- the claim system is complicated and off-putting
- the rates are not very high (and combinations are not always additive)
- patients miss out through diffidence, embarrassment or ignorance.

Housing and disabled people

The Disabled Persons Act requires local authorities to consider the housing needs of registered disabled individuals and to provide assistance with structural alterations and adaptations (e.g. ramps, rails, adapted bathrooms, widened doorways).

References

Brown G, Harris T. *Social Origins of Depression*. London: Tavistock Publications, 1978.

Cartwright A, Anderson R. *General Practice Revisited: A second study of general practice*. London: Tavistock Publications, 1981.

Davey A, Smith G, Barley M, Blane D. The Black report on socio-economic inequalities in health 10 years on. *Br Med J* 1990;**301**:373–7.

Delamonthe T. Social inequalities in health. *BMJ* 1991;**303**:1046–50.

Eachus J, Williams M, Chan P et al. Deprivation and cause, specific morbidity: evidence from the Somerset and Avon survey of health. *BMJ* 1996;**312**:287–92.

Friedman M, Rosenman R. *Type A Behaviour and your Heart*. New York: Knopf, 1974.

Holmes T, Masuda M. Life change and illness susceptibility. In: Dohrenwend B.S. & Dohrenwend B.P. (eds) *Stressful Life Events: Their Nature and Effects*. John Wiley, New York, 1974.

Holmes T, Rahe R. The social readjustment rating scale. *I. Psychosom Res* 1967;**11**:213–18.

Leach J, Ridsdale L, Smeeton N. Is there a relationship between a mother's mental state and consulting the doctor by the family? *Fam Pract* 1993;**10**:305–11.

Lynge E. Occupational mortality in Norway, Denmark and Finland (1971–5). In: Committee for International Cooperation of National Research in Demography (ed) *Socio-economic Differential Mortality in Industrialised Societies*. Paris, WHO, 1981.

Martikainen PT. Unemployment and mortality among Finnish men 1981–5. *BMJ* 1990;**301**:407–11.

Moser KA, Fox AJ, Jones DR. Unemployment and mortality in the OPCS longitudinal study. *Lancet* 1984;**ii**:1324–9.

Office of National Statistics. Income and wealth. National statistics online: www.statistics.gov.uk (accessed 2008).

Office of National Statistics. Population ageing. National statistics online: www.statistics.gov.uk (accessed 2008).

Palmer G, Carr J, Kenway P. *Monitoring Poverty and Social Exclusion*. York: Joseph Rowntree Foundation, 2004.

Stroebe M, Schut H, Stroebe W. Health outcomes of bereavement. *Lancet* 2007;**370**:1960–73.

Tudor Hart J The inverse care law. *Lancet* 1971;**i**:405–12.

Watt GCM. All together now: why social deprivation matters to everyone. *BMJ* 1996;**312**:1026–9.

White A. Internal practice audit. Academic Primary Care Meeting, 2008.

Zola I. Pathways to the doctor: from person to patient. *Soc Sci Med* 1973;**7**:677–89.

Zollman C, Vickers A. ABC of complementary medicine: Users and practitioners of complementary medicine. *BMJ* 1999;**319**:836–8.

Appendix III – Med forms

FOR SOCIAL SECURITY AND STATUTORY SICK PAY PURPOSES ONLY
NOTES TO PATIENT ABOUT USING THIS FORM

You can use this form either:

1.   For Statutory Sick Pay (SSP) purposes - fill in Part A overleaf. Also fill in Part B if the doctor has given you a date to resume work. Give or send the completed form to your employer.

2.   For Social Security purposes -
To continue a claim for state benefit fill in Parts A and C of the form overleaf. Also fill in Part B if the doctor has given you a date to resume work. Sign and date the form and give or sent your Local Social Security Office QUICKLY to avoid losing benefit.

NOTE: To start your claim for State benefit you must use form SC1 if you are self-employed, unemployed or non-employed OR form SSP if you are an employee. For further details get leaflet 18202 (from Social Security Local Offices).

Doctor's Statement

In confidence to
Mr/Mrs/Miss/Ms ....
I examined you today/yesterday and advised you that
(a) You need not   (b) you should refrain from work
    refrain from
    work   for*†...

                              OR until...

Diagnosis of your disorder
causing absence from work ....
Doctor's remarks

Doctor's   Date of
signature   signing

Form Med 3

NOTE TO DOCTOR*† *See inside front cover for notes on completion*

Notes for the MRCGP: A curriculum based guide to the AKT, CSA and WBPA, 4th edition. By K. Palmer and N. Boeckx. Published 2010 by Blackwell Publishing, ISBN: 978-1-4051-5724-7.

Med 5

FOR SOCIAL SECURITY AND STATUTORY SICK PAY PURPOSES ONLY

Special Statement by the Doctor

In confidence to
Mr/Mrs/Miss/Ms ....

(A) I examined you on the

following dates...................

....

....

and advised you that you
should refrain from work

....

from...............to.................

Diagnosis of your disorder
causing absence from work

Doctor's remarks.

(B) I have not examined you but, on the basis of a
recent written report from -

Doctor .... (Name is known)

of ....

....

....(Address)

I have advised you that
you should refrain
from work for a ....

....

Doctor's
signature

Date of
signing

The special circumstances in which this form may be used are described in the handbook "A guide for medical practitioners."

Form Med 5

PATIENT TO COMPLETE PARTICULARS ON REVERSE

Med 5 001137 07/01 SPSL

Med 4

Doctor's statement

Do not use this form for people claiming Statutory Sick Pay

To the doctor We are assessing your patient's eligibility for incapacity Benefit and other state benefits under the all work test. Please fill in the following statements.

In confidence to   Mr/Mrs/Miss/Ms _____

Main diagnosis
(be as precise as possible)

Other diagnoses

Doctor's remarks
(Including comments on the disabling effects of the condition .... progress. Accuracy and detail will avoid requests for completion of a medical rep........)

To the doctor While the all wor.... st .... arried out, we need some evidence that your patient should refrain from their usual ....ation..... information you give here will not be part of the all work test.

I am issuing the ..lo.. ng statement based upon the current guidance to certifying medical p...ti..oners. I examined you today / yesterday and advise you

☐   that y.. ne.. no.. refrain from your usual occupation.

☐   that you sho.. d refrain from your usual occupation

for _____ (period).

or until _____ .

Doctor's
signature _____ **Date** ___ / ___ / ___

Stamp

Med 4

Med 6

Doctor's statement

In confidence

To be filled in by the doctor. Please use BLOCK CAPITALS.

To   **The Manager**   **DO**

Patient's surname   Mr/Mrs/Miss/Ms

First names

Address

Postcode

National Insurance number
if known

I have been issuing medical statements to this patient who is under my care. I have been recording a 'Vague' diagnosis on the statements. This is because, in my opinion, to record the actual diagnosis may be harmful to my patient.

Please send me a medical report form so that I can give you additional information, including the actual diagnosis of the disorder suffered by this patient.

Doctor's signature

Date   /   .

Stamp

Please send this form to your patient's Social Security office. The address is in the phone book. Look under SOCIAL SECURITY or BENEFITS AGENCY. Do not send this form to Benefits Agency Medical Services.

You can get more copies of this form from your Health Authority or Health Board.

Med 6

RM 7

Doctor's statement
In confidence

To be filled in by the doctor. Please use BLOCK CAPITALS.

To **The Manager** _____ **DO**

Patient's surname   Mr/Mrs/Miss/Ms _____

First names _____

Address _____

_____

                              Postcode _____

National Insurance number if known

I have been issuing medical statements (form **Med 3**) to this patient who is under my care. Please could you arrange for a doctor from the Benefits Agency Medical Services to give an opinion on their ability to carry out their own occupation.

Please send me a medical report form so that I can give you additional information.

Doctor's signature _____

Date _____ / _____ / _____

Stamp

Please send this form to your patient's Social Security office. The address is in the phone book. Look under SOCIAL SECURITY or BENEFITS AGENCY. Do not send this form to Benefits Agency Medical Services.

You can get more copies of this form from your Health Authority or Health Board.

RM 7

Mat B1

MATERNITY CERTIFICATE

MAT B1

Please fill in this form in ink

Name of patient

TO THE PATIENT
Please read the notes on the back of this form ▶

Part A

Fill in this part if you are giving the certificate before the confinement.

Do not fill this in more than 14 weeks before the week when the baby is expected.

I certify that I examined you on the date given below. In my opinion you can expect to have your baby in the week that includes ..../........./.......

We use week to mean the 7 days starting on a Sunday and ending on a Saturday.

Part B

Fill in this part if you are giving the certificate after the confinement.

I certify that I attended you in connection with the birth which took place ..../........./....... when you were delivered of a and [ ] children

In my opinion your baby was expected in the week that includes ..../........./.......

Date of examination ..../........./.......

Date of signing ..../........./.......

Signature

Registered midwives
Please give your UKCC PIN here

Doctors
Please stamp your name and address here if the form has not been stamped by the Family Practitioner Committee.

SPECIMEN

DS 1500

Doctor's Report for Disability Living Allowance, Attendance Allowance or Incapacity Benefit to accompany your patient's claim under Special Rules

THIS IS NOT A CLAIM FORM   Patient's copy

Surname

Other names

Date of birth   /   /

Address

Part 1 - Condition

What is the diagnosis?   Other relevant diagnoses?

Date of diagnosis?
/   /

Is the patient aware of their condition and/or prognosis?

YES ☐   NO ☐

If not, please tell [ ] address of their representative

Part 2 - Clinical Features which indicate a severe progressive condition (For example: rate of progression, recurrence, staging, tumour markers, CD4 count and viral load, bulbar involvement respiratory and/or heart failure etc.)

Part 3 - Treatment

Please give details of relevant past or current treatment with dates **including response** (if not palliative, please state)

Is any other intervention or treatment planned which may significantly after progression of the condition?

Declaration: the person filled above is my patient. This is a full report of their condition and treatment. I have read and understand the notes on the completion of this form and I am satisfied that the form is appropriate. I am the patient's:

☐ Registered General Practitioner

☐ Hospital or hospice consultant

☐ _____

Signature

Your name

Phone number

Address or FHSA stamp

Date
/   /   DS1500

Appendix IV – The RCGP Curriculum map

For information on this see: www.rcgp-curriculum.org.uk.

1.	Being a general practitioner
2.	The general practice consultation
3.1.	Clinical governance
3.2.	Patient safety
3.3.	Ethics and values-based medicine
3.4.	Promoting equality and valuing diversity
3.5.	Evidence based practice
3.6.	Research and academic activity
3.7.	Teaching, mentoring, clinical supervision
4.1.	Management in primary care
4.2.	Information management and technology
5.	Healthy people
6.	Genetics in primary care
7.	Care of acutely ill people
8.	Care of children and young people
9.	Care of older adults
10.1.	Women's health
10.2.	Men's health
11.	Sexual health
12.	Care of people with cancer and palliative care
13.	Care of people with mental health problems
14.	Care of people with learning disabilities
15.1.	Cardiovascular problems
15.2.	Digestive problems
15.3.	Drug and alcohol problems
15.4.	ENT and facial problems
15.5.	Eye problems
15.6.	Metabolic problems
15.7.	Neurological problems
15.8.	Respiratory problems
15.9.	Rheumatology, musculoskeletal and trauma
15.10.	Skin problems

Notes for the MRCGP: A curriculum based guide to the AKT, CSA and WBPA, 4th edition.
By K. Palmer and N. Boeckx. Published 2010 by Blackwell Publishing,
ISBN: 978-1-4051-5724-7.

Index